Communication & Professional Competencies: A Guide for Surgeons

Distributed by: Cine-Med, Inc.
127 Main Street North
Woodbury, CT 06798
(203) 263-0006

ISBN: 978-0-9788890-1-2

Notice: Our knowledge in clinical sciences is constantly changing. As new information becomes available, changes in treatment and in the use of drugs or medical devices become necessary. The authors and the publisher of this volume have taken care to make certain that the doses of drugs, uses of medical devices, and schedules of treatment are correct and compatible with the standards generally accepted at the time of publication.

All doctor, patient and hospital names used in this book are fictitious.

Printed in Canada

Acknowledgments

There are those who have been major forces in our personal and professional lives – and as a result, in the development and design of this book:

Our children: S. Patrick, Brooke and Bret Tristan Morin & Christopher, Patrick and Courtney Lang, who traveled throughout the world on our scholarly endeavors providing us with encouragement, humor and feedback.

Our friend: Helen Lang, for her patience with late night, family and weekend interruptions and for her wise counsel and continued support.

Finally, our sincerest gratitude to the staff at Cine-Med and especially to our editor, Mary Panagrosso, for her modeling of professionalism and clear, concise communication throughout this project.

Pamela A. Rowland and Nicholas P. Lang

About the Authors

Pamela A. Rowland, PhD

Dr. Rowland was graduated with distinction and summa cum laude from the University of Connecticut, publishing her first book that same year. She completed her MA at the Pennsylvania State University combining her interests in computer science, statistics, and education to develop more objective methodologies to study physician-patient communication. She completed her doctorate in communication studies at the University of Massachusetts followed by clinical faculty appointments at Brown, Tufts and Dartmouth Medical Schools. For more than 25 years, Dr. Rowland has been teaching interpersonal skills to residents and assessing the behaviors of clinical faculty. As a behavioral scientist, her research focuses on variables that affect success on oral boards, patient satisfaction and interviewing techniques. She is Director of the national course, Clinical Performance & Oral Examinations in Surgery. She recently assumed the position of Director, Office of Professional Development at Dartmouth Medical School. Dr. Rowland is an affiliate member of the American College of Surgeons.

A nationally recognized expert in communication, she assists clinical faculty, residents and students improve their performance in a variety of clinical and professional settings. She is the recipient of the 1977 Rhode Island Business and Professional Woman Award, the Connecticut 1992 Matrix Award for her work in the communications field and the 2004 Outstanding Teacher in Surgery Award from the Association for Surgical Education.

Nicholas P. Lang, MD, FACS

Dr. Lang was graduated from the University of Arkansas for Medical Sciences (UAMS) and completed his surgery residency at UAMS and the affiliated Veterans Administration hospital. After two years at the National Cancer Institute, he returned to Little Rock to join the faculty of the department of surgery and the staff at the VA hospital. For more than 13 years, Dr. Lang's clinical research has been funded by grants from the NIH, EPA, and the VA. For more than ten years, Dr. Lang has been involved in teaching physician-patient communication at both the VA and university hospitals. These activities led to his recognition by his peers as an accomplished surgeon, researcher and educator who focused on patient centered quality care as well as quality education and research.

He was elected to the position of President for both the Association for Surgical Education and Southwestern Surgical Congress. Until recently, he was chief of staff at the Central Arkansas Veterans Healthcare System in Little Rock and professor of surgery in the division of surgical oncology, department of surgery, College of Medicine at the University of Arkansas for Medical Sciences. Dr. Lang is currently Chief Medical Officer, University of Arkansas for Medical Sciences Medical Center, professor of surgery, professor of radiology and professor of physiology and biophysics in the College of Medicine at the University of Arkansas for Medical Sciences.

Drs. Rowland & Lang have collaborated on multiple communication research publications and skills workshops at national meetings in surgery. They have been co-directors of Clinical Performance & Oral Examinations in Surgery, designed for surgeons who were having difficulty with oral board examinations. As part of an American College of Surgeons Task Force, they helped to design, implement and teach the course: Surgeons as Effective Communicators: Sharpening Skills for Critical Moments. This book delivers the knowledge of the editors and chapter authors in a practical and understandable way that can lead surgeons toward improved communication and professional performance.

Table of Contents

Contributors

Lori A. Alvord, MD, FACS
Dr. Alvord is an Associate Professor of Surgery and Associate Dean for Students & Multicultural Affairs, Dartmouth Medical School. She is also the first woman Navajo surgeon.

Francis X. Aumand III, MSA
Mr. Aumand has 30 years of law enforcement experience and is Director, Division of Criminal Justice Services, Vermont Department of Public Safety and Chairman of the Board, SEARCH, Inc., the National Consortium of Justice Statistics and Information.

LD Britt, MD, MPH, FACS, FCCM
Dr. Britt is Brickhouse Professor and Chairman of the Department of Surgery at Eastern Virginia Medical School, member of the Board of Regents of the American College of Surgeons and Chair of the Residency Review Committee.

Kenneth W. Burchard, MD, FACS
Dr. Burchard is Professor of Surgery and Clerkship Director, Department of Surgery, Dartmouth Medical School.

Jeffrey L. Clothier, MD
Dr. Clothier is Associate Professor of Psychiatry and Behavioral Sciences at the University of Arkansas for Medical Sciences and Associate Chief of Staff for Mental Health at Central Arkansas Veterans Healthcare System.

Nicholas P.W. Coe, MD, FACS
Dr. Coe is Professor of Surgery at Tufts University School of Medicine and Director of the Office of Medical Education.

William P. Fiser, Jr., MD, FACS
Dr. Fiser is Assistant Professor of Surgery in the College of Medicine at the University of Arkansas for Medical Sciences. He is the Medical Director of the Arkansas Regional Organ Recovery Agency.

Muhammad Jaffar, MD, FCCP
Dr. Jaffar is Associate Professor of Anesthesiology and Surgery, at the University of Arkansas for Medical Sciences and Co-Director, Anesthesiology Residency Program and Director of the SICU, Central Arkansas Veterans Healthcare System.

Joseph Jensen, MD, FACS
Dr. Jensen is Associate Professor of Surgery, Director of Surgical Education and Residency Program Director at the University of Arkansas College of Medicine

Nicholas P. Lang, MD, FACS
Dr. Lang is Chief Medical Officer, University Medical Center and Professor of Surgery, College of Medicine at the University of Arkansas for Medical Sciences.

Barry M. Manuel, MD, FACS
Dr. Manuel is Associate Dean, Professor of Surgery at Boston University School of Medicine.

James M. McGreevy, MD, FACS
Colonel (Dr.) McGreevy is Professor of Surgery and Program Director at the University of Utah. He is Commander of the 419th Medical Squadron, US Air Force Reserve, Hill Air Force Base, Utah.

Marcene R. McVay, MD
Dr. McVay is a resident in Surgery at the University of Arkansas for Medical Sciences.

Joseph Melino, MDiv
Mr. Melino is Claims Director at Lifespan Risk Services, Rhode Island Hospital in Providence, RI.

Linn Meyer, BA
Linn Meyer is Director of Communications for the American College of Surgeons.

Charles Mock, MD, PhD, FACS
Dr. Mock is Associate Professor in the Departments of Surgery and Epidemiology at the University of Washington. He is a Staff Surgeon at Veteran Affairs Puget Sound Health Care System.

Richard W. Moore, JD, CPCU
Attorney Moore wrote this chapter when he was President of Pro Mutual based in Massachusetts.

Mohammed M. Moursi, MD, FACS
Dr. Moursi is Professor of Surgery and Chief of Vascular Surgery, Central Arkansas Veterans Healthcare System and Past President, Islamic Center of Little Rock, AR.

Tyler Otten, BS
Captain Otten is a commercial pilot with Delta Airlines and an F-16 Instructor Pilot in the 419th Fighter Wing, Hill AFB, Utah. He was graduated from the Air Force Academy with a BS in Human Factors.

David W. Page, MD, FACS
Dr. Page is Professor of Surgery and Surgical Clerkship Director, Baystate Medical Center, Tufts University School of Medicine.

Thomas T. A. Parrino, MD, MBA, FACP, CPE, FACPE
Dr. Parrino is Chief of Staff, Veteran Affairs Medical Center, Palm Beach, Florida and Clinical Professor of Medicine, University of Florida College of Medicine and the University of Miami School of Medicine.

Deborah Peltier, MD
Dr. Peltier is an Associate Professor of Medicine, Dartmouth Medical School and a Staff Physician at the Veterans Administration Hospital, White River Junction, Vermont.

Victor E. Pricolo, MD, FACS
Dr. Pricolo is Professor of Surgery and Director, Division of Colon & Rectal Surgery at Brown Medical School.

Brenda Richardson, MD
Dr. Richardson is Managing Partner of Harmony First, LLC and a member of the Board of Directors, Pro Mutual Group and Massachusetts Medical Society. She is past president of Medical Staff at Addison Gilbert Hospital, Massachusetts.

Pamela A. Rowland, PhD
Dr. Rowland is Research Associate Professor in Community & Family Medicine and Surgery. She is also Director, Office of Professional Development at Dartmouth Medical School.

Ajit K. Sachdeva, MD, FRCSC, FACS
Dr. Sachdeva is Director, Division of Education, American College of Surgeons and Adjunct Professor of Surgery at Feinberg School of Medicine, Northwestern University.

Parvis J. Sadighi, MD, FACS
Dr. Sadighi is Professor of Surgery, University of Massachusetts Medical School. He is Emeritus Chairman and Program Director, Department of Surgery, Berkshire Medical Center, Massachusetts.

Kaleem Sayyed, MBBS (MD), MPH
Dr. Sayyed is Assistant Professor, Boozman College of Public Health, Health Policy & Management; Assistant Professor, Clinton School of Public Service and a University of Arkansas for Medical Science TOKTEN Fellow, United Nations Development Program and consultant, National Center for Cultural Competence, Georgetown University.

D. Matson Sewell, CPHRM, MPH
Ms. Sewell was Risk Manager for the Dartmouth-Hitchcock Alliance and Clinic facilities located in New Hampshire, Vermont and Massachusetts. Now she is a Custom Account Executive, Patient Safety/Risk Management with The Doctors Company in California.

Samuel D. Smith, MD, FACS
Dr. Smith is Chief, Division of Pediatric Surgery, Arkansas Childrens Hospital.

Stephen R. Smith, MD, MPH
Dr. Smith is Associate Dean of Medicine, Professor of Family Medicine at Brown Medical School with focus on the Virtual Curriculum.

Joan M. Teno, MD, MS
Dr. Teno is Professor of Community Health and Medicine at Brown Medical School and Associate Director of the Center for Gerontology & Health Care Research at Brown Medical School.

Mary R. Wimberly, RN
Mrs. Wimberly has a BS in nursing and a Masters degree in health services management. She is the lead care coordinator for the Home Telehealth program at the Central Arkansas Veterans Healthcare System.

Communication as a Lifeline: A Foreword

L.D. Britt, MD, MPH, FACS, FCCM

Perhaps there is nothing taken for granted more than the science of communication. Speaking a language or even being eloquent in discourse is not necessarily tantamount to effective communication. No learned person would likely debate the importance of possessing an adequate fund of knowledge. However, effective communication is, at least, as essential as a substantive knowledge base. In many arenas, ineffective communication can lead to disastrous results. The medical profession is one such arena where there is little, if any, margin for errors. In a landmark publication, the Institute of Medicine reported that there are as many as 44,000 to 98,000 deaths per year resulting from errors. Along with attributing this to system failure, suboptimal communication is also a major determining factor.

It is unacceptable for poor communication to be a component of the "quality chasm" which separates the quality of American health care that is possible, appropriate, and deserved from that which currently exists. Approximately a third of the adverse licensure actions decided by state medical boards is attributed to unprofessional conduct, with lack of or inappropriate communication often being the underlying problem. Even root-cause analysis of closed claims in legal cases confirms that ineffective communication plays a pivotal role.

Effective communication skills are not just verbal. In fact, the impact of nonverbal communication is 55% as compared to verbal or the vocal message. Of the nonverbal components, eye contact is, perhaps, the most important. The importance of nonverbal communication became quite evident when the first televised debate (the Nixon - Kennedy debate) was analyzed. Although the majority of television viewers felt that Richard Nixon had clearly lost the debate, the radio listeners who were polled felt that Nixon had won! This discrepancy was due to the fact that the television viewers were able to see the perspiring and obviously uncomfortable Richard Nixon during the debate.

The editors, Pamela Rowland, Ph.D., and Nicholas Lang, MD, expertly cover this and many other aspects of communication. This comprehensive textbook is unparalleled in its ability to specifically address both the art and science of communication. The highly qualified authors cover the full spectrum of the communication competencies in various situations and different settings, including emphasis on physician etiquette and professional image, cultural adaptability, disclosure of adverse outcomes, the communication skills required for organ/tissue procurement, and many other relevant topics. This textbook not only highlights communication needs in the steadily evolving medical environment, but provides the essential tools necessary to sharpen health care awareness and enhance delivery, consequently reducing medical errors.

I commend the editors and their contributors for unveiling this inaugural edition of the mastery of communication. It can, undoubtedly, be considered the definitive word on the principles of effective verbal and nonverbal communication.

Developing Communication Competency In Surgeons: A Recipe for Success

Pamela A. Rowland, PhD

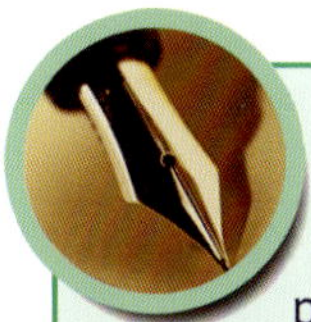

Mrs. Appleby is a 65-year-old female who has had hypertension for 10 years and is being treated with two antihypertensive medications. She is seeing her primary care surgeon today for a scheduled follow-up related to her blood pressure control. Two days prior to the visit, she mentioned to her husband that she thought she felt a lump in her left breast. Her husband repeatedly reminded her to mention this to the surgeon.

As soon as she arrives at the surgeon's office, a nurse measures her blood pressure (130/80 mmHg) in the waiting room and then escorts Mrs. Appleby to the examination room. After a wait of at least 30 minutes, Dr. Franklin arrives saying, "Good to see you again. Today is a teaching day. I know you won't mind if I have these two students sit in with us. So, how are you doing? I see your blood pressure is great today. Feeling good? Fine."

Mrs. Appleby says softly, "Well ... yes."

"Good, good," Dr. Franklin says as he flips through the chart. He turns slightly toward the students and explains that, "This lady has had hypertension for 10 years. Sometimes it's as high as 180/120 mmHg. It took a while to find a regimen that was consistently effective. But, Lopressor and Diltiazem have been very effective." He turns to Mrs. Appleby and says, "Glad you're doing so well. I think we can wait six months to see you again." As he stands and reaches to open the examination room door for the students, he turns and says, "Oh, say hi to your husband for me."

Studies show that often patients file complaints against surgeons because they failed to communicate effectively, not because they weren't effective "surgeon technicians." There may be times when patients and their families will maintain unsatisfactory relationships simply because they believe that the need for a "surgeon technician" is more important in certain situations (e.g. trauma) or that they have no alternative due to their third party plan or location. Therefore, it is unwise to believe that patient longevity implies that a patient "likes" a surgeon. Often it simply means that the patient "tolerates" the relationship. The purpose of this chapter is to outline simple communication behaviors that will improve "surgeon rhetorician" skills and thus improve surgeon-patient-student-colleague relationships.

Every surgeon makes mistakes, but not everyone gets sued or spends time in risk management offices responding to complaints. The difference — effective communication skills.

THE SURGEON COMMUNICATOR

In most current legal depositions, the plaintiff will answer the required preliminary question:

"When did you decide to sue Dr. Christopher?"

with a response such as:

"I got angry when he didn't care about my husband (or parent, or child, or me), and just did nothing."

Usually the anger is focused on a communication issue and not the technical competency of the surgeon. It is commonly accepted that all surgeons make mistakes, but not all get sued. The difference often is whether the "surgeon technician" successfully employs "surgeon rhetorician" skills.

The undisputed father of the science of rhetoric is Aristotle. He consistently argued that the only reason people bother to talk with someone is to create some sort of change: either behavioral or cognitive and ideally both. When applied to surgeon-patient interactions, some goals of surgeon rhetoric become clear. The best "surgeon rhetoricians" are able to:

- Discover information during patient interactions that is not already in the chart and could not be discovered any other way than through meeting face-to-face.
- Know what change (cognitive/behavioral) they want to occur as a result of the interaction before they leave the patient.
- Persuade the patient or family members to attempt change.
- Accurately predict what the patient will remember about the encounter (the residual message).

> **What and how you do, as well as what and how you communicate, are both major factors separating success from failure.**
>
> ***— NP Lang***

The professional survival of surgeons in the United States today depends greatly on the development of their personal and public rhetorical skills. These skills and competencies help to develop integrity, self-confidence, knowledge, self-control, adaptability and oral communication. They are necessary to engage in dyadic interactions with patients, peers, small groups such as committees, journal clubs, interviews and meetings with patient family members or administration and legal representatives. Such skills also clearly influence evaluations in case presentations, mortality and morbidity conferences, and journal and research presentations and success on the certifying examination for the marginal candidate.

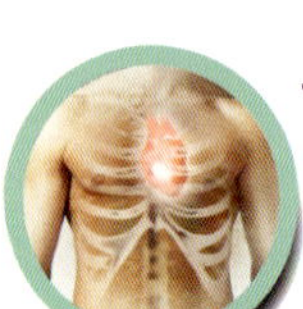

The Anatomy of Communication Competency

Too often surgeons proceed under the fallacy that patient satisfaction is determined at the end of the encounter, not at the beginning. They may believe, incorrectly, that if they 'reimplant' the severed finger, 'salvage' the spleen, or 'control' hypertension, anything else that occurs may be forgiven.

However, modern research has indicated that within the first few minutes of the initial interaction, people decide the competency of the surgeon and whether to continue or terminate the new relationship.

WHEN THINGS GO WRONG, SURGEONS SHOULDN'T ASK WHAT HAPPENED AT THE **END** OF THE INTERACTION; THEY SHOULD EXAMINE WHAT HAPPENED IN THE **BEGINNING**.

Spending more time on those first few minutes can save surgeons hours later. Often, surgeons think the interview has ended and begin to leave the room. Then as they are opening the door, the patient utters, *"Oh, by the way ...."* and lists a significant problem. If this happens often, a surgeon should examine how he or she communicates with patients in the first few minutes of the encounter.

"Joseph?" The triage nurse craned her neck through the window, peering around the waiting room. "Is there a Joseph...something, I can't pronounce the last name. Joseph, who is 76 and has hemorrhoids, please come to the desk."

The silence in the waiting room was thick with anticipation, broken only by the couple weeping in the corner and the drunk snoring on one of the trestle benches. No one stirred.

The nurse groaned, muttered something under her breath, and vanished back into the clinic hallway. Moments later, she reappeared in the doorway with obvious annoyance and strode into the waiting room. She confronted an elderly man standing by the exit door.

"Aren't you Joseph?" she demanded, glaring at him.

Slowly, he turned to face her. "My name is Dr. Budzynkiewicz. What is yours?"

The first five minutes in an initial outpatient interview should include the following behaviors as the absolute minimum of middle class courtesies in the outpatient setting:

1. The provider's introduction includes the use of honorifics.

(Mr., Mrs., Prof., Dr., Officer, Professor)

"Hello, Mrs. Jones, I'm Dr. Smith."

2. Eye contact is established.

3. A handshake is offered.

4. Both persons are speaking, listening, and beginning conversation.

Initial impressions (first few minutes) are critical. Damage caused then may never be repaired.

Diagram of an idealized reciprocal dyadic communication system in the outpatient setting.

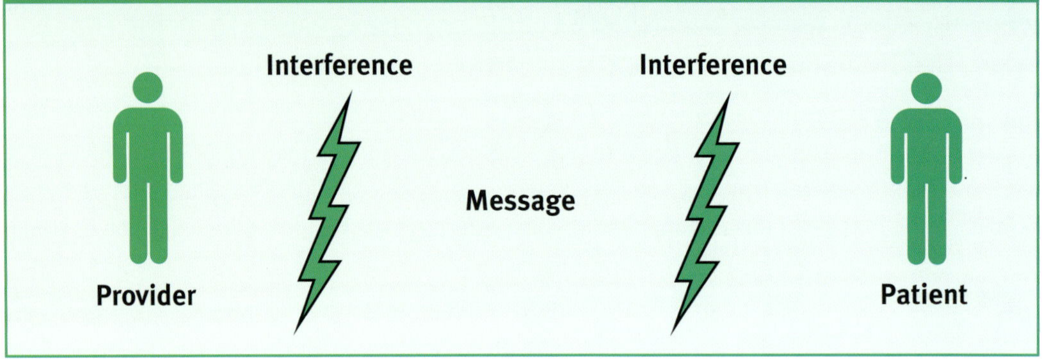

While many will argue that the use of first names by health care staff is better for patients, there simply isn't any evidence to support that assumption. In fact, there is more evidence to support that the use of honorifics with initial encounters will display respect and professionalism. It is the patient who has the power to ask to be called by his or her first name, not staff members.

Aaron Lazare, MD, Professor of Psychiatry, agrees with the above, stating that, "professionals seeing adult patients for the first time should refer to them by their proper titles and last names. Calling new patients by their first names forces a level of intimacy to which the patient has not agreed. It also assigns to patients a lesser status, since they are generally not expected to refer to the physician by his or her first name. Asking patients how they would like to be addressed puts the burden on them to anticipate what the professional would like to hear. Changes in the way the professional and patient address each other should be initiated by the patient and/or negotiated as the relationship evolves."

Such minimal courtesies help establish rapport and professionalism. However, surgeons can further improve the basic atmosphere for communication in a number of ways. For example:

1. **Place nametags on the right side in the outpatient setting, NOT the left pocket.**

   Often surgeons put the nametag on the left pocket of their lab coat or sports jacket pocket and assume that patients will remember their names after only one introduction. However, patients often leave and only recall "the older doctor," "the one with the beard," or "the short doc," and the name is lost. When the nametag is worn on the right collar area instead of the left pocket, it makes it easier for the person to hear and read the name at the same time that the handshake is initiated with the right hand.

2. **Eliminate the 'cattle call' approach.**

   Eliminating the "cattle call" approach to locating patients in waiting areas is another way to improve communication. Rather than shouting a patient's name from the clinic entrance, surgeons or their representatives should go 'to the patient.' If necessary, some physical assistance should be offered. A "follow me" or "heel" technique does not help the relationship in the waiting area. Instead of returning from the waiting room in silence, surgeons/staff members should be encouraged to use that time for some type of conversation. Saving time saves money.

Most Common Greeting Patterns in the United States		
Cattle Call	Person stands at clinic door, shouts patient name and retreats into clinic	Most common across the US
Heel Technique	Person enters clinic slightly, calls name, turns to return to clinic and expects patient to 'heel'	Still considered 'clinic quality' care approach
Business Class	Person enters waiting area, stands, calls name and waits for patient to come to her/him, some conversation and walks into clinic	More often seen in private offices, higher end HMO's
First Class	Person walks into one section of the clinic and says patient name loud enough only for that section, and repeats in other waiting areas until patient is found.	Goes to the patient rather than patient going to her/him

3. Watch and listen.

Surgeons can also use the first few minutes to watch and listen for information they can use later in developing a realistic plan for their patients. In addition to identifying specific patient problems, a surgeon should be able to determine the following:

1) The patient's attitude toward the surgeon;

2) Patient's attitude toward illness; and

3) Attitude of simply being in a medical setting –all within the first few minutes.

VERBAL COMMUNICATION

Adjust Vocabulary Level

During medical school and residency training, a surgeon probably learns at least an additional 100,000 new words, the equivalent of a new language. This information is continually expanded as new pharmaceuticals are developed, new procedures perfected and new techniques designed. Therefore, one surgeon skill that is vital is the ability to translate complex information on many different levels. For 11 to 16 years surgeons-in-training are asked to regurgitate information on a post-graduate level to peers and colleagues. Residents may be asked to explain to a student the main pathophysiologic differences between gastric and duodenal ulcers and their therapeutic implications. Or a student may be asked to state the main indications for lower extremity revascularization by an attending. Then, in the latter years of training, they are expected to translate this complex information to clinic patients at a middle or junior high school level, similar to that of most newspapers. Once technical competency is mastered with peers, the continuing challenge is to adjust the presentation appropriately to a new patient audience.

For example, a resident should be able to do the following:

- Discuss the treatment options with a 42-year-old woman who has recently undergone an excisional breast biopsy. Pathology report reveals a 2cm infiltrating ductal carcinoma. She has no clinical evidence of metastasis. She is a high school English teacher with a master's degree.
- Discuss indications for repair, risks, anesthesia options, and expected recovery period with a 78-year-old man with a large symptomatic inguinal hernia. His PMH include COPD, two previous MIs, HTN, and A. Fib. on Coumadin. Before he retired, he was an international pilot for Delta.
- Discuss different surgical techniques of cholecystectomy (laparoscopic vs. open) with a 45-year-old woman who has symptomatic cholelithiasis, demonstrated by ultrasound. She has had a previous appendectomy and two C-sections. She runs the Before/After School Program in the local community.
- Discuss different treatment options, risks, and possible complications with a 68-year-old man who has a rectal carcinoma at 5cm from the dentate line. He is otherwise healthy and has no evidence of metastases. He still works at his family-owned hardware/lumber store.

Surgeons constantly practice speaking in "technical" terms to faculty, colleagues, and staff. During training, feedback is immediate, but patients are reluctant to ask for clearer explanations when their surgeon misses what they need. Obviously, practice with observation is best, but using computer word processors to evaluate vocabulary level is also solid quantitative feedback. Most vocabulary in outpatient public hospital settings will measure at a fourth or fifth grade level for patients and fifth or sixth for experienced faculty. The goal is not to be exactly the same, but to speak on a level playing field.

Surgery is now a team sport.

Surgeon Translator

Surgeons should never assume that the explanation of cholelithiasis developed for Mrs. Greenan will work with most other patients. Mrs. Greenan has her own unique ideas of how the world works and so the approach used for her will miss the mark at least half of the time with other adults. Patients may be and often are bright, but not up-to-date on specific medical subjects. This is a *surgeon-translator* skill that constantly needs practice. However, the better the conversation surgeons have with patients in the beginning few minutes of the interview, the easier it is to develop this vocabulary adjustment skill.

Develop Conversational Skills

Social scientists have supported a variety of stereotypical personality types across surgeon specialties that vary from warm and caring to cold and authoritarian. But, they have noted that across all specialties there is a pattern of social immaturity in young surgeons. Perhaps the isolation from those in other disciplines throughout their prolonged education accounts for this. Often this is manifested in a lack of conversational skills appropriate for their age and training. Yet professionals who depend on interviewing as a means of data gathering will argue that the best interviews are simply good conversations. They have developed the skill of conducting a natural give and take continually throughout the exchange, even with complete strangers, rather than a list of 55 direct questions that sound like an interrogation. Therefore, nascent surgeons should seriously focus on developing this skill early in their training as a way to:

- Get to know new patients, staff and family members;
- Meet new colleagues at social gatherings;
- Meet new professionals at professional meetings;
- Interview more comfortably, and;
- Reduce stress associated with not having developed such skills prior to entering a specific setting.

The Chinese developed a method to make surgeons more "conversational" with the 'people' by forcing all young medical students to live and work with the peasants for one year during their training. However, in the United States, we isolate our medical students for four years from nonphysicians, then semi-isolate them for five to eight years more with health care teams and maintain a prolonged adolescence for up to the age of at least 31 when board certification becomes available. Often, all outside commitments are on "hold" until residency is completed, socially isolating residents even more.

As time becomes shorter, carry the Week-in-Review Section from the Sunday newspaper with you. Your goal should be to finish it by the end of the week. This will broaden your attempts at conversation with others outside your work experience.

Control Fluency

The greatest presentation of a plan to patients can be destroyed if the surgeon's speech is peppered with 'junk' words or 'habit' phrases known as vocal segregates.

Eliminate Vocal Segregates

Surgeons should not pepper their speech with the following:

"um"	"uh-huh"	"you know"	"absolutely"
"and ah"	"uh"	"for sure"	"right"
"and um"	"ah-huh"	"wicked"	"OK"

Habit Phrases

Habit phrases are those words used so often that they lose their meaning. Basically, they function on a normal curve. If they are used occasionally, naturally they do not present a problem and add to an oral versus regurgitated speaking style. Habit words are often regional in nature and most are based on a casual speech style that doesn't belong in the adult outpatient setting. No one goes to a surgeon to establish a casual relationship. Therefore, casual speech in the surgical setting can lead to conflict.

When a patient asks a surgeon about how to care for a child's persistent ear infection, and the surgeon says,

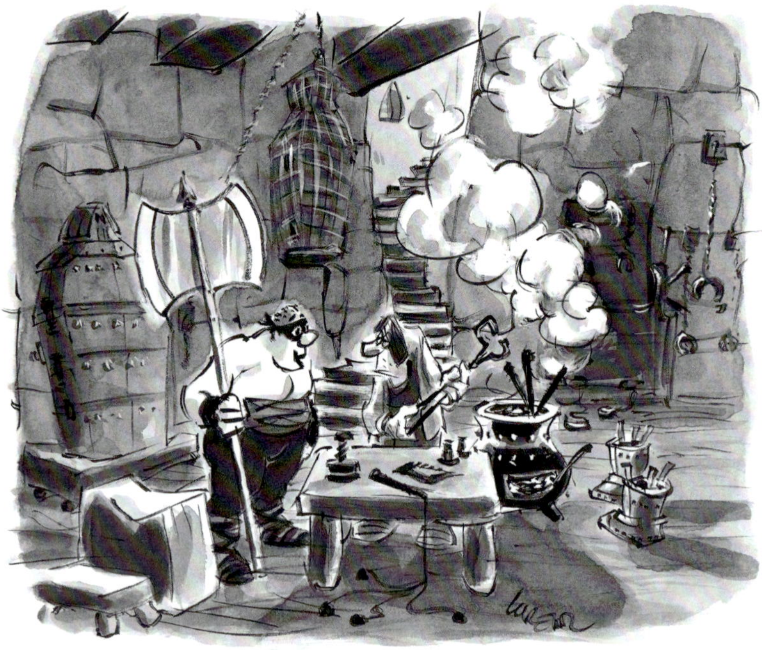

"I was afraid it was bursitis, but it's only repetitive stress injury."

"Well, um, ah, well, ah, we, um I mean, ah, you could try...well, maybe I'll.."

The parent will wonder about the surgeon's credibility, even if the correct information is buried in the utterance. When a patient asks a surgeon about how an operation went and he hears,

"Well, ah, I, um, think, ah, hmm, most everything went, ah, um, alright...ahh..."

and couples the response with a slow rate of speech, there will be problems! The patient will question the confidence and integrity of the hesitating surgeon and wonder what may have gone wrong. If the surgeon appears 'young' to the patient, then the conflict is even harder to overcome.

In studies that focused on case presentations and surgery oral examinations, young surgeons whose speech contained 'junk' words and 'habit' phrases and indirect eye contact did not do well, even though their content was appropriate. When residents presented the same information without these types of words, their scores improved.

The 'safe' approach is to use formal speech in formal settings, business speech in business settings and casual speech in casual settings. This is another form of reciprocal behavior.

When someone cries from room to room during the oral examination, the examiners question the surgeon's confidence and control of emotions. Crying with others after a death is acceptable. Consistent clearing of the throat during conversation indicates that the surgeon/patient is uncomfortable with the discussion. Laughing while saying something unkind does not negate the message. It could be considered a form of harassment.

Inappropriate behaviors for a surgeon			
A form of harassment			
Emotion	Tiredness	Rude	Zero tolerance
Laughing	Sighing	Belching	Yelling
Crying	Moaning		
Clearing of the throat	Yawning		

While mildly chuckling and smiling, "...well Mary do you ever think you'll be able to be a real surgeon since you're only 5 feet tall?"

Demanding on-call schedules and balancing personal needs drains on everyone's energy levels. Often surgeons get calls from nurses, residents, and other providers when energy levels are being tested. The listener hears 'sighs' and 'moans' across the telephone line and interprets them as "not caring," "you're disturbing him," and "what you're asking isn't important," when the lack of energy is pushing the behavior, not the question.

To resolve this behavior, *without chemical intervention*, simply:

1) Recognize that you're not your best and; then
2) When listening—turn the receiver upside down; and
3) When talking, hold the microphone in front of your face. Continue to repeat this process until the conversation is completed.

Grammar: Talk the talk - 'Surgeons' Grammar

A surgeon's use of grammar and vocabulary have a tremendous impact on the audience, whether it be a board examiner, jury, other physicians, and even patients.

Although most listeners will have the ability to understand what you are trying to say whether your grammar is at the tenth grade level or that of a ten year old, poor grammar may influence their perception of your intelligence. This can not only have a negative impact on juries, but also influence your colleagues whom you depend upon for referrals and promotions.

Language	
Common Jargon	**Better choice**
different than	different from
to 'follow up'	just avoid jargon
what type of surgery?	what operation did he have?
die from	die of
etc, so on, so forth, and the like	such as, including
like we just mentioned	as previously stated
irregardless (not a word)	regardless
whether or not	whether
graduated	were graduated from
married	were married
followed up over five years	followed for more than five years
if I was	if I were

Grammar Common Errors

Accept vs Except

The American Board of Surgery accepted his argument.

All of the variables entered into the multiple regression analysis contributed to the outcome except resident salaries.

Affect vs Effect

His affect was a signal to his colleagues that he might be depressed.

The increase in hormone levels had a large effect on the spread of metastatic disease.

Allude vs Elude

To mention indirectly

Dr. Brown alluded to the fact that he was ready for retirement.

Elude means to escape understanding

The reason he wasn't invited to the conference eluded him.

Among

Refers to one item in a group

Only one interviewee among this group seemed sincere.

Between

Use with 2 or more independent items

There wasn't a difference between the chemotherapy in any of the protocols.

Anybody

Can be interchanged with everyone

Means an unspecified person

Any body

A noun referring to a singular human body (alive or dead)

The lab was not able find any bodies that were fresh.

Anymore

Refers to time

Residents don't do parathyroids anymore.

Any more

Used with a noun or indefinite pronoun

The journal didn't need any more submissions for the special issue on liver transplants.

Anyone

Refers to any person

Anyone can apply for an HHS grant.

Any one

Used to refer to one part/person of a group

Any one of these toxins could have made him susceptible to cancer.

As

Used as a conjunction; it should be used before phrases and clauses

Just as Tom mentioned, we need to pay attention to the ABSITE scores of the candidates.

Cheap

Implies an inferior quality. If you are referring to the costs related to medications, instruments, or quality of care, "less expensive" is the better choice.

Lie

To place or put –
Past tense – *laid*

Lay

(people) rest or recline

Past tense - lain

Like

A preposition that means "in a similar way"

The PGY-2 acted like an adolescent.

Assure

To state in a positive way; provide confidence

I assure my patients that I will do my best.

Insure

Make certain; guard against financial risk

We insure our residents for any disabilities as a result of their work.

Ensure

Means to make certain; similar to insure

When you ligate the vessels, ensure that you've identified the nerves.

Can

Means the ability to do something

Chief residents can take vacation any time of the year except June.

May

Means a request for permission or indicates a certain likelihood

Dentretic cells may hold the answer for combating certain types of cancer.

Farther

Means physical distance

Further

Refers to time

Examine

Patients are examined

Evaluate

Conditions and disease are evaluated

Optimal

Don't use as a noun; means more favorable

Optimum

Used as a noun

Rational

An adjective meaning someones ability to reason

Rationale

A noun meaning the fundamental reason

The rationale behind our expansion plans for the ED was based on population shifts.

Signs

An indication of the presence of a disease or disorder, especially one observed by a provider, but not apparent to the patient.

Fever is a sign of an infection.

Symptoms

Applies to people

The symptoms included fever and a rash on his abdomen.

Symbols

Represent something. Do not look like what they represent. Letters are symbols.

Oral Style

Can't, don't, won't.

Written style

Cannot, do not, would not

Datum

Singular and only one result

Data

plural

Sharpen Articulation

It is a common expression that "Speech is caught, not taught." Organs and muscles synchronize in a millisecond to produce speech without any formal training, yet it is one of the more important skills humans possess. Speech announces a tremendous amount of information to listeners. Most surgeons take for granted that somewhere along the way in their medical training, they assimilated or 'caught' the appropriate skills to "talk" like a surgeon.

"Speech is caught, not taught."

One of the most common mistakes in articulation is the elimination of the endings on words. Endings such as "ing," "ed," and "t's" are often not pronounced, especially when anyone is tired. "T's" are often not pronounced regardless of their order in a word. However, not pronouncing these sounds can effect the listener's perception of the surgeon's intelligence. "Going" becomes "gunna," "Long Island" turns into "Longuyland," "wanted" sounds like "wan Ed." Certain regions in the United States switch words ending in "a," to "er" ("idea vs ideer"). The more surgeons swallow or eliminate the endings of words, the less intelligent they sound. What may be perfectly normal in one area of the country may clash with acceptable, professional speech in another.

Medicine and surgery were once local markets. Today, they are not just statewide, regional, or national – they're global. Therefore, your communication skill set must recognize this broader audience to be successful.

Patients may travel from Kuwait, New Zealand or Dallas to see you for your specific expertise. Surgeons sound more intelligent when their speech is clear and easy to understand. Slack or sloppy speech may reflect an uncaring attitude toward the listener (patient, staff or students). This does not mean that accents have to be eliminated or changed as long as they don't interfere with communication.

Speakers of English as a second language can review lists designed specifically to focus on common problems associated with their native tongue and standard English.

Adjust Volume

Clearly, in communication the listeners are the judges. If Mrs. Merrill didn't hear what her surgeon said, then he didn't say anything. If the examiners at the American Board of Surgery Certifying Examination didn't hear the candidate say that he would have ordered a test, then it wasn't ordered.

The listener's problem with hearing becomes the speaker's responsibility. Surgeons must adjust their volume for the listener. If surgeons notice that while they are talking to someone in a dyadic situation, the listener is focusing attention on the surgeon's mouth and not on the eyes, this may indicate that the listener is having difficulty hearing what is being said. (Note: Occasionally part of lunch left on the front teeth may also produce this reaction.) This may be due to loss of hearing or difficulty adjusting to an accent. To improve the situation, surgeons should increase their volume, slow their speaking rate and aim for crisper articulation.

During training, young surgeons may become aware that older faculty members are speaking too softly and it becomes difficult to hear descriptions over the sound of equipment. It is not rude for the young trainee to ask for repetition; students and residents are there to learn.

Verbal Behaviors to Adjust		
Intensity	Too soft	If the preceptor – oral examiner – or jury can't hear you, they question your competence
	Too loud	Your message may be ignored and the focus may be on your intimidating manner
Pitch	Too high	Message may be ignored because pitch is annoying – gender specific
	Too low	Loses listener interest
Extent	Too drawn out (drawl)	Listeners assume your cognitive processing is also slow
	Too fast	Listeners assume you are 'pushy'

Develop Residual Messages

Modern communication theory states that in oral interactions (surgeon-patient), persons only retain approximately 4 to 5% (residual message) of what they hear without some form of repetition.

In the surgeon-patient interaction, surgeons need to influence and reinforce a specific residual message for each patient visit, whether it's an initial hour or 10 minute follow-up. All gall bladder patients shouldn't get the same message, nor should all pregnant women. The residual message may be the same at every visit or may vary across visits.

In stressful situations, the retention may be decreased.

Otherwise, the patient will choose messages randomly from all of the topics discussed and miscommunication can occur. The skilled surgeon decides what the most important residual message is for each encounter and reinforces it appropriately for each patient. To test for the residual message, surgeons should ask themselves, "If Mrs. George goes home and her daughter asks her what the doctor said, what will Mrs. George say?" The response should be one simple sentence or the residual message. A good surgeon will know what that sentence will be. Some sample residual messages might be the following:

- "Check my glucose levels daily."
- "Walk at least to the end of my driveway every day."
- "Change my dressings twice a day."
- "Take this pill if I feel chest pain."

METHODS TO REINFORCE THE RESIDUAL MESSAGE

1. Use stylized redundancy

Saying the same thing in many different ways. Simply repeating 20 times, "I really care about you, Mrs. Slade" doesn't accomplish much and would seem silly to the patient. Instead, surgeons could effectively emphasize 'CARING' messages in such ways as the following:

1. Providing examples that the patient can relate to;
2. Changes in vocal variety, rate, and volume;
3. Sincere eye contact;
4. Asking questions that indicate you're listening;
5. Appropriate humor; and
6. Anecdotes or anything else that will work with this patient.

A surgeon should have some concept of what style or persuasive methods will work with a patient after an initial conversation. The better the conversation, the better able the surgeon is at communicating the key residual message.

2. Select an organization to reinforce the residual message

When surgeons talk to a family to enlist their support, to obtain consent or to inform, the interaction needs some structure. Although the content may vary tremendously, there are methods to help in the organization of a surgeon's remarks. The first step is to decide if the goal is to inform or persuade. This decision determines the structure.

GOAL: TO PERSUADE

You have a better chance of reaching your goals if you follow sequential steps throughout a conversation or professional presentation.

Step One: ATTENTION

Gain the attention of the person(s); patient, family members or staff. Relate your statements to their situation by mentioning the importance of the treatment, surgery, follow-up, medication. Make a startling statement, ask a question, tell a story or use a media aid (heart, inner ear model).

Step Two: NEED

Let the patient know that this is a problem that needs attention. Demonstrate evidence in a way that will relate to this person's values or experiences. By the end of this step, the patient should be so concerned about their problem that they are prepared to hear the solution.
"Mrs. Jones, you said you want to attend your granddaughter's wedding next spring. Well, if you..., then you probably can."

> **"No one goes to a surgeon to establish a casual relationship."**
>
> ***PA Rowland***

Step Three: SATISFACTION

Simply present a solution(s) to the problem. Present the treatment plan and show how it will work for them. Be sure to adjust the details about the plan, along with alternatives, so that the patient or family member is able to understand.

Step Four: VISUALIZATION

Present the benefits of your plan. Discuss how the patient will profit from your plan. Make the patient/spouse/child see how much better the patient's condition will be once the plan is adopted.

Don't assume that patients, whether employees or families of surgeons who are patients, understand the system/process. If you don't take time to explain how your system works, they will second guess and draw conclusions such as "I have to wait longer for my test because I'm not rich."

Step Five: ACTION

Once the patient/family is convinced the plan is beneficial, call for action. Say exactly what the patient should do and how to do it. Give the patient the address of where to go for physical therapy, or the name of the surgeon that the patient should see next Friday morning. Finally, end with a statement that reinforces both what your and the hospital's commitment is to the patient and what the patient's commitment is to this process.

GOAL: TO INFORM

When presenting *new* information to a patient, family member, or at a professional meeting, there are three easy steps to follow:

Step One:

An opening statement(s) to introduce the topic.

Step Two:

The physician should repeat the residual message in a variety of ways (stylized redundancy throughout the body of the speech). The surgeon may use stories, anecdotes, humor, or analogies that work for the particular patient, family member or group. Adjust the vocabulary for that audience.

Step Three:

The surgeon summarizes what has been said. New information is not introduced and the final message is kept short. Remember the **KISS** technique – Keep it Simple Surgeon!

Regardless of which structure the surgeon follows, there should be sufficient pauses to allow for interruptions by the patient seeking clarification.

Surgeons should:

- Check for understanding throughout the interview, not only at the end;
- Watch the listeners, not the patient record, and listen for clues about how you are doing.

If you can't learn to look at patients, you may as well communicate via e-mail.

Nonverbal Communication

Communication can be crudely classified in two ways: verbal and nonverbal. Throughout this text, verbal refers to what is heard, while nonverbal refers to all messages other than words.

Surgeons are effective communicators when they are able to

- Define their goals (whether to persuade or inform); and
- Accurately predict their patient's residual messages.

It is critical to note that if the nonverbal behavior of a surgeon conflicts with the verbal, all other efforts may have been wasted. Therefore, surgeons need to closely examine their nonverbal communication with different patients, staff and family members.

It is important to note that verbal and nonverbal communication are not independent parts; just different sides of the same coin. Even though everyone's cognitive framework processes them differently, they work together to arrive at meaning for both the surgeon and the patient.

Communication MUST vary by the setting
Patient registration
Operating room
Emergency department
Outpatient setting
Bedside
Hallway encounters
Certifying examination
Clinic setting
Courtroom setting
Social settings

Acceptable behaviors may not be written, but by observing them in different settings, surgeons can learn acceptable versus unacceptable behavior for a particular setting and culture. Part of the learning process in medicine is discovering these rules throughout medical school, residency, and fellowships. A person whose normative behavior is unacceptable for a particular setting is often labeled "immature," "young," "unsophisticated," or "naive." For example, a fourth year student is expected to arrive on time and in proper dress for a patient interview and to know that the center chair at M&M's and Grand Rounds at a specific hospital is for the department chief.

Few behaviors, if any, are universal. What is interpreted by most Americans as friendly is often viewed by others as rude and crude. Even within the United States, rules of courtesy vary (Southerners use of "sir" and "ma'am"). It is the responsibility of professional surgeons to understand the meaning of specific nonverbal behaviors for the culture within which they are practicing. The only universal negative nonverbal behavior that we are aware of is "vomiting on another person.

The following areas describe the effects of common types of nonverbal communication:

Proxemics:

- the environment;
- patient, staff and surgeon use of territoriality (i.e., seating preference);
- violating personal, interpersonal and impersonal boundaries.

Kinesics or Body Language:

- gestures;
- touching (tactile communication) both towards self and with patients and staff;
- body movements; and
- posture in specific settings.

Vocal Cues:

- voice on personality characteristics;
- judgments regarding emotions;
- response-time latency (< or > 2-3 seconds);
- hesitations;
- repetitions; and
- use of silence.

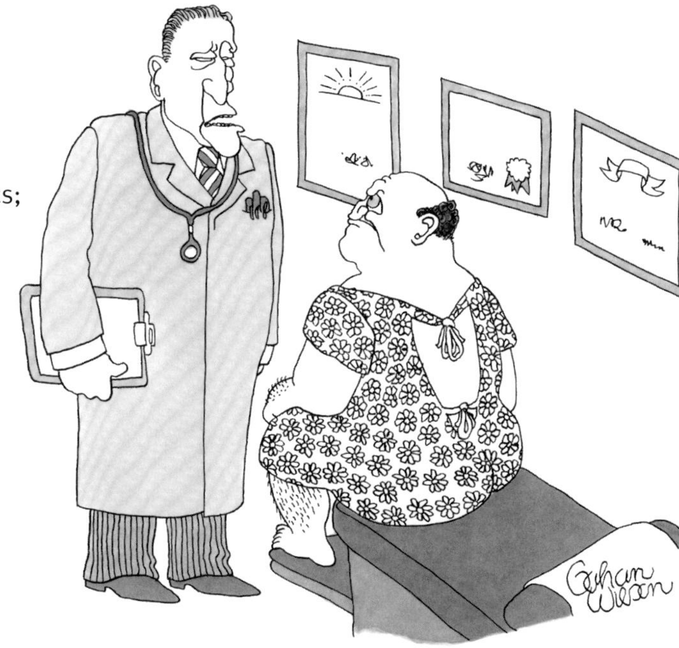

"Humiliation is a very important part of the process, Mr. Keifer."

Facial Expressions, when used for:

- feedback;
- definitely culturally bound;
- in dyadic (surgeon-patient); and
- small group interactions (family, conferences).

Professional Image or Artifactual Communication:

- clothes;
- hair;
- body image;
- odor(olfactics); and
- "tools of the trade."

Initial impressions are quick to form and difficult to change - even in the light of new information.

Temporal

How time communicates (e.g., whether surgeons see a need to be "on time").

Each one of these areas may be communicating different messages at the same time. However, the focus should be on the overall message. In the American culture, research has shown that some areas differ in importance. For example, Americans focus more on the eyes for clues.

Situations arise for which a behavioral approach to nonverbal communication is helpful. Incorporating a checklist may help isolate weaknesses in nonverbal communication. For example, residents whose notes are clear and presentations are concise but who seem to frequently make the attending angry should examine their nonverbal behavior.

Proxemics

Surgeons' offices immediately communicate the roles and attitudes expected from everyone in a given encounter, including the patient, student, resident, surgeon, and surgeon's staff. One impression, either positive or negative, is formed after multiple "mini" impressions are created.

Color

Color communicates a variety of impressions. Although specific colors communicate age by the popularity of the color (1992 green; 1990 mauve), research has shown color communicates general emotions. Certain colors seem to be more calming than others.

Office Settings

The minimum requirement for an office setting is a desk and two chairs. But it is the physical arrangement and type of furniture that indicate several things to the patient or family members. The size and comfort of a chair indicate how long the person in that chair is expected to stay in that area and the status of persons in the encounter. As someone advances in the hospital hierarchy, the quality of furniture and amount of space between speakers usually increases.

Often surgeons in managed care settings have little control over the decor of rooms they need to use as they talk with patients, their families and colleagues. While it is ideal to remove barriers between speakers, that is not always physically possible in a hospital setting or a clinic room that is shared with multiple surgeons and other health care providers. However, there are some guidelines for different situations that will improve the amount and quality of communication.

In hospital rooms with more than one bed, surgeons and students should choose to stand with their backs to the wall, rather than between beds, so the patient doesn't feel the entire population of the room is in the audience.

In dyadic situations, sitting at right angles will increase the amount of communication. Sitting directly opposite each other may seem authoritarian and decrease the amount of communication.

For small group discussions, a circular seating pattern produces the best communication flow. This seating pattern allows all members to maintain eye contact equally with all other members in the group. For example, if the surgeon is directly opposite the family group, the eye contact is maintained equally and the leadership role of the surgeon supported. If, however, the nurse is directly opposite the family members and the patient, leadership roles are not as well defined and the amount of communication may increase.

At rectangular conference tables, participants should try for equal spacing between all members to increase the amount of communication. There are many possible seating patterns. Each position indicates surgeons' attitudes toward their patients, students, residents, family members or colleagues. The power seat is located at the end of the table and will limit interactions. Sitting at the head of the table automatically puts the surgeon in the leadership position. If the patient or family member is directly across the table from the surgeon, the conversational flow will not be as great as it would if the participants are seated at right angles to each other. To increase the amount of verbal interaction, surgeons should sit at the middle of the table.

The key is to identify the goal of the interview before selecting a seating pattern. There are times when the surgeon's position of authority needs to be emphasized, but there are other times when it is most helpful to reflect a role of reassurance and team cooperation. Surgeons should remain flexible and make deliberate choices and not take the only seat left in the room.

The modern surgeon must speak not only in dyadic (one-on-one) situations, but often in small and large group situations. In both, surgeons are usually expected to assume the leadership role, keeping in mind the rules for personal space and appropriate touching.

Types of Space	
Personal space	Physical contact to 18 inches
Casual-personal	1-1/2 feet to 4 feet
Social-consultation	4 – 12 feet for impersonal business
Public	12 feet to the limits of sight and sound
The topic and space must be consistent. If not, there is conflict.	

The topic under discussion dictates which type of space (personal, casual, social, or public) is appropriate. In some situations, the violation of personal and public space is obvious. Surgeons who speak to the hospitalized patient about the patient's "personal" health from the "impersonal" doorway are violating the rules of nonverbal communication. Patients can feel humiliated when something such as their weight, which they consider personal, is talked about in social-consultative space.

Conversely, surgeons who speak to colleagues with too little space between them can promote resentment and distrust. Females may suspect males, or visa versa, of unprofessional behavior if they simply speak to them without enough space between them. Males or females may interpret another's sexual preference simply because of speaking distances being too personal for the setting or topic. Males and females will often put barriers (e.g., charts) between them to prevent others from invading their space. Colleagues will place pens, books, folders, coffee cups, or coats on conference tables to enlarge their space and 'stake out' their territory. Patients will do the same in waiting areas. Space is often equated with power. They may ask strangers to "hold their seat" in crowded waiting areas while they talk with a receptionist.

To prevent a person from getting "too close," we can unconsciously "stab" them with our pens or pencils.

Kinesics

Gestures can enhance or distract from what surgeons are saying. There are cultural stereotypes among the American population that vary from speaker to speaker. This may range from the White Anglo-Saxon/little movement to the Italian/constant movement. However, there are some basic premises that need to be followed:

- A gesture cannot substitute for the verbal message on the telephone.

  The surgeon may nod constantly to what the patient is saying on the telephone. But, by not saying something like, *"Yes, that's a good idea, keep it up,"* the now anxious patient may conclude, *"The surgeon didn't say anything. He just said he'd see me at my next appointment."* A short verbalization of the nonverbal would have prompted reassurance and patient compliance.

- Gestures below the waist are distracting.

  The patient needs to focus on what the surgeon is saying. If, when speaking, the surgeon fidgets with pocket change, the stethoscope, or a watchband, the patient's eye will follow the movement and not focus on what is said. Gestures above the waist and away from the body are most effective when you are speaking. The patient's eyes follow movement. You always want your listeners to focus on your face and what you are saying.

- Arms or hands close to the body can be interpreted as defensiveness.

  Closed versus open positions may signal to patients or colleague that they shouldn't approach someone to speak or that a surgeon may be quite judgmental. There may be times when this is appropriate. However, when asking patients to express a concern or answer questions about something they might find embarrassing such as their sexual activity, open positions (hands apart) may invite conversation, while arms folded across the chest may restrict it. In addition, patients, peers or family members may interpret a closed, hands-in-lap, or "praying" position as indicative of a lack of confidence or judgment. Residents who immediately put both hands behind their back when presenting at M&Ms look as though they are ready to be handcuffed.

Tactile Communication

Touching is probably one of the most primitive forms of communication. Surgeons begin to learn the rules of touch in infancy and continue throughout their personal and professional development. The appropriate "feel" of the liver or breast tumor must be learned along with the appropriate touching behaviors of children, elderly, and ethnic groups within patient populations.

The amount and kind of contact in dyadic encounters varies considerably with the age, sex, setting, and relationship of the surgeon-patient or surgeon-staff member. If, in the patient's perception, any surgeon touched him or her inappropriately for any of these reasons, conflict will develop and the patient will no longer be paying full attention to the encounter. Also, if a child or female reacts abnormally to what the surgeon considers appropriate touching, the surgeon should look for signs of physical abuse.

During the initial stage of an outpatient interview, middle class courtesies are extended. When surgeons initiate the handshake, this signals confidence and an acceptance of the patient. It is appropriate in the United States for female surgeons to extend a right hand first to her patients, whether male or female. It helps reinforce her role and project a feeling of confidence.

There are moments when touching colleagues seems appropriate. However, peers and attendings are never supposed to touch each other in anger (zero tolerance). Handshakes are safe methods for starting and ending a conversation. A touch above the waist on the top of the shoulder is acceptable to most Americans if used to quietly get attention. Hugs between members of the opposite sex are 'safer' if permission is asked by simply saying, "May I give you a hug?" before actually hugging a student, resident, staff member or attending.

There are moments when touching patients is appropriate outside of the physical examination. For example, reassurance and encouragement through touch is the least any surgeon can offer when the prognosis appears extremely grim. The ethical (and medico-legal) responsibilities regarding truth-telling should be mitigated by the commitment to support the patient psychologically. In this context, specific actions such as acceptable body contact and even non-traditional medical techniques may offer hope and support.

Posture

The surgeon's posture can indicate an attitude toward the patient and the encounter.

In addition, the degree of relaxation needs to be interpreted from posture. For example, leaning forward usually is interpreted as being alert and attentive. Leaning too far forward could be read as a threat. Leaning back can indicate a state of relaxation, or a casual encounter. When combined with open arms at the side, the degree of relaxation increases. However, seeming too relaxed for the topic can be labeled "cocky" or "uncaring" by the patient or the patient's family. This behavior is not usually appropriate for surgeons.

Surgeons who face patients directly while speaking (shoulders parallel) will be perceived as paying full attention to the encounter.

No one goes to a surgeon to establish a casual relationship.

Patients prefer surgeons who seem to be paying full attention to the encounter. Although the degree of relaxation obviously varies according to the setting (e.g., pediatrics vs. trauma rooms), patients or family members in the outpatient setting prefer to have surgeons turn to face them when they are being spoken to. The habit of standing or sitting with legs apart is influenced by the sex and status of the speakers and listeners. For males and females, conflict arises when a more alert posture is not used with persons of higher status.

Vocal Clues

Certain decisions that patients make regarding surgeons' credibility are made from the voice alone. Sometimes a surgeon is well received simply because he or she speak well. This has been shown not only in public speaking situations, but in case presentations of medical students and on oral examinations. Conversely, if the style of the surgeon is distracting, the listener misses part of the content.

In general, there are some perceptions that are associated with specific types of voices (feminine, masculine, intellectual). There are professionals available to work with students/surgeons to change

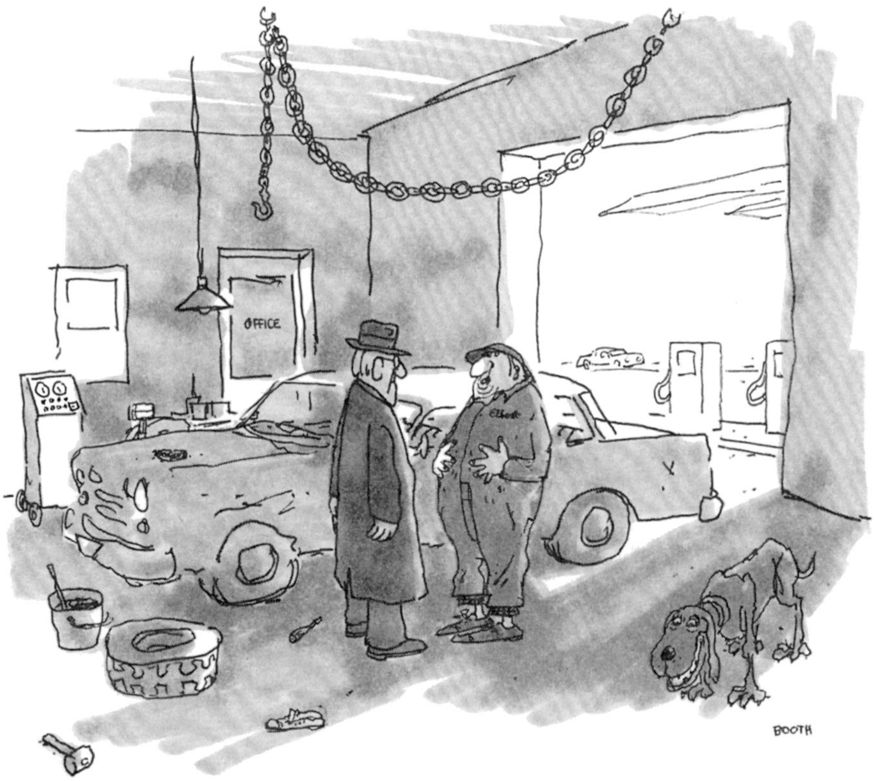

"If I were a surgeon, Mr. Ferguson, which I ain't, and your car was my patient, which it ain't—except that it is, in a funny sort of way; that is, if you want to look at it like that; you know what I mean—and you was her husband, I'd have to say, 'Sir, your wife is going to need a valve job.' "

negative aspects of their voice quality. These include stereotypes of regional accents and social class. Certain accents are associated with prestige. Specific voices are determined to be more "masculine," "feminine," "smarter," "older," or "younger" than others and conflict arises when the perceived image doesn't match the voice. When a surgeon projects a professional image, the voice aids in supporting or distracting from that image for specific audiences. Everyone should attempt to speak differently (formally-casually) to different audiences. Surgeons need to learn to adjust pauses and pitch when under stress as well as to control for volume and rate. All are important in speaking with peers, patients and families and in presenting at conferences.

Pauses

In social situations, most people will respond to a verbal utterance within 2 to 3 seconds. Lengthened response time latency (>2–3 seconds) tends to create anxiety. For example, a student meets with his faculty advisor and asks, *"How well did I do on the written exam?"* If the response is silence for five seconds, he knows he didn't do well. Likewise, when a patient asks, *"How am I?"* and the surgeon doesn't respond within 2 to 3 seconds, the patient begins to worry. Courtroom lawyers are very good at using this technique. By lengthening the response time, they create anxiety for the witness and because of the discomfort, the witness says something unpracticed. This technique of lengthening the response time is useful for surgeons having difficulty getting a patient to elaborate on a story. When the patient stops speaking, the surgeon continues to look engaged as if there is more to come. By not talking, the surgeon can get the patient to elaborate and perhaps provide additional information.

On the other hand, because surgeons are uncomfortable with silence, they sometimes tend to fill the silence with vocal segregates such as *"you know," "um," and "ah,"* rather than simply pausing to collect their thoughts. This may be because surgeons are afraid that someone else will begin speaking and they will lose control. However, patients may interpret this as a lack of knowledge and preparedness. These phrases may simply be habit phrases (e.g., 1990's *"absolutely"*). If the people with whom surgeons associate use these phrases often, they will begin to also. Although frequently regional, such speech patterns are associated with immaturity and unprofessional behavior and should be controlled or eliminated in the professional setting.

Rate

Rate of speech tends to indicate the level of relaxation.

Most people tend to increase their rate of speech when under stress, although a small percentage will become painfully slow. Lazare argues that sometimes people in a lower status will increase their rates when speaking to someone they perceive in a higher status in an attempt "to fit everything in."

Rates are regional.

Persons from rural areas tend to speak at a slower rate than those from urban or suburban areas (the "country boy" vs. the fast-talking "city slicker"). Occasionally, someone who isn't from an urban area will have a faster rate because their parents came from an urban setting and passed their language patterns on to their children.

Conflict

Conflict can occur when one speaker has a slower rate and the other has a faster rate. The faster speaker can become irritated with the slower-rate speaker and the slower-rate speaker may resent feeling rushed. Therefore, it may be helpful for surgeons to concentrate on slowing their overly rapid rates in dyadic situations to avoid creating stress for listeners. Usually during the first few minutes a comfortable rate is negotiated between speakers.

Facial Expression

Most Americans initially focus on the face for nonverbal cues. Multiple emotions are blended from the presence or absence of color, hair, and moisture, the direction and intensity of the gaze, the type of smile, and movement.

Color

Surgeons have learned that specific colors on certain areas of the face indicate health, both physical and emotional, or attractiveness of females and males. For example, the presence or absence of red in the eyes, nose and lips are indicators of health. The intensity of red on the lips can indicate attractiveness. The color blue in the eyes and on the eyelids may be attractive to some, but indicates poor health when in the lips, skin or nasal passage. Green can indicate injury if on facial skin or attractiveness if placed on the eyelids. Yellow can be added to eye color through make-up, but can indicate poor health if found in the skin.

Hair

Hair styles and their attractiveness can vary, but the presence or absence of hair on the face can indicate femininity or masculinity. Hair is acceptable in the eyebrows, but is perceived as masculine above a women's lips, or on chest, nose and ears. Again, attractiveness isn't the issue—conflict is and may distract the listener from the message.

Moisture

Moisture found near the eye socket is acceptable, but indicates a change in emotion when it tears and flows from the eye area. Moisture observed in the nasal passage, on the forehead or on cheeks may indicate a change in health status. Moisture leaking from the mouth may indicate, for an adult, a health alert.

Eye Behavior

Americans will tend to focus on someone's eyes when they want feedback and to establish an interaction. Customers in busy restaurants are constantly trying to catch the eye of the waiter and waiting rooms are full of people looking to establish eye contact (ocular contact) with the receptionist. When surgeons walk into an emergency waiting room, everyone focuses on the surgeon's eyes to see if she looks back at them. When people decide to look back into the eyes of someone who is already looking at them, this indicates that both parties are willing to begin an encounter.

Staring

Staring or focusing, on one space for an extended period of time can be interpreted as aggressiveness. Desmond Morris in *The Naked Ape* relates this to biological backgrounds of animals staring at each other before the attack. The eyes lock and the nostrils open (nasal flaring).

Offices

When surgeons arrange their seats in their offices at right angles with patients, it is easier to prevent the "staring" stereotype and to reduce aggressive modes. As patients and surgeons move farther apart in distance, each can comfortably increase eye contact (ocular contact) without appearing aggressive. In a higher status/lower status relationship, it is important to maintain eye contact with the higher status person to give the impression of alertness, respect and attention.

With Patients

Likewise, it is critical for surgeons to initially look their patients in the eye when speaking with them. This will be one indicator of whether the patients understand what is being said. Too often, surgeons are looking in the patient's chart or screen while saying, "Any questions?" The patients may be verbalizing the word "yes," while their bodies are shouting "no" with head movements from side to side, foot movements and hand wringing.

Closings

Business Cards

If a surgeon hasn't done so before this point, the interview can be closed by presenting a business card personalized in some way for each patient, family member or colleague. It can be as simple as circling the office number or writing the name of the surgeon assistant or nurse on the back. But it also presents an opportunity to write down the residual message for that patient or colleague (i.e., pharmacy for BP check–Wed; call to discuss paper). Patients or colleagues will be more likely to retain a card that has been personalized in some way.

Handouts

If the surgeon is giving patients any preprinted materials, it will help to personalize the sheet by saying something like, *"Mr. McKee, I want you to try exercises #5, 6, 8, and 9.."* rather than simply handing the copy to them.

Ending

Surgeons need to remind patients that they have listened. Adding something from the first few minutes will tie the conversation together at this point. For example, it is simply good conversation to say things like, *"Good luck getting your boat in the water!" or "Remember, I'm only a phone call away,"* or *"I hope you enjoy your granddaughter's wedding."*

Behavior breeds behavior.

Changing Behavior

Adults learn to change through practice of new behaviors. Frustration occurs when too much change is demanded too quickly. It is important to understand that optimal change occurs when only one or two behaviors are identified and adjusted at a time. It is unrealistic to ask a resident to speak 'better' when 'better' has not been operationalized for that resident. Instead, a realistic approach would be to suggest, "Eliminate saying *'umm,' 'like' and 'ah'* consistently throughout your case presentations." Then when this task is accomplished, it would be possible to add a new behavior such as asking the resident to "look at the attending when speaking."

STEPS TO CHANGING YOUR BEHAVIOR

Adults progress through four specific steps when learning new skills/behaviors. First, they are **unconsciously incompetent.** They don't know that they aren't able to do something. They just assume they can. For example, all adolescent males just know how to drive a car – unconsciously incompetent.

In the second stage they are **consciously incompetent**. They try this behavior and realize that they don't have the ability yet.

With practice, they learn to perform this new behavior or skill, but they have to focus so that they become **consciously competent**. They need to think about adjusting the mirrors, seats and seatbelts before they drive.

Every time we learn a new skill as an adult, we go through these steps.

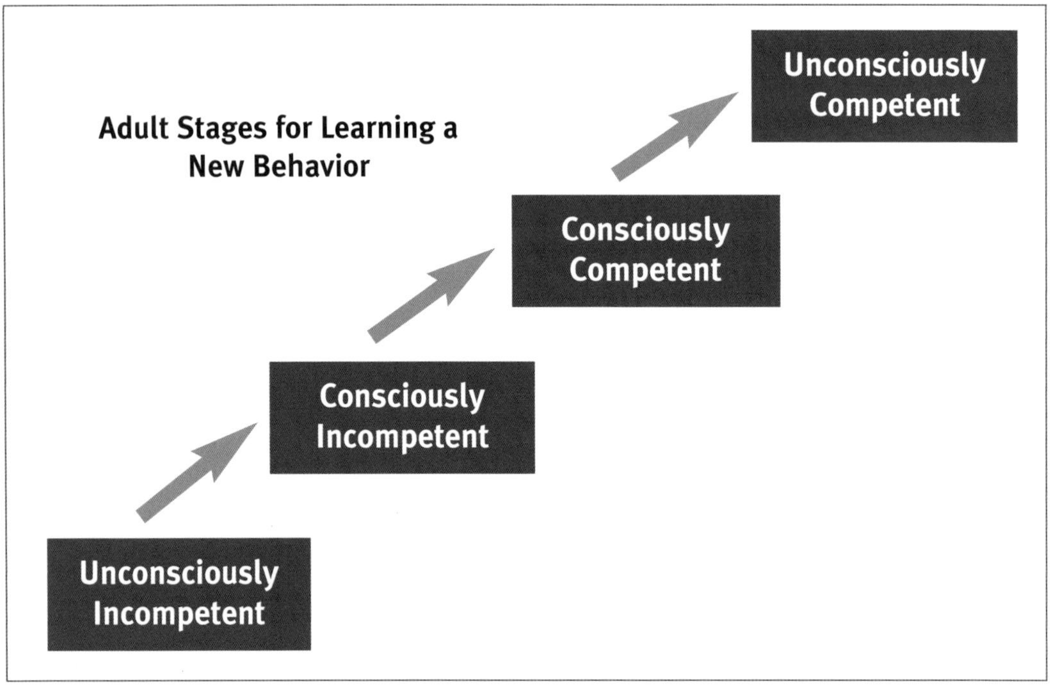

Finally, through continued practice, they perform the skill with comfortable confidence and reach stage four, **unconsciously competent**. It is important at this point to reevaluate behavioral change at three weeks to see whether positive change has occurred. If it has, then surgeons should sequentially travel through the steps again with a new behavior.

All of the behaviors and variables discussed in this chapter are setting-specific and must be altered in importance depending on the topic, setting and listener. In every setting the desired residual message should be identified and delivered consistently across all behaviors and variables.

The following chapters discuss in detail safe methods for approaching a variety of communication interactions that surgeons encounter throughout their professional career.

No patient or family ever complains of the surgeon being too supportive, speaking too clearly or delivering a message that is too consistent.

NP Lang

SELECTED REFERENCES

1. Andriole D, Rowland PA. Communication Apprehension in the Third Year Clerkship. Acad Med. 1999.
2. Barth RJ, Rowland PA, Mott LA, Burchard KW. Communication Effectiveness Training Improves Surgical Resident Teaching Ability. Am J Surg. 1997; 185:516-519.
3. Burchard KW, Rowland PA. Assessing the Communicative Skills of Surgeons: A Behavioral Approach. Acad Med. 1990; 65:274-276.
4. Burchard KW, Rowland PA, Coe NP Garb J. Interrater Reliability in Oral Examinations. Acad Med. 1995; 70(11):91-93.
5. Burchard K, Rowland PA, Berman N, Hanissian P, Carney P. Clerkship Enhancement of Interpersonal Skills. Am J Surg. 2005; 189(6):643-646.
6. Coe NP, Rowland PA, Garb J. Factors Affecting the Validity of the Oral Examination. Curr Surg. 1992; 49:459-464.
7. Coe NP, Rowland PA, Garb J. Communication Skills in Oral Examinations: A Description of Techniques for Identifying and Modifying Poor Communication Skills. Curr Surg. 1995; 52(1):42-46.
8. Coe NP, Rowland PA. Comparative Evaluation of Educational Methods in Surgical Residency Training. Arch Surg. 1995; 130:1022.
9. Edward T. Hall, The Hidden Dimension, New York: Doubleday; 1969.
10. Goldberg RJ, Novack D, Rowland PA, Landau C, Wartman S. Toward A Competent Psychiatric/Behavioral Science Curriculum for Primary Care Residents. Psychosomatics. 1989; 30(2):213-223.
11. Lang N, Rowland-Morin, PA, Coe NP. Identification of Communication Apprehension in Medical Students Starting a Surgery Rotation. J Surg. 1998; 176:41-45.
12. Lazare A. Shame, Humiliation, and Stigma in the Medical Interview. Arch Intern Med. 1987; 147:1653-1658.
13. Lazare A. Shame, Humiliation, and Stigma in the Medical Interview. In: Lipkin M, Putnam SM, and Lazare A. eds. The medical interview: clinical care, education, and research. New York: Springer-Verlag; 1995; 341.
14. Morris D. The Naked Ape, New York: Dell Publishing Co., Inc; 1967.
15. Pontes M, Pontes N. Variables that influence consumers' inferences about physician ability and accountability. Health Care Manage Re 1997:22:7-20.
16. Rowland PA, Batchelor A. Women Physicians: Dressing for the 80s. JAMWA, Nov-Dec 1987, 42(6):183-185.
17. Rowland PA. The Eye of the Beholder. JAMWA, 1988, 43(2):33-34.
18. Rowland PA, Carrol JG. Verbal Communication Skills and Patient Satisfaction: A Study of Doctor-Patient Interviews. Eval Health Prof, 1990, 13(2):168-185.
19. Rowland PA, Burchard KW, Garb J, Coe NP. Influence of Communication by Surgery Students on Their Oral Examination Scores. J Acad Med, 1991, 66(3):169-171.

20. Rowland PA. Communication Skills: A Rationale for Surgeons. Focus on Surgical Education, 1995, 12(2):15-18.
21. Rowland PA, Coe N, Lang N, Greenberg G, Reed W, Spence R, Burchard K. The effect of improving communication competency on the certifying examination of the American Board of Surgery. Am J Surg, 2002, 183:655-658.
22. Rowland PA,Coe NP, Burchard KW, Pricolo VE. Factors Affecting the Professional Image of Physicians. Curr Surg, 2005, 62(2). 214-219.
23. Ryan VerBerkmoes. Physician Fashion: It Pays to Dress Well. AMA News, 1988, 31(19):27-28.

Before the Interview Plan

Setting (check one only)

- ☐ outpatient clinic
- ☐ bedside
- ☐ emergency room
- ☐ other
- ☐ outpatient office
- ☐ waiting room
- ☐ patient's home

Topic: ______________________________

Goal of the interview: (circle one) inform persuade

Residual message: one simple sentence ______________________________

____

____

Professional Image: Physician Credibility

Victor E. Pricolo, MD, FACS;
Pamela A. Rowland, PhD

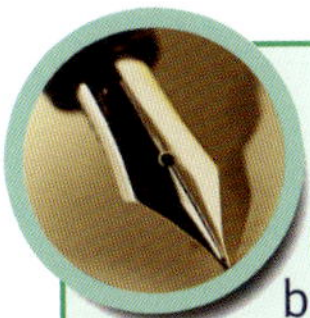

The deposition had just started and the plantiff's attorney calmly asked the plaintiff the usual demographic information: where she was born, educational background, legal address, and marital status. He then slipped in, "Mrs. Carter, could you please tell me what you remember about the morning of September 9th?"

"My OB arrived at the hospital to meet me at my bedside on Saturday morning...about 10 AM. I still remember that he had jeans on and...a short sleeve shirt. I couldn't see his shoes well when he was talking to me next to my bed, but when he left the room I could see that he had sneakers on. I had just seen him yesterday in his office and he didn't look like this. He said he would induce labor and be back later.

I should have known right then that he just wasn't focusing on me and what was going on. They said he wrote in the chart later that I had normal blood loss. How could I and then need 2 pints of blood the next day? He just wasn't paying attention to me..."

A small grin appeared on the attorney's face. He knew from experience that he could convince a jury—casual dress means casual attitude.

– Anonymous patient

"The physician must have a worthy appearance; he should look healthy and be well nourished, appropriate to his physique; for most people are of the opinion that those physicians who are not tidy in their own persons cannot look after others well. Further, he must look to the cleanliness of his person; he must wear decent clothes and use perfumes with harmless smells. The physician must have a certain degree of sociability, for a morose disposition is inaccessible both to those who are well and to those who are sick."(1)

Hippocrates (460-370 BC) eloquently describes the impact of personal appearance on professional image and the effects of behavior on physician credibility.

The image projected by physicians in their first encounters with patients has intricate and complex implications in the patient-physician relationship. In general, the "first impression" that a patient develops of a newly-met physician will have a profound effect on the faith and trust upon which any patient/physician relationship must be based. It will affect the physician's ability to obtain a complete medical history, to perform a thorough physical exam, and to recommend diagnostic tests and therapeutic interventions. It will influence the patient's compliance with the physician's recommended treatment and ultimately the outcome of the patient's illness.

If a good result is to be expected, appearing credible and convincing becomes as necessary for the physician as advising the proper treatment. It impacts the physician's ability to effectively communicate a message of sincere concern for the patient's condition and of competence in diagnosing, preventing and treating disease. Regardless of the results, this message may also significantly reduce the likelihood of malpractice litigation on the patient's part.

On a larger scale, image influences the physician's reputation with colleagues, nurses and other health care professionals, hospital and university administrators. All of these individuals are not only potential patients themselves, but also are likely to make remarks to patients and their relatives about the physician's ability. A patient hearing encouraging and reassuring comments about a physician by other health care professionals who see that physician in action every day, will strengthen the patient/physician bond and enhance the patient's optimism about the chances of recovery.

If you want people to treat you like a surgeon, start by looking and acting like a surgeon.

The professional image of physicians is clearly influenced by several variables that can be physician-related, patient-related, and environment-related. The physician should have an understanding of image potential and adapt it, as necessary, to different situations.

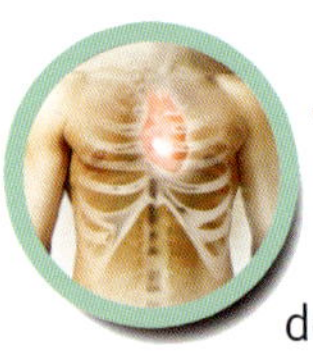

THE WHITE COAT

Should a physician wear a white coat or regular clothes in the adult setting? What does a white coat mean? What does it symbolize? How is it perceived by patients?

D.W. Blumhagen published a very detailed review on the effects of the white coat on a physician's image.(2) The white coat has become the most easily identifiable symbol of the physician in modern society and is a formidable nonverbal communication tool. Its role goes far beyond the practical virtue of being easily laundered and more easily changed than street clothes.

The introduction of aseptic surgery and the development of ever more complex diagnostic and therapeutic techniques could only be performed in an increasingly sophisticated hospital setting. By the end of the 19th century, a renovated faith in scientific discoveries changed the public perception of the hospital from *"a place where people die"* to *"a place where people heal."* Since the beginning of the 20th century, hospital physicians in the United States have been wearing white coats.

The concept of a uniform for physicians had profound symbolic implications. The color choice was probably motivated by several considerations. White symbolizes life as much as black symbolizes death. Moreover, white has been interpreted as a sign of purity. In a medical setting, this concept can be seen as both proof of ethical integrity, sexual indifference and innocence, superhuman power or initiation into the mysteries of the healing arts.

The patient's expectation of a physician goes well beyond the medical knowledge and competence that are the result of years of education and special training. The white coat implies the kind of moral integrity and commitment to universal ethical values generally enunciated in the Hippocratic oath. Patients are expected to allow their physician access to the most remote recesses of their mind and body in the name of medicine. This unique privilege can be properly exercised, without disturbing

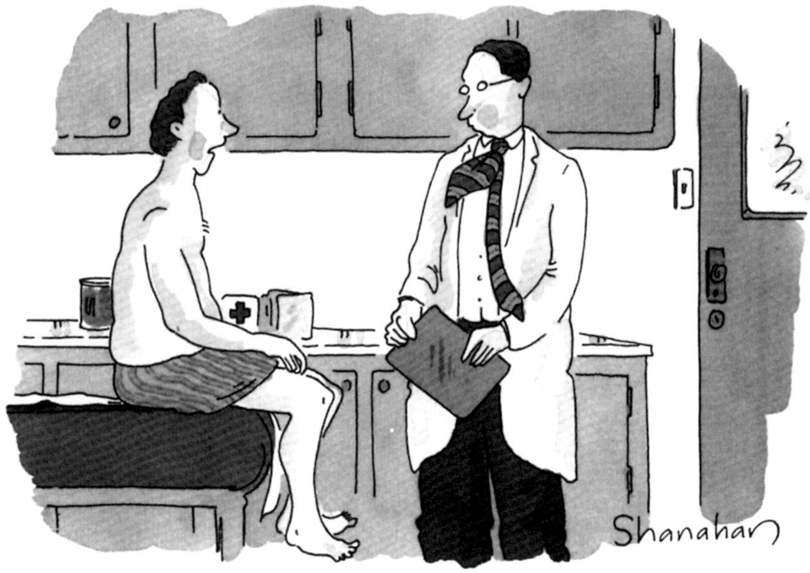

"And would you be performing the actual surgery?"

the patient's comfort and confidence, only if the environment and the physician's clothing and behavior are perceived as absolutely professional.

The white coat may also be perceived as an authoritarian symbol. The traditional patient's blind faith in the physician's competence

"Whatever you say, Doc; you know best!"

is becoming rare in clinical practice. With the development of mandatory second opinions by third party payors, extensive media coverage of physicians' mistakes, and information about hospital and physician "rankings" in different areas of the country, patients are being encouraged to question their physicians' professional qualifications. The public is constantly being reminded of the fact that "there are bad physicians out there." Clearly, it has become all the more important for a physician to give an impression of competence and reliability to a modern patient population that is not only much better informed through access to the internet and media blitzes, but also more suspicious. In this context, the physician may have to relinquish the typical authoritarian role

"Trust me, I am a physician!"

and assume the role of the more skillful partner in a team fight against disease.

The first question in establishing these roles then becomes: "Does a white coat imply competence and inspire confidence or is it too formal, creating a barrier between physician and patient?" The results of a questionnaire on this topic distributed to 200 patients at the University of California, Irvine, Medical Center clinical settings were published in 1988. (3) Of the respondents, 44% felt that a physician's credibility is influenced by clothing. The remaining 55% denied the value of appearance, emphasizing friendliness, openness and medical expertise. Both groups, however, agreed on the importance of neatness and cleanliness for physicians. Only 39% were in favor of white coats as a symbol of professionalism, while 86% stressed the importance of a visible physician's name tag. One problem with this study is the inability to investigate the effects of single variables (white coat, name tag, etc.) on a patient's perception. In other words, the 55% of patients who denied the importance of a physician's appearance may simply not be aware of it, and the 39%/61% split about white coats may represent the degree of overall patient satisfaction with their own medical care at the center. The other problem is that this study focused only on resident physician attire or those still in training and only on return patients.

VARIATIONS ON THE PHYSICIAN'S UNIFORM

Each medical specialty may place a different emphasis on clothing and the white coat in particular. As the white coat became increasingly perceived as a mark of authority, physicians and nurses in psychiatry chose to wear less formal street clothes as a more likely way to put their patients at ease.(3-4) In pediatrics, where the person in the white coat may be feared as the one licensed to inflict pain even in the presence of maximal parental protection, the use of pastel colors, funny stickers on beepers, and small bears or squirrels climbing on stethoscopes are used to distract, amuse and reassure children. However, a study in pediatrics found that children between 6 and 12 years of age with little or minor medical history preferred a physician in a white coat. Those with more extensive medical history preferred more informally dressed physicians.(5)

Surgical patients are literally asked to place their lives in the hands of a surgeon whom they may have never met before. As much as the internist's recommendation plays a major role, the surgeon's image assumes a dramatic importance during this process. No one goes to see a surgeon to establish a casual relationship. Patients have to make a decision to relinquish control and enter a temporary deathlike state (general anesthesia) to allow another person to heal them through a controlled and illuminated injury (surgery). Therefore, if surgeons project a casual attitude through their attire, patients may become suspicious. They need someone with optimal motor skills, hand-eye coordination, neatness, precision and meticulousness in surgery and will inevitably look for such clues in the surgeon's clothing and behavior. After the surgeon has successfully completed the operation, meeting the patient's family in "scrubs," complete with hat and a hanging mask, may actually convey the message.

"I didn't want you to worry one extra minute, so as soon as I finished the case, I came right out to reassure you that everything has gone well!"

However, meeting the surgeon at a 1PM appointment in the outpatient office with scrubs may convey a disorganized, negative impression.

Because the relationship with a surgeon may be brief before a procedure, the role of dress, behavior and communication shall assume exaggerated importance in the course of the relationship.

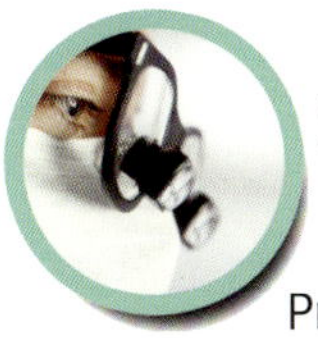

STUDIES ON PHYSICIAN APPEARANCE

The patient-physician relationship, in any setting, should never be a casual one. Proper physician's attire makes a strong nonverbal statement to support the physician's attitude in this setting.

Colt and Solot in 1989 published the results of a survey of 190 emergency department patients and 129 medical specialists from Oregon and Pennsylvania.(6) In this survey, 73% of physicians and 43% of patients attributed importance to physician's appearance. While 49% of patients thought physicians should wear white coats, 19% disapproved of scrub suits. Patients were more tolerant than physicians about casual dress. Despite this, there are frequent examples of the adverse impact of casual dress for some occasions.

Gjerdingen et al. analyzed responses from 404 patients, residents and staff physicians from Minnesota and Wisconsin on male and female physicians' professional appearance.(7) In general, positive responses were associated with traditional clothing items, such as dress, shirt and tie, dress shoes and nylons, white coat and name tag. Negative responses were elicited by blue jeans, scrub suits, athletic shoes, clogs and sport socks, prominent ruffles and dangling earrings on women, and long hair and earrings on men.

Dunn et al. interviewed 200 patients from Boston and San Francisco. Sixty-five percent of respondents said physicians should wear white coats; 27% believed physicians should not wear tennis shoes; 52% said no to blue jeans; 37% said yes to neckties for male physicians; and 34% believed female physicians should wear dresses or skirts.(8)

Major et al. found a relationship between surgeons' appearance and mannerisms on a surgery service and patients' perceptions of the quality of medical care received. In this survey, most agreed that surgeons should wear white coats and that blue jeans were not acceptable.(9)

Decisions on a physician's attire may be influenced also by the tradition of the institution. In most academic hospitals in the Northeast, attending physicians and senior residents wear long white coats, while interns and junior residents wear short coats. At Northwestern University, residents wear light blue, fellows wear gray, and only attendings are finally "allowed" to wear white, the color of accomplished autonomous competence. At the Mayo Clinic, on the other hand, trainees such as residents and fellows wear white coats, while attendings (consultants) are expected to wear formal or semiformal street clothes with a visible name tag.

Regardless of whether a white coat is worn, studies show that several other physician clothing items are very visible, and are certainly just as relevant. Unfortunately, several of the above mentioned studies were conducted by questionnaire, asking hypothetical questions about different clothing items, rather than actually showing real examples. This may have influenced the respondents' ability to be unbiased toward their own prior experience.

Weekends are not 'casual' to the surgery patient.

BEYOND THE LAB COAT

Deviations from the expected conservative business attire can, in some cases, result in damage to the surgeon-patient relationship. This risk increases with new patients.

The professional image of a physician can influence both the patients' and peers' perceptions of that physician's credibility.(9) When physicians and patients were asked to rate actual slides of practicing male and female physicians of varying age on different aspects of professional image, the perceived age of the physician did not effect the rating on credibility. However, specific aspects of clothing that were present or absent did affect where the physician was rated on a scale of professionalism. In parallel research on the effect of image and dress on ratings of case presentations, the professional image did affect the scores students received on case presentations and supported additional research on the effect of image and success on oral examinations in surgery.(10,11)

Basically, the "safe" image for young physicians in the United States today closely resembles many of the guidelines set forth in conservative business communities.(12,13) Although there are variations to these guidelines, these formulas help ensure young physicians that there will not be anything in their attire to distract from what they are saying. Since it is important for those in the specialties to get referrals from their peers, addressing professional image requirements may aid in

Safe Items for a Professional Image in Adult Outpatient Settings

Male

Shoes	tied, leather, no sandals
Tie	conservative; tied with a dimple
Pants	no jeans
Shirt	collared
Jewelry	no earrings, business watch, wedding band
Socks	color should blend with color of pants
Belt	leather, same color as shoes
Hair	style conservative for age; clean, not matted
Hygiene	Americans are expected to bath daily; good oral hygiene; no body odor
Jackets	layering with either labcoat or suit jacket
Age	not a factor

Female

Shoes	closed toe, no sling-backs, no sandals
Skirts	conservative length, not ankle length
Stockings	natural colored
Jewelry	only one earring per ear; business watch, wedding band
Blouse	conservative cuts front/back, avoid ruffles
Hair	shoulder length or above, natural colors
Hygiene	Americans are expected to bath daily; good oral hygiene; no body odor
Jackets	layering with either labcoat or suit jacket
Age	not a factor

building respect throughout the medical community for future practice. Studies in the nursing profession also argue for professional image to project trust in a competitive health care environment and differentiate health care roles.(14-15)

What physicians wear in their office is symbolic to the patient of what their attitude is toward the patient, the setting, and the interaction on that day. Although there are degrees of flexibility, there are some basic checklists that are "safe" for the young physician.(16,17)

Safe Items for a Professional Image in an Oral Examination Setting

Males

Shoes	tied, leather
Tie	conservative; tied with a dimple
Suit	business suit
Shirt	formal collar, not button down that is worn with a sports jacket; long sleeve only with suit; should be 1/4 inch longer than jacket arm length
Jewelry	no earrings, business not sports watch, wedding band only
	no bracelets, chains, piercings
Socks	color should blend with color of pants
Belt	leather, same color as shoes
Hair	conservative for age
Scent	no cologne
Deodorant	not only is body odor offensive to many Americans, but you don't want the examiners to see you sweat
Tatoos	not visible
Fingernails	groomed, no polish
Symbols	avoid academic, religious and political symbols that may offend or draw attention away from your performance
Glasses	business, not sporty, no self-darkening lenses
Age	not a factor

Female

Shoes	pumps with heel
Suit	business suit, conservative length skirt
	avoid light pastels or white; avoid an 'all black' look
Stockings	natural colored
Jewelry	only one earring per ear that doesn't move; business not sports watch, simple necklace, if appropriate
Blouse	avoid high collar
Makeup	natural
Fingernails	well groomed, light-colored polish or clear
Symbols	avoid academic, religious, or political symbols that may offend or draw attention away from your performance
Hair	shoulder length or above, natural colors
Scent	no cologne or perfume to distract
Deodorant	not only is body odor offensive to many Americans, but you don't want the examiners to see you sweat
Tattoos	not visible
Glasses	business, not sporty, no self-darkening lenses
Age	not a factor

The communication premise, ***"It is difficult to change initial impressions, even in the light of new information,"*** cannot be overemphasized. Once credibility as a physician has been established, perhaps more variety is tolerated by patients and peers.

Safe Behaviors for a Professional Image in a Business Setting

Gentlemen:

Unbutton the suit jacket with your left hand when you sit down.

Button the suit jacket with your left hand as you rise, and extend your right hand for a handshake.

Ladies:

Choose a jacket in which you can sit comfortably without major unbuttoning. Do not choose a jacket that must be unzipped before you sit. Someone will be watching.

Choose a skirt in which you can sit comfortably, without exposing your inner thighs.

Safe Items for a Professional Image in Business Casual Settings

Business casual is:

1. Region specific
2. Work-site specific

Ask the organization that is hosting the event what they mean by business casual. Or, ask your host to define business casual. Nothing can be more embarrassing than to arrive unprepared.

Casual for men may mean:	**Business casual for men may mean:**
Jeans	Sports jacket with jeans
Tee shirt	Sports jacket, no tie
Sandals, no socks	Summer suit, no tie
Shirts, no collar	Sports jacket, shirt without collar
Shorts	Sports jacket with knit collared shirts
Casual for women	**Business casual for women**
Sundress	Suit with pants
Shorts	Dress
Beachwear	Skirt and blouse
Jeans	Jeans with sports jacket
Sleeveless shirts with pants or skirts	Open toe shoes
Sandals	Sling back shoes

BEHAVIOR AS PART OF IMAGE

Patients expect much more from their physicians than cold knowledge or competence. A computer or a book could provide that with less danger of errors of omission. If dress is accepted as a powerful nonverbal communication tool in the very first moments of the physician-patient encounter, a physician's behavior throughout the meeting is of critical importance.

A physician should convey a sense of compassion and confidence that things are going to be all right. According to the patient's personality and level of knowledge, a variable amount of time is needed to do this, but it will greatly reduce anxiety and positively influence the patient's outlook. Empathy should, however, be mitigated by competence, and role identification should be clear.

A. C. Celsus (first century A.D.) described the emotional detachment necessary for a surgeon:

"A surgeon ... must be compassionate so that he wishes to cure the patient ... but not to the extent that he is moved by his cries either to go faster than is desirable or to cut less than is necessary; he must do everything just as if the cries of the patient cause him no emotion."(18)

The importance of this emotional detachment to maintain the necessary clarity of mind and judgment explains why it is considered unwise for physicians to treat relatives or loved ones.

CONCLUSION

A physician's image is more than a facade. It is a mirror of competence, expertise, compassion and commitment. The risks of not paying adequate attention to the implications of personal appearance on the psychology of patients, relatives, nurses, colleagues, patients' families, or juries can have negative consequences on the physician's overall reputation and professional success.

Remember that 'casual' dress may be linked to 'casual' behavior or 'casual attitude.'

REFERENCES

1. Hippocrates, 460-370 BC.
2. Blumhagen DW. The Doctor's White Coat - The Image of the Physician in Modern America. Ann Intern Med. 1979; 91:111-116.
3. Friis R, Tilles J. Patients' Preferences for Resident Physician Dress Style. Fam Prac Res. 1988; 8:24-31.
4. Ninstein LS, Stewart D, Gordon N. Effect of Physician Dress Style of Patient-Physician Relationship. J Adol H Care. 1985; 22:456-459.
5. Zwart DL, Kimpen JL. The White Coat in Pediatrics: Link Between Medical History and Preference for Informally Dressed Physicians. Nederlands Tijdschrift voor Geneeskunde. 1997; 141(42):2020-4.
6. Colt HG, Solot JA. Attitudes of Patient and Physicians Regarding Physician Dress and Demeanor in the Emergency Department. Ann Emerg Med. 1989; 18:145-151.
7. Gjerdingen GK, Simpson DE, Titus SL. Patients' and Physicians' Attitudes Regarding the Physician's Professional Appearance. Arch Intern Med. 1987; 147:1209-1212.
8. Dunn JJ, Lee HT, Percelay JM. Patient and House Officer Attitudes on Physician Attire and Etiquette. JAMA. 1987; 257:65-68.
9. Major K et al. Attitudes regarding surgeons' attire. Am J Surg. 2005; 190:103-106.
10. Rowland-Morin PA, Burchard KW, Garb J, Coe NP. The Influence of Communication by Surgery Students on Their Oral Examination Scores. J Acad Med. 1991; 66:169-171.
11. Burchard KW, Rowland-Morin PA, Coe NP, Garb J. A Surgery Oral Examination: interrater agreement and the influence of rater characteristics. J Acad Med. 1995; 70(11):1044-46.
12. Coe NP, Rowland-Morin PA, Garb J. Factors Affecting the Validity of the Oral Examination. Curr Surg. 1992; 49:459-64.
13. Malloy JT. The New Women's Dress for Success Book. New York: Warner Books; 1996.
14. Mangum S, Garrison C, Lind C, Hilton HG. First impressions of the nurse and nursing care. J of N Care Quality, 1997, 11(5):39-47.
15. Davidhizar R, Shearer R. Improving your bedside manner. J of Prac Nursing. 1998; 48(1):10-40.
16. Rowland-Morin PA, Batchelor A. Women Physicians: Dressing for the 80's. JAMWA. 1987; 42:183-185.
17. Gjerdingen GK, Simpson DE. Physicans' Attitudes about Their Professional Appearance. Fam Prac Res. 1989; 9:57-64.
18. Celsus: De Re Medicine. Cited in Bevan, PG: The surgeon as teacher, counsellor, and politician. Ann Roy Coll Surg. 1974; 55:143-46.

Physician Professionalism:
More Than Book Smart

Brenda Richardson, MD
Pamela A. Rowland, PhD

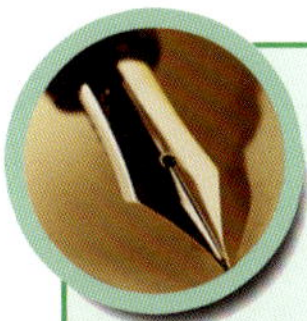

British Physicians, 1770:

"Haughty, rapacious, careless, and often brutal in his manners."(1)

American Physicians, 1998:

"What manners?"(2)

For years the United Kingdom's schools in London, Edinburgh, and Dublin were the medical Mecca for the entire world. Physicians from these schools were anchored only to the wealthy classes who could afford to attend. They wore uniforms of the privileged marked by wigs, canes and top hats.(3) However, the practice of medicine in the American colonies did not mirror that of the Europeans. Most learned through apprenticeships and few had books(1700—1800's). Medical degrees with their automatic gentleman status from across the ocean were envied.

The advent of curative (1940's) rather than supportive medicine, coupled with the formal training and licensing of physicians in the United States (1860+), changed the status of the American trained physician dramatically. No longer the tolerated second cousins of medicine, American-trained physicians are now envied for their cutting-edge expertise. Unlike their counterparts elsewhere in the world, admittance to medical school in the United States today requires superior performance in an undergraduate degree program. What seems to have been lost, at least according to consumers, is the 'gentlemanly' status that went with the awarding of medical degrees. It cannot be assumed that an undergraduate education produces gentlemen and gentleladies for society or that medical school training simply adds to the scientific training of these young minds. Modern medicine is searching for a happy medium between scientific knowledge and the necessary social and professional behavior of physicians.

The purpose of this chapter is to provide 'safe' guidelines for developing the manners and etiquette of surgeons in the United States.

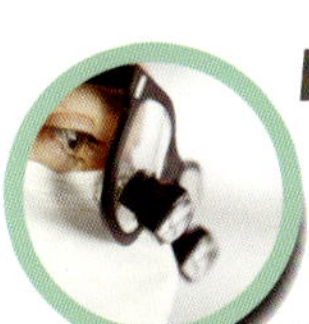

MANNERS

Manners (both good and bad) are the ways in which people convey meaning to others. All humans are born with manners; typically, they are bad. People are born egocentric: demanding attention, with no regard for time of day or night, and little attention to the needs of others. Through a learning process, this changes over time. Humans still have needs, but through the miracle of education and good upbringing they acquire good manners and the ability to contribute to others' lives.

The lexicographical definition of manners is "social conduct or rules of conduct as shown in prevalent customs."(4) Further, manners are described as "habitual conduct or deportment." "Etiquette" is defined as the conduct or procedure required by good breeding or prescribed by authority to be observed in social or official life. Perhaps it is safe to say that a well-mannered person generally is bound by the rules of etiquette and uses discretion when applying them. Put another way, manners are the packaging of the product (message) which the truck (communication) is trying to deliver. Many good products are rejected by the consumer because the packaging is weak or offensive. Good packaging makes for better reception.

So, what is meant by "physician manners?" Often when patients refer to the treatment they received by a surgeon or staff member, they are referring to that person's manners. It makes sense for surgeons to invest the time to learn or improve their manners. Those who practice, teach, or are learning the art of medicine will find that paying attention not just to the message but to the way it is delivered can:

- improve patient care;
- increase satisfaction with care provided;
- improve surgeon satisfaction; and
- improve the surgeon's position with students, peers and superiors.

Manners are a distillation of common sense, kindness, and knowledge. There are many times that the proportions of these three elements are uneven, but the result, when good, is usually described as "good manners." There are many people who get by with a little common sense and even less knowledge, but if they are kind, it carries the day. The same three elements of manners apply just as much in the professional engagement in physicians who, after all, are humans treating and working with other humans.

As mentioned earlier, manners can be divided into manners and etiquette. Etiquette, the "mechanics of manners," (11, 12) can then be subdivided into social and business etiquette.

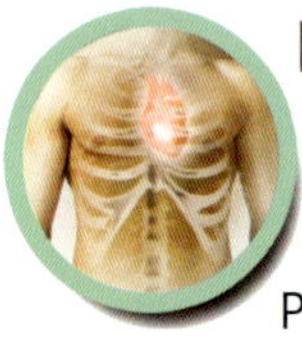

ETIQUETTE

Some people confuse manners with etiquette. While it is difficult to have good manners without some knowledge of etiquette, etiquette alone will not carry the day. Physicians who only understand etiquette can come dangerously close to being perceived as "oiling their way across the floor."(23) The socially aware know that the difference between the etiquette literate and caricature is sincerity. Phonies, even polite ones, are easy to pick out. However, physicians must brush up on etiquette. There are many ways to do this.

There is a tradition in medicine of ***"See one, Do one, Teach one."*** This may be applied to etiquette as well. (12,15) In addition to the many good reference books on the subject, there are also online services. (12,13,14) There are schools which actually teach manners and etiquette to adults if their families and schools neglected to review these skills. Finally, if students and residents don't feel that they know what to do in a particular circumstance, they should simply ask. It is a weakness to never admit doubt. That is what permits many of the abuses seen in the patient-physician relationship, as well as professional relationships. (5, 6,16) Experts tell us such behavior is not merely rude, it can be dangerous and lead to serious liability for the practitioner. (5,6,10) Sometimes young physicians-in-training may feel that they have plenty of time to learn these things, or that they don't apply to them since they are smarter than anyone else in their group.

A young senior resident at a community hospital who, for the most part, was a competent clinician, exhibited one problem. In the physician, lounge he insisted on throwing fruit peels into the garbage can located at the end of the sofa, usually at a time when two physicians would be talking between him and his target. This did not seem to bother him, and he just kept on throwing the skins and interjecting comments into their conversation. He continued with this behavior even when a senior physician was present who had been asked to consider including him in his practice upon graduation. The older physician was a good observer and had noted on other occasions that the younger man was equally annoying in other settings. For instance, he would always be late for grand rounds and then announce his arrival by walking to the front of the room, obliterating the screen. The senior physician was so offended by this young man's seeming insensitivity to his surroundings that he decided he could never have him in his practice.

This technically competent young man may have well been helped by a structured program of etiquette training.

Etiquette also involves learning about the proper behavior for the surroundings. Another name for it is cultural literacy. (17, 18, 19) It may be argued that it is only respectful to try to understand the cultural imperatives of patients and colleagues. No doubt this is true, but physicians will also find it useful to learn the significant elements of the etiquette as it applies to other cultures, particularly if a great deal of time is going to be spent in that culture or with people from a specific culture. For example, it is rude to offer things to Indians with the left or "unclean" hand or to insist on wearing your outside shoes beyond the doorway when you enter a Japanese home.

ELECTRONIC MAIL: E-MAIL

Surgeons are often required to write in patient records and send e-mails, even though they might prefer to nod.

There are some guidelines that apply to surgeons and e-mails.

E-mails do not convey emotion well. They do not convey personality.

E-mails should be short. Recipients will be annoyed with you if you attach cute pictures of emotion icons and nonprofessionally necessary pictures that will greatly increase download times. Make your e-mail short, objective, sticking to the facts – no emotions or threats. Although

> **"Never write what you can say; never say what you can wink; never wink what you can nod."**
>
> —Unknown

others, especially adolescents, may find grammatical errors and abbreviations acceptable, use your computer's spellcheck before sending.

There is no privacy with e-mails. There will be an employee somewhere, at some time, who has kept a copy. Attorneys armed with subpoenas can collect information from a computer server that will hold comments you made about another professional years before. E-mails are not postcards; they are billboards.

Most institutions have policies regarding use of their systems. Do not download any information from sites that might not be considered 'professional' by others or attach items from those sites with any of your hospital or office e-mail.

TOPICS OF CONVERSATION TO AVOID

It is a given that certain topics risk offending individuals. It is the reason people who want safe topics are advised never to talk about money, politics, or religion. People should never assume that someone else feels the same way on an issue or cares as much or as little about it as they do. Unless the stated purpose in being in a particular situation is to discuss one of these topics, it is better to avoid them. For example, it is rude for a physician to talk about money with patients or colleagues.

> A senior cardiac surgeon, respected for his medical judgment and speed, often offended his staff. During long bypass procedures, he debated with his assistant about how much they were probably earning per minute. The surgical technician harvesting the vein never looked up, nor did any of the operating room nurses add to the conversation. The circulating nurse simply raised her eyebrows.
>
> PA Rowland 1997

Sex

Sex is another off-limits topic with patients or staff members. Patients may tell surgeons about their sex problems, but a surgeon's sex life is not the issue. It is never safe to become personal about sex. For the purposes of the professional relationship, surgeons avoid the topic. This is a very dangerous subject. Not only is it impolite to discuss sex casually, it can result in disciplinary action that is often cited in state medical review board reports.

> **A married male surgeon and some nurses from the OR decided to go out for dinner on a weekend. This behavior is usually acceptable for those who celebrate good work together. However, when the nurses decided that after dinner they would go to the local adult club, the surgeon should have excused himself. Instead, he joined them.**
>
> **The next week, he was the center of gossip at the nursing station and in the OR.**

Religion

Religion is a deeply personal matter. It is also illegal to ask potential employees, students, residents or fellows what their religious beliefs are, or what their family members practice.

INTRODUCTIONS

Surgeons should always be first to introduce themselves in a room, whether it is a treatment room, staff lounge or lecture hall. This alleviates any possible embarrassment if, as is likely, not everyone in the room knows the surgeon by name. Once the surgeon has made that introduction, it is important to acknowledge and be introduced to the others in the room. Surgeons should act as though they care about the others who are there.

Use of Honorifics

Another reason surgeons must be introduced or need to introduce themselves is to give the patient a clear indication of their status (physician or student) and what they would like to be called.(12) They should not be insulted if a youngster calls them "Joe," rather than "Dr. Jones," when they introduced themselves as "Joe." If a surgeon wants to be called Dr. Jones, that's how he should introduce himself. Similarly, upon first meeting someone, it is best to use an honorific (e.g., Mr., Dr., Mrs., Miss) rather than to assume it is acceptable to use the person's first name. This is particularly true when addressing older women (12) and women from unfamiliar cultures.

Surgeons are always on-stage in their communities.

In Colt and Solot's study, 96% of physicians addressed patients by their last name or title, even though 43% of the patients said they preferred being called by their first names.(20) In Dunn's study, 40% of patients wanted physicians to address them by first name, but only 10% of patients would address their physicians by their first names.(21) In Rowland-Morin's study, reciprocity of behaviors (honorifics) between the physician and patient in an initial interaction produced improved patient satisfaction. (22)

SOCIAL VERSUS BUSINESS ETIQUETTE

Numerous references point out that many good messages are lost in delivery by the lack of understanding of the proper business etiquette. (12) For example, surgeons should be sensitive to the fact that when in dyadic (one to one) or small group rounds, a staff physician may be quite happy to be called 'Jim.' It is quite different, however, to refer to him as 'Jim' during grand rounds with visiting professors in attendance. Similarly, senior persons show superior knowledge of etiquette and respect when they afford dignity to students or younger faculty by referring to them formally at

---

Reciprocity (of style, vocabulary, honorifics, etc) improves communication and satisfaction.

The Chief of Oncology at a large Canadian hospital clearly remembers the night his son was born. He assumed he was well known and very respected throughout the medical community. Finally, he said, he was told to come in to see his wife by the medical student who said, "George, you may come in now."

a meeting. Dr. Margaret Hill at Women's College in Toronto was a beloved teacher for many reasons, but her ability to make a youngster feel great by simply referring to them as "Doctor" in rounds or seeking their opinion at grand rounds was renowned. There is a time and a place to be familiar (5, 12,17) and a similar time and place to be formal. It is important to know the difference.

Dr. Mason had a patient who had just been diagnosed with a relatively rare, but life-threatening ocular malignancy. She had known the patient for many years, and felt quite concerned about the prognosis. The patient was a 60-year-old teacher who was an intelligent, concerned individual trying to gather information in order to evaluate her treatment options. She had been referred to a tertiary hospital by the original consultant on the case to see a senior physician specializing in the treatment of ocular malignancies. Indeed, the physician enjoyed a global reputation for scholarship. The patient had asked Dr. Mason to come to the consultation, as she felt nervous and wanted her input later.

On the appointment day, the patient, her husband and Dr. Mason arrived at a very busy office. The office staff was very pleasant. After some time the patient was seen. Dr. Mason sat in the exam room with the family while the patient was seen first by the fellow and then the attending. The fellow was a nice person who tried to explain the problem, but did not ever actually smile or address the patient by name. When the patient asked a question he said, "You will have to ask Dr. Pratt." Usually this was said with the head down or the eyes covered. When Dr. Pratt arrived, he did not introduce himself and never once called the patient by her name. Further, he never acknowledged that others were in the room. When the patient asked why one treatment over another, Dr. Pratt said, "What a stupid question. We would never be talking about this in a reasonable situation." He closed his eyes and sniffed when Dr. Mason interjected, saying that she did not think it was a stupid question at all, but one which must be answered. Dr. Pratt reiterated his experience many, many times. He told the patient when she would be treated and said that she must make up her mind quickly. He knew best.

The couple knew that the information was substantially correct because they had done a great amount of research as well, but they felt that if there existed another treatment option, or if there were other sites, they would go there—not because they felt Dr. Pratt was incompetent, but because they felt that his behavior was rude and arrogant.

Dr. Pratt could have enlisted the support of Dr. Mason had he tried to engage her as a colleague rather than treating her like a pest. Perhaps, more importantly, he would have understood that Dr. Mason has the ability to severely impact the flow of future consults to him. She also has the ability to lobby for the development of parallel services which would quickly rival him. Finally, although it is a subtle thing, Dr. Pratt would have been able to accomplish what he really did want. He would have preserved his reputation as the leader, not just in technology in his field, but as a true leader in his profession by positively influencing the patient and her team to seek the best treatment. No one doubted his skills, but the visitors were sad and unhappy with his manner.

In the language of process improvement and quality improvement,(4) could the process represented here have been changed to improve the outcome, which in this case is the provision of information resulting in optimum care? It probably could have in the Mason case. The meeting would have been shorter because the patient's anxiety would have been dispelled rather than heightened. The fellow would have received better information from the patient had he engaged her with polite behavior. The fellow would have improved his standing with this professor, if that were one of his goals. The patient would have been less anxious, and more confident about her decision, which would have reduced the delay in treatment by several days. Dr. Pratt would be assured that his position as the leader were safe had he taken the time to listen to the questions elicited by his fellow, and the visiting team.

> Dr. Wharton was a young surgeon who had been asked to speak at a nurses' meeting. He stunned the group by showing up on time and thanking the nurses for their attendance. He also thanked them for showing him every kindness in the time that he had been at the hospital. He said that he could not tell them how much he appreciated this and that he looked forward to spending the rest of his career at the hospital. The room was quiet for a whole minute.

What did Dr. Wharton do right? Just about everything. His performance was truly the synthesis of kindness, common sense, respect and knowledge of etiquette. He did not "oil his way across the floor."(23) There was no doubt that he was being sincere. He did the simplest thing; he said "thank you" as he looked at the assembled group.

In addition to appearing on time and being appropriately dressed, Dr. Wharton not only presented a very professional talk on AIDS, but he also delivered information about himself. After the talk he answered every question in a respectful manner, and when he did not know something, he admitted it. It was a very good performance. After the meeting, one of the nurses commented that she had come to the meeting because she had heard that he was good, and that now that she had attended she would have no trouble recommending him to others. Was the product delivered? Was it received well? Yes. He had enhanced his reputation with them, and by adding that he hoped to stay there for the rest of his career, he had reinforced their feeling that their hospital and community were solid.

Finally, unlike Dr.Pratt, he had taken the time to understand his audience. Dr. Wharton was from "out of town." He did not assume, as Dr. Pratt did, that since the audience had come to him they had to listen to what he had to say and would accept his recommendations without question.

Surgeons need safe and simple ways to meet the requirements for having good manners, that is, exhibiting kindness, common sense, respect, and understanding in our interactions with colleagues and patients. (2,5,6, 14,15)

"There is always time for courtesy."
Ralph Waldo Emerson US Essayist and Poet

KINDNESS

Although organized medicine has taken a high profile in the fight against domestic abuse,(24) it has been said that surgeons have a bad habit of "eating their young" trainees. Intellectually, surgeons know that this is wrong from every perspective, yet it could be argued that the traditions of training border on the abusive.(6) What can this be doing to the present and future leaders of the medical profession? Young trainees soon learn to ***"kiss up and beat down."*** They see their faculty as all-knowing and certainly all-powerful. Why not model their behavior after them? The opposite response is to lose the lesson the professor is trying to give in his message and discount all he legitimately has to offer because of the offensive manner. Everybody loses, and it is not just a short-term loss. The resident gradually turns into his teacher, repeating the behavior once he is the professor and training his interns and medical students the same way. The institution loses because those trainees and younger staff leave or harbor ill feelings for the rest of their careers. It has been argued that one has to "be cruel to be kind." However, simple courteous acts of kindness should be practiced in every possible situation and especially in a teaching environment.

Kindness

1. Look into someone's eyes when talking to them. It is a lot harder to be negative with the connection that eye contact establishes.(6) Physicians should teach what Osler knew—that listening to the patients will tell them the diagnosis.
2. Think before you talk. Remember the old parable of the gossip who was sentenced to shake a down pillow into the wind and then try to pick up the now scattered feathers. Once the words are out, like the feathers they are gone. (5,6, 12,15,25)
3. Senior physicians may remember that they were at that age and stage once. Students should remember that they will be at that age and stage someday. (6,26)
4. Take someone and their comments and concerns seriously. Never laugh at a question asked in earnest. Never snort or huff as Dr. Pratt did when asked questions. (6,14)
5. Pay attention and react to the sociology of the institution(s) where you work. Pretending to be isolated, as if on an island, only works when you want to be detached. If the institution/colleagues perceive your apparent desire to get away, they may not be amused. (17,18,19)
6. React. Remember that both the physician and patient are human. Therefore, as Buckman tells Canadian medical students, emphasize that physicians should act as though they are receiving bad news from a neighbor. It is a courteous and necessary thing to do.(25)
7. Try to understand what the patient or colleague is saying.(5,6,5,19,25)
8. Be honest.(8,10,14,25,26)

RESPECT

Surgeons need to respect patients, peers, students, and colleagues by paying attention to them. A basic sign of respect is to acknowledge that everyone's time is valuable. Surgeons should attend the meetings they say they will. If they cannot be there on time, they should call to let someone know. This requires a degree of flexibility when setting up meetings. It may be unrealistic to always expect meetings with other professionals to fit into personal schedules. When there are problems with a scheduled time, concerns must be voiced at the scheduling. It is poor behavior to not show up or to insist on a change later.

Everyone attending the meeting should be prepared. It is insulting and rude to come to a scheduled meeting unprepared. It does not make a difference whether the meeting is grand rounds (5,12) or pre-op rounds.

Most surgeons attend a variety of national, regional and specialty meetings. The decision of which to attend annually involves balancing clinical responsibilities, staffing, budget and family needs. However, once a surgeon has been elected or appointed to a position within an organization, that surgeon is expected to attend the entire meeting. The executive committees within an organization usually assign working groups or academic papers to be presented throughout the meeting. Inviting someone who is not an officer within the organization to present on the last hour of the last day of the meeting and not have most officers of the organization present is not polite. It signals to the last participants that their work is not valued.

"Dressing for success" (17,19,27) has become a familiar phrase for Americans. In terms of manners, dressing for success means appropriateness. Dr. Pratt dressed perfectly. He was clean, neat, and he was clearly identified by a name tag, which was a good thing since he never said who he was. Dr. Wharton appeared at his meeting also appropriately dressed. He looked as though he cared about his appearance for the meeting.

COMMON SENSE

There is a saying in the "quality improvement" literature, "Do the right thing at the right time." (4) This seems so sensible, but too often the "right thing, wrong time" approach to medicine seems to be the case:

- The patient was given a suppository in the presence of visitors.
- The patient was asked sensitive questions in the waiting room.
- The attending asked the residents to alter their meeting time, because he did not want to alter his golf game [even though he knew they were expected at another meeting].(28)
- The senior resident asked the junior resident to take an extra night of call so that he could do something else, even though he knew she had a newborn at home.
- The patient was asked if she was "going to keep it" or get an "abortion" after receiving bad news from an amniocentesis.

All of the surgeons in situations like these would be viewed as having bad manners. At the very least, an attempt to indicate an understanding of the underlying situation should be made. This can be done with comments as simple as:

> "Gee, Mary, I know that the baby is home now, and I appreciate your need to get home, but do you think we could revisit the schedule for next week? If not now, could we do it tomorrow?" (12) or,
>
> "Could I ask you all to leave for a moment, since I must speak to your dad."

A good strategy is to mentally ask the same question to yourself before doing so to others so you can imagine some of the same pressures of the other person. If the question doesn't seem appropriate to you, it is not likely to be well received by the audience.

SUMMARY

Finally, why should surgeons care about all of this? Many hours and dollars are being spent on the effects of proper communication on medical care and outcomes.(4, 5, 6, 26) Manners, whether good or bad, will affect the outcome of the communication. Even such simple gestures as learning to say **"please"** and **"thank you"** can have a positive impact. Physicians should listen to themselves talking to and with their patients and colleagues. They should care about what they say and how they say it.(14,15,12) Good surgeons care enough to learn the rules of etiquette for wherever they are. It is an investment in the most important asset they have—themselves. (29) They will be better surgeons, not just a better liked one.

"Good manners will open doors that the best education cannot."(30)

Clarence Thomas

US Supreme Court Justice

REFERENCES

1. Stratling M. John Gregory (1724-1773) and his "Lectures on the Duties and Qualifications of a Physician," Wellcome Library for the History and Understanding of Medicine. MedSecoli. 1997; 9(3):455-75.
2. Gilbert S. Forget about bedside manners, some doctors have no manners. New York Times. 1997: Dec 23;Sect. C:7.
3. Starr P. The social transformation of American Medicine. New York: Basic Books; 1982.
4. Webster's Ninth New Collegiate Dictionary. Springfield: Merriam-Webster; 1993.
5. Blumenthal DR and Scheck AC, editors. Improving clinical practice. Total quality management and the physician. San Francisco: Jossey-Bass Publishers; 1995.
6. Corney R, Developing communication and counseling skills in medicine. London and New York: Tavistock/Routledge; 1991.
7. Roter DL, Hall JA, Doctors talking with patients/patients talking with doctors. Improving communication in medical visits. 2nd ed. Westport, Connecticut and London: Auburn House; 2006.
8. Buetow S. Four strategies for negotiated care. JR Soc Med. 1998; 91(8):454.
9. Miyah NT. The power of compassion: Truth-telling among American doctors in the care of dying patients. Soc Sci Med. 1993; 36(3): 249-264.
10. Gertis M, Edgman-Levitan S, Daley J, Delbanco TL. editors. Through the patient's eyes. Understanding and promoting patient-centered care. 2nd ed. San Francisco: Jossey-Bass Publishers; 2002.
11. Leaman TL, Saxton JW. Preventing malpractice. The co-active solution. New York: Plenum Publishing Corporation; 1993.
12. Lancaster H. Managing your career. Workday etiquette: Know the right fork and watch that E-mail. The Wall Street Journal. 1998: April 21; Sect. B:1.
13. Post P. Emily Post's etiquette. 17th ed. New York: Harper Collins; 2004.
14. Claiborne C. Elements of etiquette: A guide to table manners in an imperfect world. New York: William Morrow & Co; 1992.
15. Washington G. The papers of George Washington. School Exercises: Rules of civility & decent behaviour in company and conversation. Rules of Civility Homepage. Available from: http://www.virginia.edu/gwpapers/civility/civ-tran.html [cited 6 August 1998].
16. Smith FR. Manners and conduct in school and out. Available from: http://darkwing.uoregon.edu/~joe/diglib/ [cited 11 August 1998].
17. Platt FW. Conversation failure. Case studies in Doctor-Patient communication. Tacoma Washington: Life Science Press; 1992.
18. Gropper RC. Culture and the clinical encounter. An intercultural sensitizer for the health professions. Yarmouth: Intercultural Press, Inc.; 1996.
19. Mitchell JL. Cross-cultural issues in the disclosure of cancer. Cancer Pract. 1998; 6(3):153-160.

20. Levine R. Re-learning to tell time. American Demographics Magazine; January 1998. Available from: http://www.demographics.com/publications/ad/98-ad/9801-ad/ad98016.htm [cited 6 August 1998].
21. Colt HG, Solot JA. Attitudes of patient and physicians regarding physician dress and demeanor in the emergency department. Ann Emerg Med. 1989; 18(2):145-151.
22. Dunn JJ, Lee HT, Percelay JM. Patient and house officer attitudes on physician attire and etiquette. JAMA. 1987; 257(1):65-8.
23. Rowland-Morin PA, Carroll JG. Verbal communication skills and patient satisfaction: A study of doctor-patient interviews. Eval Health Prof. 1990; 13(2):168-185.
24. Lowe F. You Did It. On My Fair Lady [DVD] Burbank, CA: Warner Home Video Columbia Records 1998.
25. Alpert EJ. Partner violence- How to recognize and treat victims of abuse: A guide for physicians and other health care professionals. 2nd ed. Waltham: Massachusetts Medical Society; 1992.
26. Goodman G. Domestic violence resources on the internet. JAMA Netsight. JAMA. 1998; 280(5):477-478.
27. Buckman R. How to break bad news: A guide for health care professionals. Baltimore: The Johns Hopkins University Press; 1992.
28. Page IH. Speaking to the doctor: His responsibilities and opportunities: selected editorials from Modern Medicine. New York: New York Times Media Company; 1972.
29. Molloy John T. John T. Molloy's new dress for success. New York: Warner Books; 1988.
30. Eagles JM, Rhind GB. Increasing handicaps in hospital medicine: Two-point cross sectional study of golfing activity among doctors. BMJ. 1997; 315:1656-1657.
31. Gillespie J. ed. Communication briefings. Volume XV, Number 11. Blackwood, NJ: Encoders Inc.; 1996.

ACTION POINTS

- Always say "please," "thank you," and "excuse me."
- Offer your hand as part of your introduction in the outpatient setting.
- Hold the door for the person behind you, male or female.
- Look the listener in the eye when you are speaking to them.
- Identify yourself to the listener.

Safe Behaviors for Professionals

Traveling to Conferences

- *Before* leaving, inquire what to wear to meetings and dinners (business casual, formal, business suits).
- Dress in business casual clothes for travel. You are representing your institution.
- Bring small bills for tipping at the airport, on arrival at the hotel, and for luggage transport.
- Remember to extend middle class courtesies to all ladies and gentlemen(colleagues, spouses) outside of the hospital (e.g. opening doors; standing when an older person/lady enters the room or joins your table).
- Collect receipts for everything.
- If you are an officer of an organization, plan to attend the entire national meeting. Leaving before the end signals to others that you don't value their time.

Dining with Colleagues at Meetings

- Introduce yourself to *all* of the other persons at your table (8 or less) before the food is served.
- Remember that your bread and butter plate is to your left—use it, but don't point out another's misuse. That is bad manners.
- Always offer to the person next to you before you serve yourself (e.g. salad dressing, wine, rolls) and then pass on.
- Always pass to the right side, never across the table.
- If you leave your chair *temporarily*, put the linen napkin over the top of the chair, or over the chair arm to let the waitstaff know you are returning.
- Put the napkin in your lap before you eat anything and keep it there until the end of the event.
- When you finally leave the table, put the linen napkin to the left of your plate.
- Pass both the salt and pepper together, even if only one is requested.
- Start with the utensils on the outside and work toward the plate.

Asking Questions at Meetings

- Always address your questions to "Doctor" even if you are good friends.
- Never assume everyone should know who you are. State your name and where you are from.
- If you are a meeting moderator use only "Doctor" or "The gentleman/gentlewoman at the first microphone" even if you know the person well.
- If you are asking the question from a stationary microphone, stand facing the speaker until he or she finish the answer. Do not ask the question, turn, and return to your seat while the speaker is answering your question.

Parties at a Faculty Member's Home

- Greet both the host and hostess upon your arrival, introduce your guests and identify their relationship to you (e.g. wife, cousins, date, daughter).
- Thank your host and hostess when you leave.
- Bring a small hostess gift.
- If your spouse cannot attend at the last minute, call ahead but still go.
- Leave before the invitation's stated finish time.
- Don't smoke unless you inquire first.
- Send a thank-you note within a week of the event if the invitation was in writing. If the invitation was via an e-mail message, an e-mail thank-you note is fine.
- RSVP – this means that you need to make a commitment. If the invitation was via e-mail, an e-mail response is all that is required. A written invitation usually lists a telephone number for responses.
- REGRETS ONLY means that you are expected to attend if you do not respond. Remember to respond before the event to help with planning and not after the event with excuses.

Casual Parties

- Ask whether the gathering is business casual or casual.
- If children are included, ask if you should bring a sitter for a wandering toddler.
- Ask if you can help by bringing something.
- Send a thank-you note within a week of the event if the invitation was in writing. Or, if the invitation arrived via e-mail, an e-mail thank-you is acceptable.

Adverse Outcomes: Successful Disclosure

Matson Sewell, MPH, CPHRM

The surgeon motions the family to a corner of the waiting room. They huddle close to her, leaning in against the noise of the television. She notices blood splatter on her shoe cover and bends to remove them. "Your husband's in PACU. He's stable now."

A redhead, one of two daughters whose names the surgeon has forgotten, holds her mother's shoulder. She asks, "What did you find?"

A laugh track from "Everyone Loves Raymond" blots out the second part of the daughter's question. The surgeon glances at their faces, wife and daughter about to need each other more than they can imagine.

The daughter repeats, "You got it all?"

Eyeing a family of four glazed before the TV, the surgeon balls up the shoe covers and folds her arms. "The problem's the size of the cancer. It invaded right into the abdominal muscles...and into the right ureter, the tube carrying urine to the—"

"Wait!" said the daughter. "You're saying he's not cured?"

"I'm saying I'm not sure. The surgery was technically difficult."

The wife frowns and grasps her daughter's hand. "Is my husband going to make it, doctor?"

"Look, the problem is I cut his ureter. I had a urologist come in and repair it. So, it'll be OK. The case was hard, everything was stuck. We lost a lot of blood."

"*He* lost a lot of blood, you mean," the daughter hissed. "My father... not you! Doctor, why don't you tell us what really happened?"

Perhaps no area of health care communication has posed greater challenge and sustained more persistent confusion than the communication with patients after adverse medical or surgical outcomes. Despite the efforts to date, those on the front lines of surgery struggle in the application of published recommendations. Many also express ongoing confusion about the terms used in patient safety and disclosure and how they can apply the communication process fairly and with integrity. Some have had the dismaying experience of attempting to follow guidelines and, despite their sincere efforts and intentions, had a backlash of consequences that felt surprising and unfair.

"...even when the standard of care was met...failed communication leads to anger, mistrust and litigation."

F. Dean Griffen, MD, FACS
ACS Closed Claims Study

Most health care providers have gone through only a handful of disclosure processes following serious and surprising bad outcomes. Most have also never been present when a mentor or colleague has met with patients and family members following clinical catastrophes. This communication process represents a very private pain that is not discussed as a learning opportunity for colleagues.

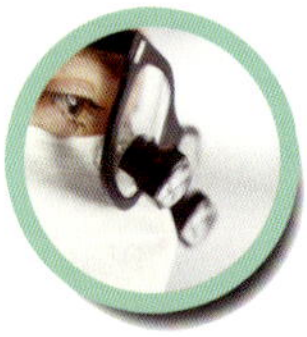

When the American College of Surgeons (ACS) 2006 Closed Claims Study examined communication failures involving surgical procedures, most were failures to communicate postoperatively, followed by preoperative, and then intraoperative.

PREOPERATIVE FAILURES

Preoperative failures by general surgeons were cited as major contributions to subsequent substandard intraoperative performance in the ACS study.

Injuring unintended organs

The surgeon caused nerve injury while removing a cystic hygroma but had not discussed this possibility with the patient, nor included the possibility in the consent form.

Operating unnecessarily

A lymph node regresses before surgery for biopsy, but the surgeon fails to visit with and examine the patient prior to surgery. No tissue was obtained.

Wrong site operation

The surgeon failed to call 'time out' to confirm that the nurse prepped the wrong leg for bypass.

Good communication in the pre-operative period can:

- Dramatically reduce intraoperative misadventure; and
- Help prevent problems in the postoperative period.

The preoperative communication failure that comes back to haunt surgeons in the disclosure process is a failure to frame the prospective surgery during the informed consent conversation. In the opening scenario of this chapter, a preoperative communication with patient and family referencing the unique challenges of the case and the complications which could be reasonably anticipated would have ensured that the family was not hearing those warnings for the first time after an operative injury had occurred.

The preoperative informed consent process provides the crucial platform from which to initiate a disclosure communication in the aftermath of an adverse outcome.

INTRAOPERATIVE FAILURES

Although not as frequent in the ACS study, problems with communication during surgery can be quite serious. In the 2006 ACS Closed Claims Study, communication problems contributed to:

- **Wrong site surgery;**
- **Retention of a foreign body;**
- **Inappropriate use of medications; and**
- **Flawed assistant surgeon or consultant surgeon interactions.**

The intraoperative communication failure that fuels family anger occurs when the anticipated surgical timeline changes significantly and no one comes to the surgical waiting area to inform family of the reason. When a communication disclosure eventually follows, the family members have already started to anticipate that medical staff will be withholding, delaying, and covering up information related to the surgery.

POSTOPERATIVE FAILURES

The standard of care dictum requires surgeons to deal diligently with the consequences of intraoperative errors and any adverse events following surgery.

Problems with diagnosis

A patient who had a ventral hernia repair calls daily after discharge. The patient is told every time that 'all is well,' but dies of a missed small bowel injury.

Problems with treatment

The floor nurse calls the surgeon with the patient's complaint of trouble swallowing the afternoon after thyroidectomy and reports normal oxygen saturation. The surgeon increases sedation without seeing the patient and the patient subsequently dies from hypoxia caused by a postoperative hematoma.

The cardinal postoperative communication failures related to disclosure involve avoidance of:

- The family;
- The case investigation; and
- Taking responsibility for any role in the adverse outcome.

Defendants (surgeons) suffered litigation because they failed to spend the time to provide the insight and satisfaction to diffuse anger and distrust.

F. Dean Griffen, MD, FACS
ACS Closed Claims Study

NON-OPERATIVE FAILURES

The competent surgeon develops the skills necessary to perform appropriate procedures during training. The safe surgeon also develops cognitive skills to judge when not to operate.

A teenager is discharged after observation for blunt trauma noting that there is no pain or complaint. The surgeon fails to confirm treatment with the nurse who had given repeated doses of pain medication just prior to the surgeon's visit.

The nurse could have reported a temperature spike that had not yet been recorded. The patient expires at home later the same day. An autopsy reveals a perforated hollow viscus.

The American College of Surgeons' Closed Claims Study (2006) as reported by FD Griffen, MD, FACS, demonstrated the failure of many surgeons to deal diligently with the consequences of intraoperative errors and other adverse events in the postoperative period.

Problems with diagnosis and treatment were numerous. Even though the basic complication in the majority of these cases was inevitable, the delay or failure to diagnose or treat that resulted from flawed communication drastically increased the severity of the complication from adverse events such as inescapable postoperative infection, bleeding, or thrombosis to totally preventable adverse events such as organ system failure, amputation, or exsanguinations.

Of the 35 cases involving failed communication during postoperative care, complications were caused or aggravated in 24 patients.

In many of these cases, the surgeons suffered litigation solely because they failed to spend the time required to provide the insight and patient satisfaction necessary to diffuse anger and mistrust.

Disclosure of Adverse Events to Patients in the Veterans Healthcare Systems

There are specific documentation steps required and electronic note types that must be used to document the disclosure to the patient or family. This policy wording may vary across facilities, but the tone and guidance ensure the critical elements are consistent across all VA hospitals. *VHA Directive 2005-049, Disclosure of Adverse Events to Patients, October 26, 2005.*

Internal reporting of adverse events and close call reports is protected from disclosure under Title 38 United States Code (U.S.C.) Section 5705. Records protected under 38 U.S.C. Section 5705, that is quality management and safety activities records, may not be subsequently used as the source of information communicated in the disclosure of an adverse event. The information communicated must come from those involved in the adverse event and from factual information in the patient's medical record.

Most centers have embraced the belief that honestly discussing the difficult truth that an adverse event has occurred demonstrates respect for the patient, professionalism and a commitment to improving care.

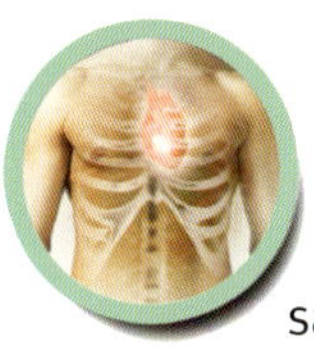

FAILURE TO COMMUNICATE

According to Griffen, the surgeons who reviewed the large set of malpractice claims said that "surgeons hear selectively." They "weigh input in favor of the best scenario, blinding themselves to reality and leading to inertia and errors of omissions." Many surgeons preferred to hear in the message that all was well, rather than probe for more facts.

The following cases represent composite scenarios spanning 15 years and 30 health care facilities in the Unites States.

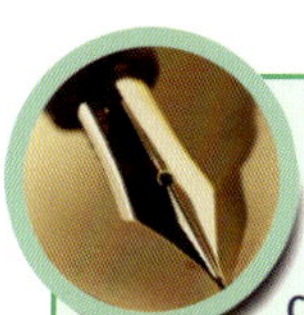

Case 1. Preventing the next patient injury

A senior surgical resident was summoned to the teaching facility's intensive care unit to insert a chest tube in a patient with a pneumothorax. The chest tube kit retrieved from central supplies was unfamiliar to him, but had the general appearance of chest tubes he had used before. After completing the chest tube insertion and withdrawing the guide-wire and sheath in his customary practice, he noted that the tip of the sheath appeared to have sheared off and was likely remaining in the patient's chest. A follow-up chest radiograph tracking the resolution of the pneumothorax indicated a tiny shadow not identified by the reading radiologist but consistent with the resident's recollection of the likely location of the retained sheath tip. Concluding that the foreign body was unlikely to embolize, the resident did not report the occurrence to his supervising surgeon or to the patient. Three days later, the same type of kit was used by another surgical resident on a patient with a hemothorax with similar results: the guide-wire sheath was sheared off and remained in the patient's chest. This time the resident reported to his chief and, based on the location of the foreign body, laparascopic retrieval was deemed necessary.

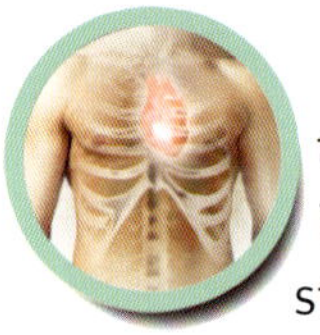

Follow-up investigation of the circumstances surrounding the two occurrences revealed the following details: The medical center's central supply division, attempting to reduce inventory overhead costs and order on a "just-in-time" basis, had run low on the standard chest tube trays. Before the next shipment arrived, the depleted stocks were replenished with a stock of trays about to reach their expiration date. The kits had been used as part of a research study and required special handling to avoid the catheter-shear experienced by the residents in the involved cases. After completing the root cause analysis, the team agreed to:

- ✔ Disclose the occurrence to both patients.
- ✔ Assure the patient that no billing would go out for the return to the operating room and an additional postoperative stay.
- ✔ Discuss with the patient, who did not have to return to the operating room, that he should have an additional chest radiograph in three months to be certain the retained body was not moving and this cost would not be billed to him.
- ✔ Include the central supplies staff in the process and implement a policy to avoid a similar future substitution in the general stores of medical devices.
- ✔ Present a continuing education program for all surgical staff emphasizing the non-punitive reporting of adverse occurrences and prevention of recurrent patient injury.

Disagreement persisted about the extent of disclosure. Some believed the second patient should be told that a similar event a week earlier had gone unreported and might have prevented his medical injury and return to the O.R. The majority argued to limit the disclosure because this additional information would offer no medical benefit to the patient and could begin conversations that might breach confidentiality related to the first patient and to their resident's performance evaluations. However, it was recognized that such information would certainly strengthen any punitive damages he might seek in a malpractice suit.

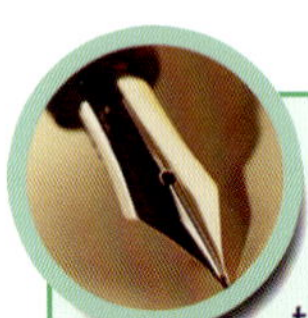

Case 2. Timing of disclosure

A vascular surgeon was notified that the instrument pack he used was found to be sub-optimally sterilized following a complex orthopedic and vascular repair on a motorcycle accident victim. On his way to the patient's room to disclose the problem—being mindful of recommendations to disclose as soon as possible, preferably within 24 hours—he notified the hospital risk management office of the occurrence. It became clear through discussion that the surgeon did not understand what sterilization failure might mean to this patient. Had she been potentially exposed to viruses including hepatitis and HIV? Would her treatment or prognosis be changed by the error? Although he felt pressured by recommendations to disclose within 24 hours, the surgeon agreed to wait to inform the patient until an urgent infectious disease consultation could be obtained.

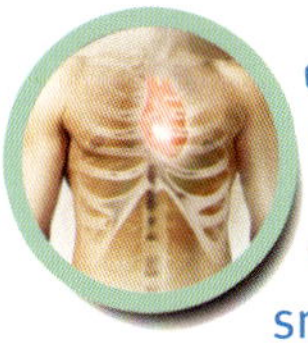

✔ The ID review found that the sterilization failure notice was issued when a Pall filter was noted missing in the sterilization unit set-up.

✔ The absence of the filter posed no risk of viral contamination, and possibly a small risk of some persistent bacterial contamination of the instruments.

✔ The patient was already on full-spectrum antibiotics for her open fracture that had been dragged through road debris and her risk of infection due to the nature of her injury dwarfed the risk due to the surgical instruments.

Following spirited debate within his section, the surgeon decided to wait and address the sterilization error only if the patient developed an infection. One member of his practice group strongly disagreed with this decision, stating that the patient had a right to know, even if this knowledge caused her additional anxiety.

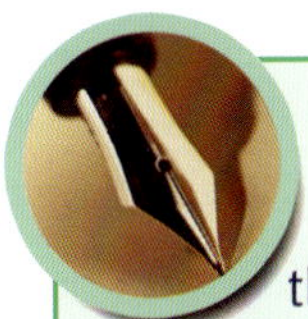

Case 3. The complexity of error

Following urgent cholecystectomy, a morbidly obese patient was moved from the PACU to the nursing floor with transfer orders including 10 units of insulin. The transfer order was written as "10u" which was read and administered as 100 units of insulin precipitating an insulin crisis from which the patient died. The surgeon promptly disclosed to the patient's husband, "Your wife died of a massive insulin overdose administered by the nurse."

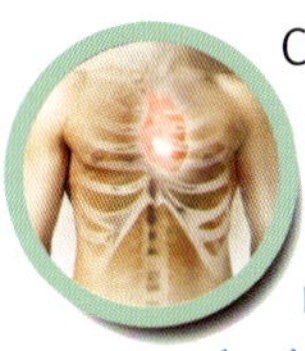

Case analysis conducted as a Sentinel Event Review found a more complex interaction of clinical failures that resulted in this patient's death.

✔ The surgeon's order using the abbreviation of "u" for units ignore violated medical staff policy implemented several years earlier to avoid abbreviations that had been found to contribute to medical error.

✔ The nurse administering the insulin was a recent nursing school graduate who had been working on a per diem basis since graduation and had minimal supervision on the involved high patient-census day.

✔ The nurse-patient ratio had been in steady decline in the facility, first due to a cost-saving cutback on staffing, and in the previous year due to nursing shortage. The facility had resorted to using traveling nurses and per diem nurses, both groups having demonstrated a higher error rate in the facility.

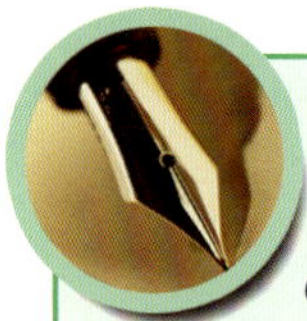

Case 4. Blind Reviews

A 67- year-old woman was referred to a cardiothoracic surgeon for evaluation of a left lower lung mass. Radiologists reading the chest radiograph had referred to a chest film taken 18 months earlier to evaluate a resolving left infiltrate. The radiologists expressed concern that they could perceive a hint of the mass in the prior film. The CT surgeon told the patient the mass was missed on the prior chest film and showed her the area of concern to his eye. The patient filed a medical malpractice lawsuit against the radiologists who read the films taken 18 months earlier.

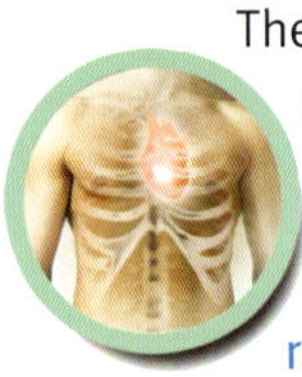

The defendant's attorney for Case 4 secured a blind review by five board certified radiologists at a regional teaching hospital. This is common in the defense of malpractice cases.

✔ In the blind review, the prior infiltrate radiograph was mixed in with routine readings. Of the five radiologists reviewing the film, not one noted any suggestion of lung mass in the infiltrate.

✔ Hindsight bias can wreak havoc on objective case reviews. Knowing the outcome can influence the perceptions of even the most experienced reviewers. When in doubt, requesting a stat review by a specialty-qualified colleague who does not know the outcome can provide much needed perspective.

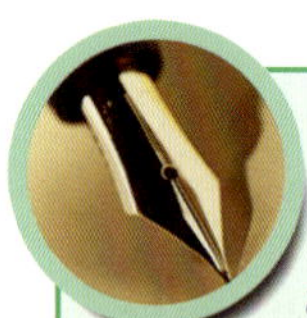

Case 5. Review of another specialty

A 42-year-old trauma patient in the intensive care unit developed signs of a "hot belly." The ICU intensivist and the trauma surgeon, who had a prior history of hostile disagreement, began an ongoing argument about management of the patient. The intensivist insisted the patient needed exploratory surgery to identify and correct the source of the evolving abdominal signs. The surgeon insisted that the surgical mortality risk in the patient's current condition exceeded 50% and he would not operate until the patient stabilized or the risk of delaying surgery exceeded the operative risks. The following day, the surgeon reassessed the patient's condition and took him to the operating room where a bowel perforation was identified and surgically corrected. The patient survived and the intensivist insisted that it was his moral duty to convey to the patient and his family that a mistake had been made to 'not operate' a day earlier.

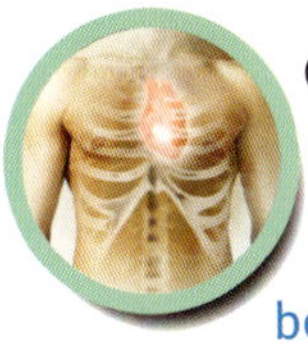

Case reviews were performed both internally and through a regional surgical quality review process. From the reviewing surgeons' perspectives:

- ✔ The pathology specimen report indicated the perforation occurred shortly before the surgery started.
- ✔ The radiographic and laboratory studies did not support operating sooner.
- ✔ No violation in the surgical standard of care occurred in this case—the timing of surgery was well within a range of reasonable surgical option, especially considering the patient's unstable condition and operative risk.
- ✔ Special care needed to be observed when a specialist insisted on conveying a disputed mistake by someone from a different specialty.

KEY POINTS FOR IMPROVING DISCLOSURE COMMUNICATION

- Ensure that care of the patient and family needs are met.
- Secure all evidence related to the occurrence for further evaluation. (e.g., sequestering equipment, sharps and refuse containers for pharmacy analysis, medication and crash cart inventory.
- Avoid erratic disclosure. Wait until you have all of the facts. Appreciate that timing, objective case review and analysis and communication style make a huge difference in the accuracy and effectiveness of the disclosure process.
- Recognize that disclosure is an organizational process that involves many others, not just one surgeon. Just as medical injury is now appreciated to involve system errors, disclosure needs to be a system process.
- Keep in mind that disclosure is not a single step or a single conversation. The patient and family's 'need to know' can evolve over time. Identifying a contact person who will coordinate ongoing communication, as needed, is pivotal for continuing to meet patient/family needs.

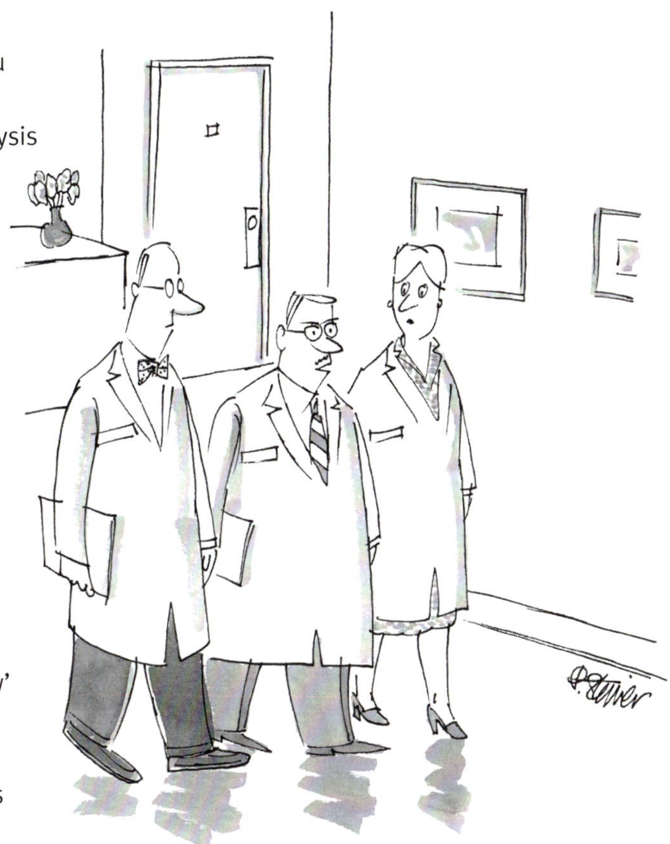

"Why carry malpractice insurance if you don't malpractice once in a while?"

REFERENCES

1. AMA's Council on Ethical and Judicial Affairs, E-8.12 Patient Information, Code of Medical Ethics: Current Ethical Opinions. Chicago. American Medical Association, 1994 (updated 2005 Oct 04). Available from: www.ama-assn.org/ama/pub/category/8497.html.
2. Barron WM. Kuczewski MG. Unanticipated harm to patients: deciding when to disclose outcomes. Jt Comm J Qual Saf. 2003; 29(10):551-5.
3. Berlinger N. Avoiding cheap grace. Medical harm, patient safety, and the culture of forgiveness. Hastings Cent Rep. 2003; 33(6):28-36.
4. Bonacum D, Houk C, Moidel BJ. Communicating about episodes of harm to patients. In: Leonard MS, Frankel A, Simmonds T, Vega KB, editors. Achieving safe and reliable healthcare. Chicago: Health Administration Press; 2004:93-112.
5. Build the public's trust by dealing openly with errors. AHA News. 1999; Aug 2:6.
6. A call for candor without fear. Am Med News. 2003; Jul 21:14.
7. Clark AP. Taking the high road: What should you do when an adverse event occurs? Part 1. Clin Nurse Spec. 2004; 18(3):118-9.
8. Cohen JR. Future research on disclosure of medical errors. Ann Intern Med. 2004; 141(6):481.
9. Condolences are fine, but be careful what you say. Healthc Risk Manag. 2001; 23(6):67-8.
10. Crane, M. What to say if you made a mistake. Med Econ. 2001; 78(16):26-8, 33-6.
11. Croteau RJ. All outcomes should be disclosed. Jt Comm J Qual Saf. 2003; 29(10):556-7.
12. Disclosure of unanticipated events: the next step in better communication with patients. Chicago: American Society for Healthcare Risk Management; 2003; May:14.
13. Disclosure requires some hard choices. Healthc Risk Manag. 2001; 23 (12):137-40.
14. Frenkel DN. Liebman CB. Words that heal. Ann Intern Med. 2004; 140(6):482-3.
15. Gallagher TH, Waterman AD, Ebers A, Fraser V, Levinson W. Patients' and physicians' attitudes regarding the disclosure of medical errors. JAMA. 2003; 289(8):1002-7.
16. Green VL. Truth-telling and the law: the bottom line of the Institute of Medicine's report on error. Obstet Gynecol Surv. 2004; 59(1):5-8.
17. Griffen FD, Stephens LS, Alexander JB, Bailey HE, Maizel SE, Sutton BH, Posner KL. The American College of Surgeons' closed claims study: new insights for improving care. J Am Coll Surg. 2007; 204: 561-9.
18. Griffen FD. ACS closed claims study reveals critical failures to communicate. Bull Amer Coll Surg. 2007; 92(1):11-16.
19. Hobgood C, Peck CR, Gilbert B, Chappelle C, Zou B. Medical errors—what and when: what do patients want to know? Acad Emerg Med. 2002; 9(11):1156-61.
20. Hoffmann PB. Revealing inconvenient truths. Managers should avoid the temptation to withhold, delay, minimize or misrepresent bad news. Healthc Exec. 2003; 18(5):56-7.
21. Kachalia A, Shojania KG, Hofer TP, Piotrowski M, Saint S. Does full disclosure of medical errors affect malpractice liability? The jury is still out. Jt Comm J Qual Saf. 2003; 29(10);503-11.
22. Kraman SS, Cranfill L, Hamm G, Woodard T. Advocacy: The Lexington Veterans Affairs Medical Center. Jt Comm J Qual Improv. 2002; 28(12):646-50.

23. Kraman SS, and Hamm G. Risk management: extreme honesty may be the best Policy. Ann Int Med. 1999; 131(12):963-7.
24. Lamb R. Open disclosure: the only approach to medical error. Qual & Saf Healthc. 2004; 13(1):3-5.
25. Lamb RM, Studdert DM, Bohmer RM, Berwick DM, Brennan TA. Hospital disclosure practices: results of a national survey. Health Aff. 2003; 22(2):73-83.
26. Larkin H. Cost drivers. Liability. Responding to patients quickly and with candor can avert costly lawsuits. Hosp Health Netw. 2004; 78(6):38-40,42.
27. Lazare A. On apology. New York: Oxford University Press; 2004.
28. Levine C. I was dead wrong. Med Econ. 2004; 81(3):59,63.
29. Liebman CB, Hyman CS. A mediation skills model to manage disclosure of errors and adverse events to patients. Health Aff. 2004; 23(4):22-32.
30. Matlow A, Stevens P, Harrison C, Laxer R. Achieving closure through disclosure: experience in a pediatric institution. J Pediat. 2004; 144(5):559-60.
31. Mazor KM, Simon SR, Yood RA. Health plan members' views on forgiving medical errors. Am J Manag Care. 2005; 11 (1):49-52.
32. Mazor KM, Simon SR, Gurwitz JH. Communicating with patients about medical errors. Arch Intern Med. 2004; 164(15):1690-7.
33. Mulholland D. Unanticipated consequences of unanticipated outcomes disclosures. J Health Law. 2002; 35(2):211-26.
34. O'Connell D, Reifsteck SW. Disclosing unexpected outcomes and medical error. J Med Pract Manage. 2004; 19(6):317-23.
35. Ott M Key considerations on drafting a policy on disclosure of unanticipated outcomes. J Healthc Risk Manag. 2001; 21(3):27-34.
36. Perspective on disclosure of unanticipated outcome information. Chicago: American Society for Healthcare Risk Management, 2001 Apr; 20.
37. Popp PL. How to—and not to—disclose medical errors to patients. Manag Care. 2002; 11(10): 52-3.
38. Porto GG. Disclosure of medical error: facts and fallacies. J Healthc Risk Manag. 2001; 2(3):67-76.
39. Robeznieks A. The power of an apology. Am Med News. 2003; 46(28):9-10.
40. Rosner F, Berger JT, Kark P, Potash J, Bennett AJ. Disclosure and prevention of medical errors. Arch Inter Med. 2000; 160(14):2089-2092.
41. Schwappach DL, Koeck CM. What makes an error unacceptable? A factorial survey on the disclosure of medical errors. Int J Qual Health Care. 2004; 16(4):317-24.
42. Talking to patients about health care injury: statement of principle. Chicago, IL: National Patient Safety Foundation. 2000 Nov 14. Available from: http://npsf.org/rc/pdf/Statement_of_Principle.pdf.
43. Telling the truth: why you should disclose medical errors to your patients. Briefings on patient safety. 2002; 3(7):7-9.

44. Volker DL, Clark AP. Taking the high road: what should you do when an adverse event occurs? Clin Nurse Spec. 2004; 18(4):180-2.

45. Weeks WB, Mills PD. Reduction in patient enrollment in the Veterans Health Administration after media coverage of adverse medical events. J Comm J Qual Saf. 2003; 29(12):652-8.

46. Wu AW. Handling hospital errors: is disclosure the best defense? Ann Int Med. 1999; 131(12):970-2.

47. Wu AW, Cavanaugh TA, McPhee SJ, Lo B, Micco GP. To tell the truth; ethical and practical issues in disclosing medical mistakes to patients. J Gen Intern Med. 1997; 12(12):770-5.

48. When things go wrong: responding to adverse events. A Consensus Statement of the Harvard Hospitals. Burlington, Massachusetts: Massachusetts Coalition for the Prevention of Medical Errors. 2006 Mar. Available from: http://www.macoalition.org/documents/respondingToAdverseEvents.pdf.

49. Rogers SO Jr, Gawande AA, Kwaan M, Puopolo A, Yoon C, Brennan TZ, Studdert DM. Analysis of surgical errors in closed malpractice claims at 4 liability insurers. Surgery. 2006; 140(1):25-33.

Cultural Adaptability: Intercultural Techniques

Lori Alvord, MD, FACS, Charles Mock, MD, FACS, PhD,
Kaleem Sayyed, MBBS, MPH, Mohammed Moursi, MD, FACS,
Muhammad Jaffar, MD, FCCP

A physician examined an elderly Native American woman at the hospital on a northern plains reservation. He explained to her that he thought she had pneumonia and needed to be admitted to the hospital. The patient indicated that she only wanted medicine and wished to go home, but the physician insisted on admission. He was puzzled as to why the woman avoided looking directly at him, but assumed that she was either depressed or trying to hide something. When the patient was eventually shown to her room, she became frightened and tried to convince the physician to change her room. As the hospital was chronically overcrowded, he saw no reason to shuffle patients around in rooms to accommodate what he perceived as a whim. The woman left the hospital without asking for or receiving any further treatment. Later, the physician learned from a local nursing aide who knew the patient's family that she had been seeing a medicine man and wished medicine to supplement his therapy with modern therapy and that she had wished to return home as a healing ceremony was being considered for the next several days. The patient had become frightened when she found out that she was being admitted to the same room in which a relative had died the previous year. She was concerned that the spirit might still be lingering in the room. After several such encounters with elderly patients, the physician learned that traditional Native Americans from that reservation do not look directly at the face of a stranger, as a sign of respect.

Knowledge, attitudes, and beliefs about the causes of diseases and their treatment may vary greatly from culture to culture. Such attitudes and beliefs are often deeply ingrained in both physicians and patients and yet neither may give much thought to the fact that the other may think differently. Cultures that have had limited contact with modern Western medicine will often have their own health beliefs and practices, and therefore it is often helpful for health care providers in Western medicine to have an understanding of the cultures of the patients they treat. Additionally, some patients may seek treatment by practitioners of modern medicine, while also using the traditional medicine of their cultures.

In an increasingly global environment, physicians and surgeons can expect to care for people from a wide range of cultures and ethnicities. The ability to provide excellent health care to these patients requires that physicians have exceptional communication skills as well as a high "cultural intelligence quotient." In this chapter, you will find guidelines for beginning the process of developing a culturally competent approach to caring for patients. Additionally, issues directly related to surgical care are addressed. It is not possible, however, to cover all the issues relevant to cultural competency in one chapter, nor can all the ways that cultures and surgical issues interact be described in a single book chapter. Instead, we aim to describe some of the more common issues that may be encountered, and provide examples from various cultures. While most of these examples may be generalized, the providers should be aware of the dangers of stereotyping.

COMMUNICATION

Verbal and nonverbal communication varies from culture to culture and within cultures. Communication that might be considered respectful and proper for one group may unfortunately be considered insulting in another. Effective intercultural communication includes an understanding of a patient's beliefs about disease causation (or a willingness to understand), and how the patient may react to the medical diagnostic work-up and the treatment plan offered. It is also important to recognize how the patient's mode of communication differs from that of the treating physician. Such differences include not only obvious barriers such as language, but nonverbal factors as well.

Culture is a difficult variable to define or recognize. Many subcultures(1) exist among any recognizable cultural group. Even within the same ethnic group, variations in socioeconomic levels, education, or life experiences can influence knowledge about science and beliefs about disease causation. There are wide variations in health beliefs, and they demonstrate the diversity that exists within cultures. The health beliefs of groups such as Latino, Navajo, Haitian, Asian and Southeast Asian, and Middle Eastern will be considered, along with methods to improve intercultural communication in the health care setting, particularly with regard to surgical concerns such as beliefs about surgery, the operative consent process, and advance directives. Some of the material discussed will be based on culture while some will be on religious beliefs.

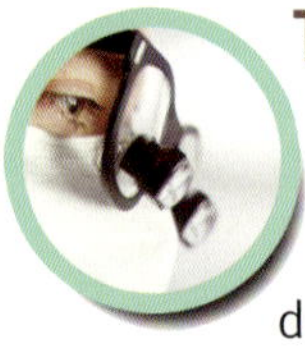

THEORIES OF DISEASE CAUSATION

Latino

One primary belief in Latino cultures is the hot/cold (calientefrio) dichotomy, which dates back historically to the Hippocratic humoral theory of disease. (2)

In this theory, the body is perceived as being in balance between hot and cold. Diseases occur when imbalances develop. Temperature plays a role, so that exposure to cold air may result in colds, arthritis, or stomach upset. Certain diseases are felt to be innate disruptions in the hot/cold balance. For example, diarrhea and ulcers are felt to be "hot" diseases. Certain foods and medicine, both traditional and modern, have hot or cold properties. Cold foods (regardless of the actual temperature at which they are served) and medicines are useful for hot diseases and vice versa. The fact that new drugs are incorporated into this schema indicates the vitality of this theory in Latino culture. Misunderstandings may arise when a recommended therapy conflicts with this balance. If patients are disregarded or criticized by the physician, such actions can lead to noncompliance and resentment.

Efforts to work with the hot/cold theory can often improve the physician-patient interaction. For example, most modern drugs, especially antibiotics, are considered hot. A frequent source of misunderstanding is the prescribing of such drugs for treatment of hot diseases such as infectious diarrhea. One way to approach this would be to recommend taking the medication with fruit juice (considered cold) to help neutralize any adverse effects of the hot substance. (2)

Other concepts of disease include caido de la mollera (sunken fontanelle), empacho, mal ojo (evil eye), and susto (shock). (3-7, 8) Sunken fontanelle affects infants with structural imbalances in the head and results in crying and restlessness. Empacho is a disorder of digestion resulting from a ball of food clinging abnormally to the intestinal wall. Susto arises when a sudden assault on the body (loud noise, unpleasant sight, emotional upset) causes part of the soul (esperitu) to leave the body. The resulting shock or susto causes weakness and loss of appetite. (4-7,8) While this concept, on first examination, may seem hard to reconcile with all opathic concepts of disease, it should be remembered that stress is increasingly recognized as a manifestation of illness, and these 'shocks' may be interpreted as a form of stress.

There are a variety of remedies recommended for these disease manifestations, some physical, some herbal, and some religious. Many in Latino communities believe that Anglo doctors do not understand these diseases, cannot treat them, and regard these beliefs as "superstitions." Some Latinos will first visit a traditional lay healer "curandero" before considering coming to a hospital or modern physician. Frequently, patients will bring medicines prescribed by a physician to the curandero for his or her opinion on whether or how they should be taken. When attempting to build rapport with Latino patients, it is helpful to ask if they have also been seeing such a curandero and if he or she had given them his or her opinion.

In addition to the curandero, the opinion of grandparents and other elders is highly valued in Latino communities, especially regarding the care of children. During the treatment of children, it is prudent to ask the parents what the grandparents think and have told them.

Hmong/Laotian

The Hmong and other Laotian hill tribes conceive of illness as a result of supernatural forces, such as the influence of evil spirits and demons. A chief cause of illness, especially among children, is soul loss, wherein fright or other highly emotional circumstances cause the soul to leave the body. Much of Hmong healing is related to guiding or calling the soul back. Another excellent source is the book *The Spirit Catches You and You Fall Down* by Anne Fadiman, which details the travails of a Hmong child and her American doctors.(9, 10)

It should be remembered that fright and situations that elicit strong emotions are also a source of stress, and since stress is increasingly recognized as a factor in many illnesses, an explanatory model that seeks to restore harmony and reduce this stress may provide elements of effectiveness.

Haitian

The predominant religion in Haiti is a mixture of Catholicism along with traditional African beliefs and rituals known as Vodun, the magical aspects of which are popularly known as voodoo. Illness is frequently viewed as spiritual in origin. Even injury such as from motor vehicle accidents is often thought to be due to spiritual causes. Frequently, such illness, injury, or other misfortune is believed to be due to the malevolence of others who have used voodoo ritual to curse or hex the victim.

A child with typhoid ileitis who developed a bowel perforation was brought to a hospital in Haiti. The perforation was repaired, but the child went on to develop an enterocutaneous fistula. The physician caring for her placed a nasogastric tube for feedings of a low residue diet. The family could not understand the need for this and thought that, as the child was progressively losing weight, she had been placed under a spell and was "possessed." They discussed this fear with the physician, who told them that no such thing was possible and not to worry about it. The family later took the child home, and the physicians lost the opportunity to continue to provide care for the child.

While patients or their families may use modern medicine, many also go to practitioners of voodoo, either as a first preference or in addition to modern medicine, to remove the root cause of the illness. Although such beliefs do not fit well with the modern concepts of disease, attempts by medical personnel to deny them or to convince patients otherwise often result in mistrust and alienation. (11)

Middle Eastern

There are now over seven million Muslims in America, and Islam is the second largest religion in the world. The Muslim population in America is very diverse, with origins in the Middle East, the South Pacific and even China. They may be assimilated to American ways, or they may maintain traditional customs, beliefs, and religious observances. Many Muslims have immigrated to the United States as professionals, but communities also have large numbers of refugees. An understanding of Middle Eastern cultures and Islamic religious practices will help providers understand current norms of Muslims living in the United States.

An important Muslim belief is that anything good or bad is from *Allah*, an Arabic word for the name of God. The disease that a patient has may be viewed as a test from Allah. The Muslim understands this and will ask God directly for help to cure the disease and to ease the pain and suffering. The end result of the disease process is due to the will of God and no one can alter that. As such, the health care provider and medicine are only tools used by God to achieve this end result. Muslims believe in the healing powers of reciting God's book, the Koran. Muslims also believe that disease and suffering may be a form of punishment for past sins committed.

Islam is the second largest religion in the world.

Asian

Among the various cultural groups discussed in this chapter, probably more variation exists among the grouping "Asian" than among any of the other groups.

Chinese communities have been well established in the Western world for generations and much has been written about their interaction with modern medicine. (12, 13) Traditional Chinese medicine is founded on the concept of the balance of the universal forces of Yin and Yang. The concepts are complex, but briefly, Yang is a masculine force represented by light, heat, and dryness, while Yin is a feminine force represented by darkness, cold, and wet. (14) Such concepts are ancient, are backed by myriad of traditional writings, and have been formally taught and passed on. Disease arises from imbalances, with balance being restored through herbal remedies and acupuncture.

Chinese patients will frequently go to practitioners of both Western and Chinese medicine for different reasons. Western practitioners are viewed as restoring health quickly but temporarily. Traditional Chinese medicine is viewed as correcting the underlying imbalances. Injections are readily accepted because of the history of acupuncture.

Southeast Asian immigrants, who have arrived more recently in the United States, are less well understood by Western physicians, and therefore miscommunication is frequent. Tremendous variation exists among this group of peoples. The mainly urban Vietnamese have more easily acculturated to the West, though of course they still face many cultural challenges. Peasant farmers from Cambodia and lowland Laos have religious and health beliefs similar to the Chinese. The Hmong and other hill tribe people from Laos have a predominantly shamanistic (use of medicine man) and animistic belief system. (14, 15)

Navajo (Diné)

The Navajo (also known as Diné) tribe is presented as representative of Native American culture. The Navajos are the largest tribe in the United States and they have received the most attention in intercultural health studies. While many tribes share similar beliefs, physicians must be careful not to generalize too widely across tribal "boundaries" as tribes have many differences as well.

A patient-physician interaction illustrates the differences doctors encounter when dealing with Native American cultures.

> A Navajo child was admitted to the hospital with osteomyelitis. A few days later, the family wanted to take the child home. The physician discussed this with them and found out that they wanted to take the child for a "sing" healing ceremony. A compromise was worked out in which the child remained hospitalized until his fever improved. He was then temporarily discharged to be taken home for two days for the ceremony, returning afterwards for the remainder of the course of antibiotics.

Attempts by practitioners to dissuade the use of traditional medicine can result in alienating patients and their families. (3,16) The above narrative illustrates how flexibility and cooperation may result in improved relations with patients and increased acceptance of Western medicine.

Traditional Navajos believe health results from a balance of natural and supernatural forces. Illness is commonly viewed as an imbalance arising from disharmony within an individual, or between an individual and their surrounding environment. The patient may view health and illness holistically, and view people, community, nature, and spirituality as interconnected and interrelated. This perspective views physical, spiritual, mental, and emotional health in unity, instead of in discrete categories. (17) A ceremony is performed by a traditional healer to restore the person back to harmony. Navajos often combine traditional healing with the use of modern medicine. These ceremonies actively employ efforts to achieve mind states that reduce stress and anxiety (which are considered minds "out of balance"); efforts to influence mind states are believed to facilitate healing, and are examples of early uses of mind-body medicine (psychoneuroimmunology).

Similar concepts of the spiritual nature of disease and its effect on treatment and recovery are held by other Native American groups. In addition to spiritually oriented ceremonies for healing, herbal and other traditional medicines are often used. Attempts to combine such treatment with modern therapy, if possible, are far more advantageous than confrontation and criticism.

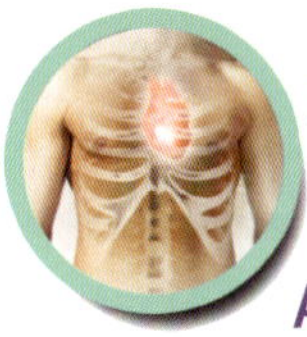

SPECIFIC PATTERNS AND STYLES OF VERBAL COMMUNICATION

Asians

In some Asian cultures, there may be a tendency to answer yes to most questions asked by a practitioner, in an effort to please the questioner and not insult him by implying that he was not understood. Practitioners may believe the patient is agreeing with them, or understands them, when in fact they do not. There may also be a tendency to deny most symptoms during the review of systems. The patients may want to deal only with the symptoms they offered. They may not wish to offer other symptoms, partly out of the belief that these other symptoms may not be related and possibly out of fear that they will be deported if found to be too ill. (14) Some Chinese families will shield patients from "bad medical news," believing that telling the patient will only make their condition worse.(18)

This preference may represent an ethical dilemma for health care providers, unless the patient elects to render decision-making to family members.(19)

Middle Eastern

Americans may consider many Muslims to be conservative by American standards, and some behaviors are assigned by gender. While men and women have specific roles, modesty is very important for both men and women in the Islamic faith. Women may wear a headscarf (hijab) as a fulfillment of Islamic beliefs, not a cultural practice. The form and extent of the hijab can also vary due to cultural differences, as noted when comparing the Arabic hijab to the more extensive ones worn in Afghanistan. Muslim women may not expose their bodies (other than just described) to unrelated individuals, regardless of gender. However, some exposure is acceptable for medically necessary reasons. Men must also maintain modesty by not exposing the area between their nipples and knees to unrelated males or females.

Muslim women make the decision to wear a hijab after puberty. The decision to wear a hijab can even vary within families. With these modesty requirements in mind, it is of crucial importance to maintain these modesty boundaries within the health care setting. Care must be taken to limit the exposure of the body to essential personnel. It is also best when dealing with a Muslim patient to strive to provide a physician of the same gender whenever possible.

Men and women may decide not to shake hands with those of an opposite gender as a religious decision. Therefore, when a health care provider approaches a patient of the opposite gender, great care must be given to extending the hand for a handshake since this could result in an awkward situation for both parties. In addition, direct eye contact between males and females is avoided by Muslims.

Premarital sexual relations, homosexual relations, and drug or alcohol use are forbidden to believers of the Muslim faith. However, this does not mean that the provider should assume these behaviors do not exist.

Cultural beliefs may also provide barriers to clear communication. For example, mental illness may be considered shameful or patients may be reluctant to disclose a sexual or drug history in the presence of family members. Such questions would challenge the honor of the entire family. Disclosure of hereditary disease or chronic disease has the possibility of bringing shame to the entire family. As a result of the importance of these cultural and religious beliefs, reassurance of confidentiality is critical to the Middle Eastern or Muslim patient. This same issue is common within many Asian and Latino cultures.

For Middle Eastern patients, physicians should initially address the entire family, not just the patient, as the family needs to establish whether they trust the physician enough to follow his or her medical advice. The patient does not make this decision in isolation.

There is a strong obligation to take care of those in different stages of the aging process. The families generally do not place elderly relatives in a nursing home.

Another very strong Middle Eastern cultural aspect that must be considered is the practice of the family to **NOT** tell the patient the correct diagnosis. This is especially true with the case of cancer. The family may want to be told first so that they can decide if they want the patient to know the true diagnosis. As with some Asian patients, this preference may result in an ethical dilemma for physicians who are trained to consider the patient as the primary decision maker for their own care. These concerns have not been fully resolved in the American health care systems, but it is best to try to obtain a balance between patient autonomy and the cultural beliefs of the family.(19)

Navajo

Navajos believe that words have great power and meaning, and that it is possible to "speak something into existence." They therefore believe that one should only speak about the future in a positive way. A casual description of potential adverse outcomes as part of informed consent or advance directives by a provider could be interpreted to mean that the provider wishes them harm, or worse. Effective providers have learned to describe the risks of procedures in an abstract way, or in reference to a third party. A health provider might say, for example: "If a person who had an illness such as yours were to have this procedure, some of the risks that could occur for them may include the following..."(20)

NONVERBAL COMMUNICATION

Variations in nonverbal communication styles may be even more difficult to discover and understand than language barriers and differences in health belief systems. There is a great tendency towards ethnocentrism in nonverbal communication. (21) Most people assume that other groups share the same stylized gestures and meaningful movements, actions which may be so ingrained as to be thought of as automatic. (21) Such assumptions persist even if a new language is learned and may include the use of body space, response to physical touch, and the use of eye contact and facial expressions. (1,21)

In health care interactions, it is important to learn the rules of protocol governing nonverbal communication for the patient's culture.

Latino

> An Anglo pediatrician in a hospital clinic was examining a Latino infant during a follow-up visit. The physician looked at the infant as he informed the family of how well the baby was doing and the importance of further visits for checkups and immunizations. Though everything had gone well on this and previous visits, the family became upset. The infant's mother wrapped the baby tighter in his blanket, at first holding him more tightly against herself, then approaching the physician, indicating that she wanted him to touch the child. The physician, feeling his personal space invaded, backed away and soon ended the visit. The family later confided to the Latino medical student who had been called upon to act as an interpreter that they were worried that the doctor was trying to inflict the infant with "mal ojo" (evil eye). The doctor's staring at the child and his reluctance to break the mal ojo by touching the child made them all the more worried. They also felt slightly insulted because they had seen the same physician several times on prior visits and thought they had a good relationship with him. But in their view, he continued to act very coldly, never closely approaching or touching either of the parents.

The above example illustrates differences both in beliefs about disease causation and in the styles of interpersonal communication between an Anglo physician and Latino patients. While there are differences among Latinos from various parts of Latin America, several deeply rooted beliefs about health are common to all. (3-7)

Mal ojo is a belief that disease results from an abnormally forceful, excessive, or covetous stare. This may be inadvertent or maliciously intentional. It mainly affects children, whose resistance is lower, and results in sudden onset of fever, headache, and crying. It can be undone by the touch of the person who caused it, as such physical touch breaks the unnatural bond. The failure of the physician in the anecdote to touch the child after staring at him aroused the suspicion of the parents that he was purposefully attempting to afflict him with mal ojo. (4,8)

Eye contact and the use of direct gaze have deeply ingrained implications and meaning in all societies. In Western society, direct gaze is considered normal for feedback and is used to open communication channels.(10) However, this is not true in many other cultures. Many Native Americans avoid eye contact as a sign of respect to a stranger, a behavior which an observer from another culture might easily misunderstand as withdrawal or avoidance. Likewise, in Latino culture, a stare that is too direct is felt to lead to disease through mal ojo. Asians also avoid direct eye contact as a sign of respect as well as recognizing authority.

Facial expression in general may also be misinterpreted across cultural boundaries. The tendency exists for Western physicians to think that Latinos show too much emotion, and that Asians and Native Americans show too little and are "inscrutable." (21) Care must therefore be taken to avoid rushing to stereotypical conclusions about the thought process underlying the facial expression.

Gestures used during the interview and the attitude toward physical exam are especially critical. Among Southeast Asians, for example, the head is considered sacred and special care should be taken during touching of the head during the exam. Contrarily, the feet are given less respect and it is considered impolite to point to the feet of another person. (14, 15).

Most ethnic groups have a particular sensitivity about examinations of the breasts and the genitals. These types of examinations should be done with the utmost of care. The visible presence of an interpreter of the opposite sex should be avoided. If the exam is not absolutely necessary for the complaint offered, it might best be delayed until subsequent visits after allowing time for better rapport to develop. (14) In case something must be done at the first visit, in any culture it is best to have a person of the same gender as the patient.

In modern Western culture, close distance between individuals' bodies is used only for intimate contact. This is not true in all cultures. Among Arabs, such close distances are used in casual conversation. A Western physician who has a patient approach too closely would tend to feel that his or her body space has been invaded and might feel offended or threatened.(1, 19) Navajos will typically not closely approach those who they do not know well.

Likewise, physical touch is forbidden in most casual Western interactions, except for the formalized handshake. This is not true in Latino cultures, where the light touch of a hand on another's arm is a gesture of warmth and consideration. Such patient-initiated contact might be off-putting to a Western physician. As the opening anecdote illustrated, Latino patients might feel that a Western physician who did not initiate such contacts was cold and uncaring. (1) Traditional Navajos, on the other hand, typically do not touch in public, or readily show outward physical signs of affection.

PHYSICAL SIGNS OF TREATMENT

Khmer (Cambodia)/Laotian

A recently immigrated family of Khmer (Cambodian) refugees brought their child to the emergency room for a prolonged febrile illness. The physician examining the patient found numerous ecchymoses on her body. She grew suspicious of the possibility of child abuse and went through the usual channels, including informing the police. After much misunderstanding between herself and the family, the physician later learned that the ecchymoses were the result of "coining," a traditional healing practice.

Among the Khmer and Laotian people, disease is felt to be due to imbalances of natural forces. Balance is restored by use of herbal remedies and a variety of dermabrasive procedures, such as rubbing the skin with a heated coin or by cup suction or pinching. Ecchymoses frequently result. As noted above, the presence of these in children has been mistaken for child abuse by some Western physicians. (14, 15) It is acceptable to ask the parents if this has been done and to let them know of the provider's knowledge. This may alleviate some fear and act as an icebreaker for the visit.

Navajo

Ceremonies of the Navajo usually involve corn pollen, and the placement of corn pollen, and other markings on various parts of the body.

REMOVAL OF BLOOD AND ORGANS

Southeast Asians

Southeast Asians frequently fear the medical practices of blood letting and surgery. Patients feel that loss of blood by venipuncture will lead to further illness. Such fears can be allayed by explaining that the blood will regenerate, specifying why the tests are needed, and forewarning when the blood will be drawn. (14, 22)

Traditional Navajo

Traditional Navajo patients may object to giving blood for diagnostic purposes and, if they agree to have surgery, will usually ask for the return of any organ that is removed. Navajos believe that body tissues or organs removed from the body retain part of the 'life force' of the person who possesses them. Body tissues may be used against that person when they are possessed by others, and could potentially harm them. (This also mirrors a medical ethics issue, as many in research fields seek Native American genetic information, and the Navajo tribe's Institutional Review Board (IRB) has rejected such requests, both on a cultural basis and from concerns regarding abnormal genetic manipulation, such as the insertion of animal DNA into plants and vice versa, which is viewed as a violation of the harmony of nature.) Therefore, when at all possible, tissues and organs should be returned to the patient after review by a pathologist. This accommodation is now fairly routine in hospitals that serve large numbers of Navajo patients. (Navajos also will wish to be buried with all their body parts, to return "whole" to their creator.)

VIEWS OF SURGERY

Southeast Asian

Surgery is especially feared, as cutting the flesh may disrupt the body's harmony, particularly if a part of the body is removed. The Hmong share the Khmer (Cambodian) concerns about surgery and blood drawing. They also do not approve of autopsies of their loved ones. They believe loss of vital organs will prevent the soul from being reincarnated and the spirit will wander about with the potential to inflict illness and misfortune upon the family. (9, 22)

There is no tradition or history of surgery in Chinese medicine, so surgery is frequently feared and avoided by Chinese patients, who feel it to be a violation of the body. Followers of Confucianism believe that the whole body must be returned at death to ensure a proper afterlife. Therefore, individuals may refuse surgery or other invasive procedures due to a concern that their body may not be whole at the time of death.(23) If such therapy is suggested to Chinese patients, it should be presented carefully and in great detail, with an explanation that nonoperative alternatives have been fully exhausted.

Navajo

Surgery is sometimes interpreted as a violation of the harmony of the body by traditional Native people. Additionally, the more technology that is used in treating patients, the more "foreign" it will feel, and the lack of familiarity combined with the invasiveness (cutting into the body) of surgery may lead to a rejection of surgery, unless the patient is extremely ill or all other means of treatment have been tried. Adding to the problem is a lack of trust of American institutions, based on a history of abuses such as broken treaties and forced relocations. However, a great many Native Americans do undergo surgery on a regular basis at Indian Health Service hospitals, and many reported that they are referred there by medicine men, particularly as a treatment for cholecystitis.

THE ROLE OF FAMILY MEMBERS

Frequently, decisions to undergo surgery in Southeast Asian patients are only agreed upon after the entire extended family has met and discussed it. This may be difficult for the physician, who must repeat explanations multiple times as more senior family members arrive and are called upon for their opinions. (14, 22) The same is true for Navajo and many Native American tribes. Muslim Arab familes are often also very involved with medical decision making for families. In such cases, it may be best to wait until immediate family members have arrived before planning meetings with family members.

DEATH AND DYING

Every culture has different beliefs about rituals and attitudes toward death. At the time of death, a Muslim is surrounded by close family members who encourage the patient to recite the Muslim confession of faith "shahada." The family washes and prepares the body and then turns it facing Mecca. The concept of modesty described above applies even when death occurs. There are religious leaders, or imams, who are called upon for all types of rituals, especially those related to washing the dead, burial, praying for the salvation of the deceased, illness, marriage, etc. The local imam will often visit the sick. During visitation, reading from the Koran is common.

Navajo

Traditional Navajo views on death include fear and avoidance, a reaction common to many cultures. The most common belief is in a multi-component spirit, with one aspect lingering near the body even after death—the good essence departs for the next world, while that which is not good, or negative, remains, and can harm the living. (24) Many Navajos no longer hold this belief, but awareness of this cultural interpretation of death may be helpful when caring for traditional Navajos.

GENERAL APPROACH TO INTERCULTURAL COMMUNICATION

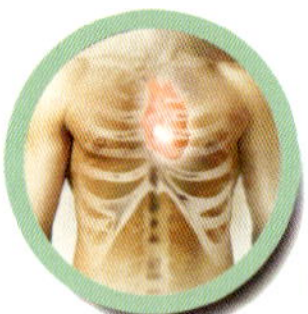

When patients from other cultures present for treatment, many of their feelings and thoughts are common to all and cut across cultural barriers. They are in pain or other discomfort and fear loss of either a body function, their life or the life of a loved one. However, when approaching patients from another culture, it is essential to realize the differences between their beliefs and those of a Western physician.

Physicians can begin by inquiring, in a nonjudgmental way, into the patient's health belief systems. An easy way to begin is to ask for the patient's perception of the disease. For example, when approaching administration of medication to traditional Latino patients, it is useful to say, "Some people believe that a food or medicine is hot or cold. Do you think so?" Many patients will have been to traditional healers in their communities. The physician should ask about any such visits, what the patients have been told and what has been recommended. The physician should try to work *with* such beliefs and practices without criticizing or belittling them. (1,11,14) This begins with informing the patient up front that the provider is open to including (if the patient wishes) the patient's traditional healing practices, so it doesn't conflict with the planned treatment, thereby allowing the patient to get better as fast as possible. Contrast the examples of the successful treatment of the Navajo child by both antibiotics and a temporary discharge for a ceremony with the Haitian patient with typhoid, whose family's belief systems were criticized or denied by the health care providers. Traditional beliefs and practices do not have to be impediments, but can be accommodated and used to benefit. (2) Acceptance of modern health care will be best accomplished when offered with respect for traditional ways. (3)

An understanding of the patient's social organization is also helpful. Most traditional societies place great emphasis on and have great respect for the opinions of elders. As alluded to in the section on Latino beliefs, asking what the grandparents or other elder members of a community have told a patient will both provide useful information and demonstrate respect. (1)

Patients frequently rely on traditional healers to explain why someone became sick and a frequent cause of dissatisfaction with modern Western physicians is that they do not provide enough explanation. (10) Such explanations may be difficult when the patient does not understand modern science and the physician does not understand the belief system of the patient. However, patients usually respond favorably to attempts at explanation of their disease and its treatment, especially if these can be geared to their level of education.

Listening to patients' stories is generally more helpful than direct questioning. Frequently, clues on areas important to the patient will surface. The physician needs to be patient and come back to seemingly unrelated issues that may have been overlooked. (1,25) The pitfalls of direct questioning during the review of systems, though necessary in many cases, should be born in mind. As noted earlier, Southeast Asians tend to deny many symptoms in such direct questioning, whereas others, such as some Haitians, may tend to answer positively to questions, hoping that more and stronger medicine will be given to them.

Beware of frequent "yes, yes" answers. Among Southeast Asians, this is a way of showing respect and represents a desire to please the questioner, rather than indicating true understanding or agreement. To overcome this, it is useful to ask patients to repeat what they have understood about their disease and the recommended treatment. It is important to remember to speak to the patient, not the translator. The translator should be in the background.

When giving lengthy explanations, break them up into short segments, especially when a translator is used, and try to assure that the patient has understood each point before moving on. Use repetition for emphasis. The physician should invite and induce discussion by the patient of alternatives for therapy.

There are interpreter services available by telephone 24 hours a day through a toll free number and access code for almost any language or dialect. An Internet search of telephone interpreter services will yield many options. Additionally, many hospitals and clinics contract with interpreter services, which may be available by telephone or in person; it is best to check with your facility to see if such services are available. The translator can participate through the use of a speaker telephone in the examination room. Although this doesn't allow for assessment of nonverbal behaviors, it is extremely helpful when no one is available to help with translation.

Interviewing Guidelines

- Recognize that the situation is bilingual and bicultural.
- Whenever possible, use professional interpreters. Do not use family members.
- Arrange a circular seating or standing environment so that the interpreter, physician, and patient can maintain equal eye contact throughout the encounter.
- Ask patients what they believe the problem is. This will give you an understanding of the patients' perspective of their illness.
- Ask patients why they believe they may have this problem.
- Watch and listen to how the patient responds to questions.
- Speak in short sentences or sentence fragments rather than in long, unbroken paragraphs. Be sure patients understand what you are telling them, and do not use "medicalese."
- Beware of patient's frequent use of "yes."

CONCLUSION

Patients from any culture present with feelings and thoughts that cut across all cultural boundaries. Pain or other discomfort and fear of loss of body function, life or the life of a loved one are terrors that transcend all boundaries.

Patients from different cultures approach disease with different explanatory models than the modern Western physician. (12, 13) They have different beliefs on disease causation and different perceptions as to how health should be restored. The physician who understands these beliefs will be better equipped to deal with the differences. It is important to realize that patient and family behavior that may seem illogical to the physician actually reflects not lack of understanding, but a reaction to what the patient and family may perceive as illogical or even dangerous. (3,26) Additionally, research in the field of the mind's influence on the body (psychoneuroimmunology) has repeatedly shown that a patient's state of mind has great influence on both the development of physical illness and on the ability of the body's physiology to heal from illness. Many practices and beliefs also act to provide support to patients, and reduce anxiety and stress, which in turn may promote healing from within. (27) Therefore, when working in an area with one or more predominant cultural groups, it is best to try to learn as much about their ideas of health and disease causation as possible, in order to allow the patient to, ideally, benefit from both their traditional beliefs and allopathic medical practices.

Finally, a caring, sincere manner is one factor which is always regarded as positive, especially across cultural boundaries where the physician does not understand the basic health concepts or customs of a patient. Fears of pain, illness and disability are common to all people, regardless of culture, and the realization that the health care provider is genuinely concerned with the patient's well-being can greatly improve the communication process. It may even be able to positively influence the healing process, both by relieving stress and anxiety and by providing a foundation for health care that is trusted and accepted by the patient.

REFERENCES

1. Kreps GL, Thornton BC. Health communication. New York: Longman; 1984.
2. Harwood A. The hot-cold theory of disease: Implications for treatment of Puerto Rican patients. JAMA. 1971; 216:1153-58.
3. Lynch L, ed. The crosscultural approach to health behavior. New Jersey: Fairleigh Dickinson University Press; 1969.
4. Rubel AJ. Concepts of disease in MexicanAmerican culture. Am Anthropol. 1960; 62:795-814.
5. Solien de Gonzalez NL. Beliefs and practices concerning medicine and nutrition among lowerclass urban Guatemalans. Am J Public Health. 1964; 54:1726-1734.
6. Simmons OG. Popular and modern medicine in Mestizo communities of coastal Peru and Chile. J Am Folk. 1955; 68:57-71.
7. Martinez RA, ed. Hispanic Culture and Health Care. Saint Louis: Mosby; 1978.
8. Quesada GM, Heller PL. Sociocultural barriers to medical care among Mexican Americans in Texas: A summary report of research conducted by the Southwest Medical Sociology Ad Hoc Committee. Med Care. 1977; 4(suppl 5):93-101.
9. Thao X. Southeast Asian Refugees of Rhode Island: The Hmong Perception of Illness. RI Med J. 1984; 67:323-330.
10. Fadiman, A. The Spirit Catches You and You Fall Down. New York: Farrar, Straus and Giroux; 1997.
11. Scott CS, MA. Health and healing practices among five ethnic groups in Miami, Florida. Public Health Reports. 1974; 89(6):525-532.
12. Kleinman A, Kunstadter P, Alexander E, Gale J. Medicine in Chinese cultures. Washington (DC): US Department of Health, Education, and Welfare; 1975.
13. Kleinman A, Eisenberg L, Good B. Culture, illness and care: clinical lessons from anthropologic and crosscultural research. Ann Intern Med. 1978; 88:251-258.
14. Hoang GN, Erickson RV. Guidelines for providing medical care to Southeast Asian refugees. JAMA. 1982; 248(6):710-714.
15. Muecke MA. In search of healers: Southeast Asian refugees in the American health care system. West J Med. 1983; 139(6):835-840.
16. Adair J, Deuschle K, McDermott W. Patterns of health and disease among the Navahos. Ann Am Acad Pol Soc Sci. 1957; 80-94: 311.
17. Culture Clues. Communicating with your American Indian/Alaska Native patient. University of Washington Medical Center. http://depts.washington.edu/pfes/pdf/AmericanIndianCultureClue4_07.pdf. Accessed 9/5/07.
18. Culture Clues. Communicating with your Chinese patient. University of Washington Medical Center. http://depts.washington.edu/pfes/pdf/ChineseCultureClue4_07.pdf. Accessed 9/5/07.
19. Aslam F, Aftab O, Janjua NZ. Medical decision making: The family-doctor-patient triad. PLoS Med. 2005; 2(6): e129.

20. Carrese JA, Rhodes L. Bridging cultural differences in medical practice: The case of discussing negative information with Navajo patients. J Gen Intern Med. 2000; 15(2):92-96.
21. Knapp, ML. Nonverbal Communication in Human Interaction. New York: Holt, Rinehart and Winston, Inc.; 1972.
22. Finck J. Southeast Asian refugees of Rhode Island: crosscultural issues in medical care. RI Med J. 1984; 67:319-330.
23. O'Hara E, Shan L. Cultural and pharmacologic considerations when caring for Chinese elders. J Gerontol Nurs. 1994; 20(10):11-16.
24. Perry RJ. Matrillineal descent in a hunting context: the Athapaskan case. Ethnology. 1989; (28):33-51.
25. Eisenberg AM, Smith RR. Nonverbal communication. Indianapolis: BobbsMerrill; 1971.
26. Putsch RW, III. Crosscultural communication: the special case of interpreters in health care. JAMA. 1985; 254(23):3344-3348.
27. Glaser R. Stress-associated immune dysregulation and its importance for human health: A personal history of psychoneuroimmonology. Brain Behav Immun. 2005; (1):3-11.

Action Points

1. Hospitals and clinics should actively translate at least the patient Bill of Rights in their practice and provide a copy to the patient.
2. Provide disease specific information in a culturally appropriate and linguistically sensitive manner.
3. Conduct regular cultural competency training in the workplace.

Oral Presentations: Polishing Your Style

Pamela A. Rowland, PhD; Ajit K. Sachdeva, MD, FRCSC, FACS;
James M. McGreevy, MD, FACS; Tyler Otten, BS

"Welcome, ah, to this week's, um, Mortality and Morbidity (M&M) Conference," said the resident at the podium. "This, ah, this is the case of a, um, 23-year-old, you know, ah, an African-American female who presents with mid-abdominal—yes, Doctor Olds?"

"Does her race contribute to your ability to make a diagnosis?"

"Well, ah, sir, I'm not, ah, sure it does. It's just, you know, a fact of the case."

"Then leave it out."

The resident eyes an older surgeon in the front row. His chairman peers at the M&M sheets without looking up. OK, he's on his own. "This woman's pain was, um, mid-abdomen at first and then, ah, it radiated, ah, to her right lower quadrant, and, you know, it became pretty steady and, ah, intensified. Her, ah, past medical history is um, non-contributory. Last menstrual period was ah, ah, it, um, was two weeks ago."

Dr. Olds: "You believe her? Did you do a pregnancy test?"

Resident: "Sir, I'll, you know, cover the labs in, ah, a moment."

He is silent and flips through several PowerPoint slides and stops at a list of labs, including a negative urine beta subunit hCG. "Ah, you know, um, the, ah, ah, white count was 18, 400 with a, um, shift," said the resident while focusing on his notes. "This, ah, supported our feeling, supported, you know, that she had acute appendicitis—"

Every aspect of the surgeon's work–patient care, interprofessional relationships, academic activities, and community education–requires the use of effective communication skills. Nearly everyone has seen a respected colleague fail to convey a vital message as a result of poor preparation or ineffective delivery. Good communication does not occur by chance. It is the end result of thoughtful planning, effective nonverbal and verbal behavior, learning through feedback and continuous practice, followed by more feedback and practice. Since the new millennium, surgeons are constantly reminded that having "good hands" is no longer an acceptable excuse for poor communication skills. The evidence clearly supports that poor presentation skills can be linked to error. The purpose of this chapter is to highlight some of the formal types of presentations surgeons encounter in training and throughout their careers and specific behaviors that can enhance these skills.

MORTALITY AND MORBIDITY CONFERENCE

The M&M Conference is a universally-recognized and time-proven educational concept that endures in spite of colossal changes in surgical practice. This conference follows a traditional format in almost all hospitals. The responsible surgeon must describe his or her patient's adverse event to a peer group. The primary purpose of this conference is education. A careful and honest analysis of adverse events by a group of experienced surgeons can be a powerful motivator for improved personal and group performance. The communication techniques used by the responsible surgeon are the most important factor in the success of this conference. Poor communication by the presenting surgeon leads to obfuscation of the root cause of the adverse event. When this happens, learning stops and the adverse event repeats indefinitely within the hospital's surgical culture. An examination of communication techniques in the aviation world can enhance communication skills for the surgeon charged with debriefing the adverse event as well as for the peer group of surgeons charged with evaluating the event. Instructor pilots (IPs) in the military use established tools in the debrief portion of military training missions. IPs perform the equivalent of an M&M after each training mission by carefully debriefing the learner. That debrief follows a format proven over decades of aviation training to improve performance: 1) reconstruct the plan, 2) reconstruct the events, 3) find the root cause of negative events, 4) generate lessons learned, 5) create a plan for the future to avoid the root cause, 6) learn and 7) press on!

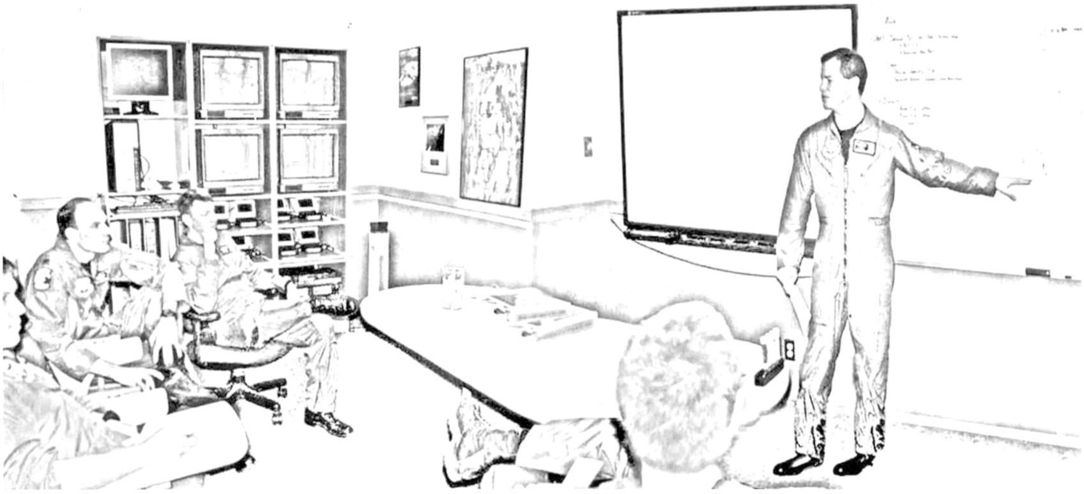

General Characteristics Of Aviation Communication

When aviators talk on the radio during flight, in the briefing room before the flight or in the bar after the flight, the language is easily recognized as pilot language. The general characteristics that are the fingerprint of this form of communication are brevity, use of terms that have a widely accepted definition, seeking loop closure (affirmation that the message was received and processed) and humor when appropriate.

In parallel, master surgeons use surgery language when presenting complex cases to their peers, with a few declarative sentences rather than several paragraphs filled with incomplete sentences, the passive voice and unnecessary information. The presenting surgeon should give an outline of the material facts only, allowing details to emerge as needed during the discussion. Brevity is perhaps the most important beginning to a successful M&M presentation which should take only 2 to 5 minutes. Brevity calls for an outline of events; the subsequent discussion can call for needed details. Excessive details hide the major point of the discussion, the search for root cause of error. Prolonged presentations distract listeners whose minds wander under the burden of a minute by minute account of a bad event. M&M communication depends upon a crisp and focused opening presentation. When an aviation briefing evolves into a lengthy event, someone usually calls out from the back of the room, "Faster and funnier!"

Master surgeons avoid local jargon. They use terms that have an established meaning accepted by the majority of surgeons in the audience. The word "peritonitis" creates a specific impression in the mind of surgeons. Saying "peritoneal signs" rather than "abdominal tenderness" presents a more detailed image for the audience. The Federal Aviation Administration publishes a list of terms and their accepted meanings to improve aviation communication. If the presenter uses a term that may not have a standard meaning, the term should be defined. Pilots often include word meanings in their briefings. Their lives depend upon a clear understanding of the mission commander's intent.

> Several years ago, a pilot was lost because the flight of four fighter jets was not flying the tactical formation briefed by the flight lead. When the jets turned to engage the enemy, a mid-air collision occurred because one of the jets was out of position.

As a result of that accident, the exact meaning of each formation was briefed before every training mission. A similar attention to detailed word meanings will facilitate communication at M&M conferences.

In aviation, communication has not occurred until the information is repeated by the listener. Certain critical pieces of information must be repeated by the pilot on the radio by regulation. Those are: altitudes, radio frequency changes and transponder codes (an assigned radio signal transmitted by an aircraft for purposes of radar identification). In a complex M&M presentation, the presenting surgeon can save time by asking for loop closure. If the audience is drifting or not following the case, the presenting surgeon should ask, "Does this make sense?" or "Do you understand what I did?" Beyond asking about understanding, the presenter may have someone "reconstruct" what was said. A listener may think they understand, but in reality may not. In the interest of time, this technique must be reserved for the critical items that must be understood to get a proper understanding of the event under discussion. Another method of loop closure is asking another surgeon if they would have ordered the same test, planned the same operation or used a different medication.
As a general rule, the presenter should speak no more than five minutes without hearing from the audience.

The best M&M conferences are dialogues and not monologues.

Appropriate humor can improve communication by dissolving barriers to communication. Anger, embarrassment, humiliation and fear are powerful barriers to learning. When discussants become angry or defensive, all learning stops. Master surgeons use humor to diffuse tense situations and level the field. Often this requires a well-timed remark aimed at self-deprecation: "At this point, I obviously was wishing I had chosen another approach!" Aviators and surgeons share many personality characteristics; a good sense of humor and an ability to play are common. Almost all aviation briefings are spiced with humor. Humor breaks monotony and brings everyone back if their minds have wandered. Master surgeons who have endured countless hours of poor M&M presentations must wish that, like pilots, someone in the back of the room had the permission to yell out, "Faster and funnier!"

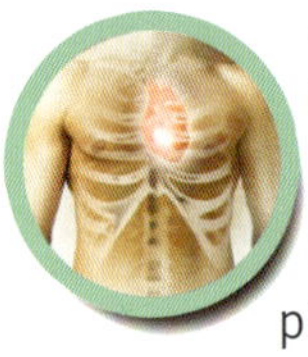

Aviation style communication can facilitate learning in the M&M conference, but more importantly, a structured debrief style discussion is potentially more powerful. Pilots in general, and fighter pilots in particular, spend a great deal of effort and time in the debrief. Since an M&M conference is a debrief, it is valuable to analyze how fighter pilots conduct a proper debrief.

Before we look closely at these phases, it is critical to observe the attitude of the participants. Fighter pilots talk of "the rank coming off" in the debrief. This phrase is indicative of an outlook that leads to honest, frank discussion and a desire to learn and improve in the future. Senior pilots do not bristle when a junior pilot questions their actions or decisions. Junior pilots are allowed to question and even disagree with the actions of senior pilots. Of course disagreements and questions must be handled respectfully, but there are no "off limits" questions or disagreements. Pilots are stereotypically the owners of significant egos. Some would claim the same is true of surgeons. Good pilots are good learners. They treat the debrief as a place to move beyond their egos and learn.

There are several distinct phases in a good debrief:

1. **Reconstruct the plan**
2. **Reconstruct the events**
3. **Find the root cause of negative events**
4. **Generate lessons learned**
5. **Create a plan for the future to avoid the root cause**
6. **Learn**
7. **Press on!**

Reconstruct the Plan

Reconstructing the plan consists of making sure that everyone understands what the plan was at the outset of the day's endeavor.

It is quickly done with a recap of the plan and a review of questions that may have arisen after the briefing or in flight that didn't get answered in the briefing. (Please take note that there is a definite structure and style to an aviation style briefing as well as a debriefing. For the purpose of this discussion we will limit our scope to the debrief's structure and style.)

There should be no questions about what the plan was before the debrief continues. If there were questions that came up in flight, they should have been answered in flight if they were substantive and could have had any effect on the outcome of the mission. There should never be unanswered questions before takeoff. Every question MUST get an answer.

In parallel, an effective M&M presentation begins with an objective, succinct summary of the case; opinion and speculation are avoided. The presenting surgeon at M&M

should quickly establish a clear understanding of his or her operative plan. The most effective way to communicate the surgical plan is in a narrative, (how the case presented and unfolded), rather than the formal History & Physical (H&P). The narrative form uses story telling which is more engaging than reading an H&P. The story follows a familiar structure:

- The problem as stated by the patient;
- The salient features of the patient's medical history;
- The physical exam findings;
- The laboratory and imaging data, and finally
- The differential diagnosis.

All this information will allow the M&M audience to critique the treatment plan, whether operative or non-operative (nota bene, non-operative is not a synonym for conservative).

Reconstruct the Events

Once the plan is clearly understood and any misunderstandings are clarified, the next task taken on by the flight lead is reconstruction of the events. This is simply "what happened." There is no discussion of why the events transpired as they did. This is critical to learning. There is no way to find root causes or generate lessons to learn without understanding what happened. The M&M scenario is simply a clear, fact-focused narrative of events and actions.

There are two general approaches to this section of the debrief. Some flight leads prefer to get all the details laid out, then identify which were positive and which were negative. Others prefer to make those distinctions as they go through the reconstruction. This section stops at identification of positive and negative outcomes. The assessment of why they happened the way they did is left to the next phase of the discussion.

The M&M presenter uses the freshly defined treatment plan as a template for an examination of the events as they actually unfolded. Once again, this requires honesty and objectivity. The presenter avoids opinion and speculation until called upon in the discussion. Aviators are brutally honest when dissecting the events comprising a failed mission. Once they agree on what happened, the learning begins.

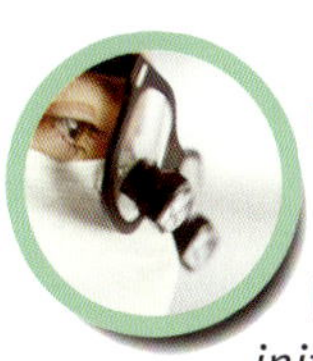

Find the Root Cause of Negative Events

An M&M conference is, by nature, a discussion of a negative event. M&M presenters should focus on the root cause for the adverse event. The root cause is the *initial* error that resulted in the cascade of events ultimately reported as a death or complication. Discovering the root causes of the negative event requires that we begin to search for the lowest level or base causes for things going poorly. Realizing that not all learning comes from negative outcomes, root causes need to be identified for some positive events as well. Therefore, it may be useful to make note of positive events and their root causes.

Root causes often take some level of effort to distill. Often, what is the apparent cause of an outcome is not always the root cause. The question that fighter pilots continue to ask is "Why?" Just as a young child can drill down to the root reason by repeatedly asking the "why" question over and over again, the aviator and the surgeon must do the same. When there is no longer another answer to the "why" question, **you** are at the root cause. Another method of getting to the bottom line cause can be borrowed from the legal community. You can find foundational causes by getting to the point where "but for" this decision or action, the outcome would have been different. The root cause is critical to generating lessons learned.

The initial error is sometimes harder to define than the proximate cause. The proximate cause is often a lesser error that accompanies the root cause or it is a lesser mistake resulting from the trail of compounding problems initiated by the root error. More experienced surgeons see root cause for error more clearly than junior surgeons because they have often committed the same errors in the past.

"Bad experiences lead to good judgment."

If the communication in the M&M is open and focused on the performance rather than the performer, the group can define the root cause for the error rather than the proximate cause, which is often the symptom of the initial problem. If the discussion focuses on the proximate cause, the complication or death will recur until the root cause is discovered and fixed. For instance, a surgeon with a high rate of leakage from bowel anastomoses might examine every aspect of stapler deployment, when the real problem is devascularization of the end segments of bowel by removing too much mesentery.

Generate Lessons Learned

Lessons learned are distilled from the discovery of root causes. By finding a way to prevent the root cause, you find yourself face–to–face with a lesson learned. Often lessons learned can be framed with the phrase "Next time I will...." The objective of the lesson learned is to increase the level of knowledge about a particular situation and what can be done to create a positive outcome when faced with a similar scenario in the future. From a broad view, it is important to note that the lessons learned are not just ways to avoid having the same negative outcome, but are vehicles that facilitate positive action to ensure a positive outcome. That may seem only a matter of perspective, but it is important to note that one perspective is narrow in focus on preventing a particular negative outcome in a particular situation while the other is broader in perspective. The broad perspective is about taking positive action to ensure positive outcomes.

Each execution error in aviation training, defined as any deviation from the plan, is turned into a lesson learned. The lesson learned identifies a future change in operations that will hopefully avoid the same error when the mission is flown again. The M&M discussion should seek a similar goal. If the discussants can focus on the performance and not the performer, the communication will address positive changes that surgeons and systems can adopt in the future. Depending upon the nature of the error, a plan for the future should be applied to individual practice, department-wide policy, or even hospital-wide best practices.

Create a Plan for the Future to Avoid the Root Cause

Plans need to be created to ensure positive outcomes in the future. This can take the form of plans or programs that need to be implemented to increase the likelihood of acceptable outcomes. In terms of plans, the debriefer must make an assessment of whether the plan was valid or not. This can be difficult to asses in some cases. If the plan was not properly executed, it is impossible to know if it was a good plan or a poor one. If it was too difficult to execute or was executed and still failed, it was probably a poor plan. Plans for the future must lend proper credence to the plans of the past and their validity.

Learn

Learning occurs as the participants dwell on the plan, events, and lessons. This can be uncomfortable for the person that has discovered that they are contributory to the root cause of a negative outcome. In an aviation debrief, pilots are asked about how they ended up being in the situation and making the decisions they did. A willingness to learn from our mistakes and "air our dirty laundry" is critical to allowing others to learn from a situation and the decision made in that situation. In the M&M conference and the aviation debrief, the desired outcome is to learn by understanding and increase the potential for success in the future.

Press On!

The future is the focus of the debrief section of the M&M conference. Both endeavors increase individual and team capability.

"It is not about who was right and who was wrong, who made mistakes and who didn't."

J McGreevy

It is about getting better at the job at hand by sharing our experiences with other surgeons.

The final phase of debrief occurs after the formal debrief. Aviators take the lessons learned and press on. The attitude about debriefing in the post debrief environment is that what "happens in the debrief stays in the debrief." That is not to say that the lessons stay there, but that any discomfort that individuals involved may have felt in the debrief stays there. The focus is on learning. Once the debrief is complete, pilots look forward to the next opportunity to excel and demonstrate their skills.

If the communication is effective, each M&M conference should create at least one plan for the future to avoid the root cause identified in the discussion. When this occurs, everyone learns!

FORMAL PRESENTATIONS

In parallel to an effective M&M presentation, an effective formal presentation is a seven-step process. However, unlike an M&M presentation, you may not know any members of the audience. Following these seven steps will increase your confidence and decrease the risk of failure in this type of presentation.

Step One is to analyze the audience. Surgeons are often requested to speak before a variety of audiences, including physicians from various disciplines, other health care professionals, hospital administrators, residents, medical students, and community groups. The presentation should be geared to the needs of the audience and planned from their perspective. A speaker can give a talk about a fascinating and provocative subject, but if it is not tailored to the needs or interests of the audience, it will have no impact. The following questions can help define the presentation content:

> **7 Steps for Preparing an Effective Presentation**
>
> 1. Analyze the audience first
> 2. Define the principle goal
>   (To inform, persuade or entertain)
> 3. Write the body of the presentation
> 4. Write the conclusion – only a summary of what has been said
> 5. Write the introduction last
> 6. Prepare the audiovisual aids
> 7. Check out the presentation environment

- How many people will be in attendance?
- What is the age and gender distribution of the group?
- What is their educational level?
- What is their current level of knowledge, skills, or attitudes relating to the subject?
- What are their beliefs or prejudices on the subject?
- What are the expectations of the group?
- What are the attitudes of the group toward the speaker?(1) And most importantly,
- What is it you want them to remember when you finish your speech?

Step Two involves defining the principle mission of the presentation. Is the goal to motivate, persuade, inform, make a request, call attention to a problem, or call for a course of action? It is very helpful to record, in 25 words or less, the exact purpose of the speech. This "purpose statement" will help focus development of the content of the speech.

What the audience remembers about your presentation two weeks later is called the residual message and should be about one sentence for a short (< 10 minute) presentation and no longer than two sentences for a long presentation (45-60 minutes). Audiences will retain approximately 4-5% of what they hear if they do not take notes. This is called the residual message. It is simply what someone remembers about the topic.

> "Jake, I got held up in the SICU, how was Grand Rounds yesterday? I wanted to hear what he had to say about gastric bypass outcomes."
>
> "Not bad – thinks we should all be doing wraps rather than just staples for closures. Improves outcomes." (Residual message)

Step Three is to write the body of the speech. This requires several substeps. Begin by writing the objectives for the presentation, clearly indicating what it is the audience should know or be able to do following the presentation. The body of the speech reinforces the residual message through a variety of examples, short stories, jokes (if appropriate), literature citings, etc.

> **EXAMPLE**
>
> **The purpose:** To persuade
>
> **The residual message:** Failure to operate within 30 minutes in hypotensive splenic injury patients will cause death.

Next, collect the relevant resource or reference materials. Then, outline the content addressing each objective.(1) This generally results in a fairly lengthy outline which must be edited. The golden rule for presentations is "less is better." The time allotted for a presentation is seldom sufficient to cover all the items on this master outline, so begin to revise the outline to cover the critical points and eliminate the less important items. Trying to fit in everything the audience might want to know usually results in a densely packed presentation, which fails to achieve its objectives and diminishes retention of information.(2)

The content for the remainder of the presentation should be properly sequenced in a step-by-step progression. One item should be linked to the next with smooth transitions. When writing out the body of the speech, the presenter should keep several speech-writing basics in mind. Oral presentations should be written in "conversational language," which means shorter sentences and simpler words than written presentations. Using first and second person pronouns like "I" and "you" will help make more of a connection with the audience. The presentation should also include some repetition (stylized redundancy) to enhance learning and retention of the material.

In structuring the content, consider if there is a need to ask the audience questions. If so, allow adequate time following each question for the audience to respond, shortening the content proportionately.

Step Four is to write the conclusion. Every presentation must close effectively to achieve a lasting impact. The conclusion should summarize, restate and highlight key concepts. It can also preview what is to follow. A "memorable statement" might be used at the end to help the audience recall the presentation in the future. Audience attention is high at the end of a presentation, so speakers use the ending to emphasize main points one more time or issue a call to action. The speech should end clearly and powerfully; it should never just fade away.

Step Five is to write the introduction. The opening is critical and should catch the attention of the audience. A speaker has only a few minutes before the audience tunes in or tunes out and should therefore utilize this precious time well. Many presentations begin with an attention-getter, which can be a quotation, a rhetorical question, a startling statistic, a story of interest, or an appropriate joke. Whichever is used, it must be relevant to the audience and the topic to be discussed. This is especially true with the use of a joke or other humorous remarks. Humor must be used judiciously and the audience's potential receptivity to humor analyzed with great care. An inappropriate joke can turn off a segment of the audience very easily, leading to the rest of the presentation falling on deaf ears. Also, a joke at the wrong time might distract the audience from the message.

After the attention step, the speaker needs to further motivate the audience. This may take several forms. The speaker might stress the importance or relevance of the topic, state why the audience should know the subject, or place the topic in the context of what they have learned or what they will learn later (previewing). Once the audience is motivated, the speaker should state clear objectives for the presentation and outline the format that the remainder of the presentation will take. The audience should know whether they can interrupt or whether they need to save questions until the end.

Since an oral presentation is written out of order from written style—body first, then conclusion and introduction—the presenter should check it in its entirety to ensure a smooth flow, making changes as necessary. Once the speech is ready to be printed in its final form, the type should be bold and legible from a distance and marks made on the manuscript to indicate pauses, interposition of slides, and other cues which will help during the presentation. Through repeated practice, the speaker should become familiar enough with the manuscript to be able to look at the audience most of the time. This is especially important for the opening set and the closure when audience attention is highest.

Step Six involves planning and preparing media aids to support the presentation. Such support can be very helpful in keeping the presenter organized, in highlighting key points for the audience, in summarizing important items, and in providing images to complement the talk. However, not every presentation needs visuals, so a speaker should carefully think through how these aids will enhance the presentation. If audiovisual support is not required for the presentation or is poorly handled, it can have a negative impact by adversely affecting communication with the audience and become a distraction.

Audiovisual Support

Audiovisual support can take a variety of forms such as computer based presentations, 35mm slides, overheads, flip charts or chalkboards, videotapes, CDs, DVDs, movies, and props.

Slides

Whether computer based or 35mm computer based presentation, slides must be carefully planned prior to the presentation. A well prepared speaker never needs to apologize for the quality of the visuals.

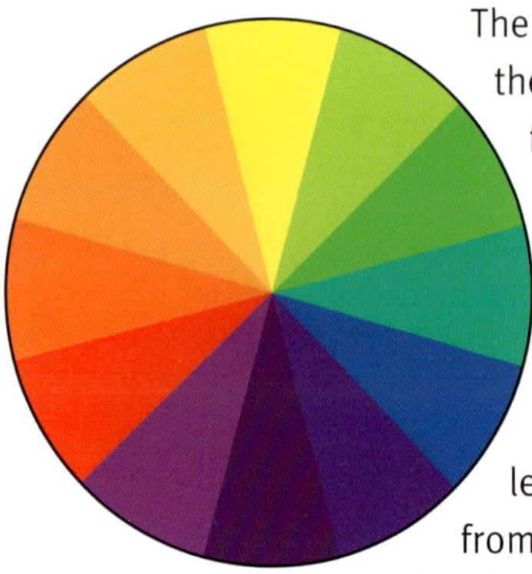

The most common slide format is the 24X36mm image on 35mm film, the standard PowerPoint presentation. They should be kept simple and uncluttered with the words legible to an entire audience with 20/40 vision. For example, Snellen letters for 20/40 vision, read from 20 feet(6.096m) are 18mm high. There is a simple trigonometry formula to determine the exact size necessary when speaking in a very large ballroom.(3) The words should be typeset or computer-generated for crisp lettering with sharp margins.(3-6) Entire typewritten pages or pages from journals and books should not be scanned, photographed or pasted onto slides. Likewise, complicated charts, tables, and graphs taken directly out of a book project poorly on the screen. Horizontal slides are preferable to vertical slides. Material on the top and bottom portions of a vertical slide tend to go off the screen when the projector lens is set for horizontal slides.

'Safe' Guidelines for PowerPoint Presentation

- Prepare your information for the person in the back corner of the room with 20/40 vision.
- Color selection: Use opposites on the color wheel for optimal visual resolution. Do not use colors that are in immediate adjacent positions on the color wheel.
- Font: Use a sans-serif upper case boldface font. Lower case or serif fonts tend to blur when seen at a distance.
- Background density: Human visual resolution is optimal with a neutral density background—neither totally black nor white. Standard diazo slides work well with their medium density background (7-9).

The use of color on slides is also very important. Slides with black lettering on a white background are not only dull, but the glare of the bright background can be distracting after a while. Computer programs for slide preparation allow an unlimited range of hue and color density for alphanumeric data, as well as the addition of graphics, banding or clustering of data, and type font variation. Standard diazo slides (white lettering on blue background) are the workhorse for slide presentations because of their medium density background. Such slides project well in rooms of various sizes and with different levels of lighting. They are soothing to view even for prolonged periods of time. However, the number of different colors on a word slide should be kept to no more than three and the use of these colors should be consistent throughout the presentation. Color selection should be based on the color wheel with the best choices residing at opposite positions on the wheel for maximum contrast. (4-6) It is important to follow these guidelines because the human eye has only limited visual resolution in darkened auditorium conditions. There are a few common sense guidelines to using slides that are all too frequently overlooked. When using slides, a speaker should show them only at the appropriate time and not leave them up longer than necessary. In order to reach out to the audience at certain times, push the letter [B] on your computer keypad to blacken your screen. The audience will then focus their attention on you. To return to your presentation when the screen is blackened, simply push the letter [B] on your computer keypad again. This is especially important for lengthy presentations in order to break up the talk and keep everyone awake and attentive.

Flip Charts

Flip charts are well suited to small groups and informal discussions. They are readily available and can be used in a dynamic fashion during the course of the discussion to jot down various ideas. Some find it helpful to use masking tape to put pages with notes around the room for the audience to refer to. There are even new flip chart pads that have a self-sticking back on each page.

Chalkboards – White Boards

Chalkboards or white boards may be used similarly but tend to distance the speaker more from the audience. Unlike flip charts, chalkboards do not generally allow progressive disclosure of previously written information.

Videotapes, DVDs or CDs

Videotapes, DVDs or CDs are especially useful for demonstrating procedures and effective behaviors, capturing the dynamic interaction between members of the health care team, including the health care provider and the patient, and even enhancing the speaker's own presentation skills during rehearsals. Videotapes are relatively easy to produce and easier to play back specific segments before large and small audiences. If you connect a VHS player to the LCD projector or run a DVD on your computer and then through the LCD player, have additional external speakers attached to your computer or the sound will not project well.

There are several disadvantages to projecting videotape or DVDs. The presenter should make sure there are enough monitors for easy viewing by the entire audience. Also, while VHS and DVD players are more readily available than other models in most teaching rooms and auditoriums, the program may need to be converted to other playback standards, especially if it is taken abroad. Videotaped or DVD segments, when digitized and inserted into PowerPoint presentations, may not be as clear as VHS videotape or CD originals.

The disadvantage of using a DVD is that although you may have cued a segment before you began your presentation, the DVD often returns to the beginning menu and your audience may be left in silence while you search for the segment again.

CAUTION: Video clips inserted into a PowerPoint presentation occasionally don't synchronize sound and visuals perfectly across different computer systems. This may be distracting to the audience.

Props

Props are helpful in demonstrating anatomy, certain types of equipment, instruments, and other objects. Frequently they can be passed around the room for closer examination, but for maximum effectiveness, their use should be limited to small groups.(8)

Multiple Formats

To increase the effectiveness of audiovisual aids, speakers sometimes alternate between formats. For example, a speaker may go from a PowerPoint to a flip chart for a while, and then come back to the PowerPoint. Or the speaker may turn off all visuals for some time to ask the audience a question. When utilized effectively, these options help keep the audience attentive.

Rehearsals

Speakers need to be very familiar with the content of their presentations. Practice will make a speaker more comfortable with the material. If the content is new and/or the session very important, such as before a prestigious national society, or the surroundings unfamiliar, a presenter may never feel totally at ease. However, a little anxiety is not always bad. If the extra energy is properly channeled, it results in greater animation which, in turn, enhances the effectiveness of the presentation.

Recording a rehearsal on audio or videotape is a very powerful way to identify strengths and weaknesses and to affect change. Practicing in front of a mirror or an experienced colleague, who can offer honest feedback, is also very helpful. Ask someone to complete a written evaluation form every time you present or practice a presentation. (See Presentation Evaluation Form.)

Step Seven empowers you to manage the presentation environment. Proper planning prior to the presentation should include checking out the physical set-up of the room where the presentation will be given. A speaker may be familiar with the room but, if not, it is very helpful to call in advance to check on the facilities available, and to clearly state any specific needs to the host.

This allows enough time to correct for something that may be missing or needs adjustment. For example, the remote microphone may need a battery, or a VHS system is in the auditorium but you brought a DVD. Perhaps the podium is huge and you need to find a platform to stand on so the audience can see you. Even if you are speaking at 8 AM and there is another event at 7 AM, arrive at 6 AM if you are not extremely familiar with the setting.

Golden Rule:
Arrive one hour before the presentation to set up. This gives you time to fix problems.

Questions to be answered during this time include:

- ➤How large is the group?
- ➤Are there objects which would obstruct the vision of some members of the audience?
- ➤Can these objects be moved or the furniture rearranged?
- ➤Is the arrangement of chairs appropriate for the session?
- ➤Is there enough space to move in front of or between the audience for appropriate interaction?
- ➤Would a U-shaped design be better than a classroom seating pattern?
- ➤Is the lectern in a good position? If not, can it be moved?
- ➤Can the lights be adjusted?
- ➤Is a laser pointer available?
- ➤Does the microphone need a new battery?

Experienced speakers arrive at the location one hour early to check these items and make any last minute changes if necessary. Except for the carpeting and wallpaper, the presenter should be able to change almost anything in the room.

Check the audiovisual equipment and try out the visuals prior to the presentation. Become familiar with the lectern and its controls. Insist on a spare bulb for the LCD projector, especially if the visuals are critical to the presentation. A duplicate marked copy of the speech will help explain the audiovisual needs clearly to the projectionist or room technician, if one is available. If you speak often, purchase your own remote control for your laptop that is wireless and inserts into your USB port. This will allow you to move around the room and not be confined to the podium.

If you are planning an interactive presentation with computer-linked keypads or audience response systems, prepare hard copy handouts in case the computer presentation doesn't function as you had expected.

Delivering an Effective Performance

A weak delivery can *destroy* the entire message. A powerful delivery is the result of effective nonverbal, verbal, and general behaviors.

Delivering an Effective Performance

1. Nonverbal behavior
   - Early eye contact
   - Animated delivery – Catch the audience's attention
   - Continued eye contact
   - Avoid distracting behaviors
2. Verbal behavior
   - Clear articulation
   - Variety and vitality
   - Effective pauses (use eye contact)
   - Avoid "aah", "uh", "ooh," "um"
3. General behavior
   - Do not lean on podium; move around
   - Do not rely excessively on notes
   - Do not turn back to audience
   - Point accurately
   - Gestures should be above the waist and away from the body

Nonverbal Behavior

The first few moments in front of an audience are critical. A speaker should make a dynamic entrance, dressed appropriately for the occasion. Walk in with confidence and poise. Establish contact with the audience for a few seconds before beginning the presentation. Eye contact with a few individuals and a smile establish an immediate relationship with the group.

Effective behavior and an animated delivery give the message impact and help highlight key points. Remember that excitement shows, and enthusiasm is infectious. Facial expressions and deliberate movements toward the audience can be extremely effective in this regard. For example, leaning forward and nodding the head displays interest and involvement. Arms and hands should be used for emphasis. Avoid standing still or keeping arms and hands restricted to one position for long periods of time.

Eye contact is one of the most effective avenues of communication. Try to make eye contact with an individual in the back of the room for a few seconds. Then move to someone in front or in the middle before going to the sides and so on. Effective eye contact can also be used to highlight a key concept. The positive impact of this powerful tool is immediately obvious from the visible response of the audience.

Avoid distracting behaviors. These include such things as excessive movement, shuffling of feet, repetitive purposeless actions (for example, twirling the cord of the remote control slide changer), and jingling of coins in the pocket. (10,12)

Verbal Behavior

Clear articulation is the hallmark of good communication. Many speakers have a tendency to drop the volume at the end of a sentence, resulting in inaudible words. Adequate projection takes practice in breathing to avoid running out of air toward the end of the sentence.

Successful speakers match the style of delivery to the message. A serious message may require a more somber tone. However, even in those situations some animation will keep the audience attentive. The tempo, or speed of delivery, should be appropriate to the message. Exceptionally fast delivery leads to incomprehensible speech. Very slow speech is the perfect sedative.

Speech must have variety and vitality, often referred to as vocal variety.(7) Monotonous speech is dull and ineffective. Changes in volume, tempo and pitch add vocal variety. Energetic speech is powerful and draws the attention of the audience to the speaker.

One of the most powerful and underutilized verbal behaviors is pausing.(8) Inclusion of purposeful and adequate pauses can be very effective. A pause of about three seconds is very appropriate between statements. Longer pauses can help a critical concept sink in or give the audience a chance to analyze something. For example, a speaker asking a complex open-ended question will need a sufficiently long pause for the audience to reason before responding. On the other hand, a speaker who asks a rhetorical question, for which no immediate response is expected, should not pause too long or someone in the audience might try to respond. A highly effective behavior is combining a dramatic pause with eye contact. This is usually reserved for special emphasis of critical items.

Avoid distracting vocal behaviors such as "aah," "uh," "ooh," and "um." These have been described as annoying auditory stimuli (AAS) or vocal segregates, and occur in presentations of even experienced speakers.(11) Reducing anxiety and replacing these sounds with pauses helps to significantly diminish the frequency of such behavior.

Accents can be very appealing to an audience, capturing their attention and thereby enhancing the effectiveness of the presentation. However, for an accent to be effective in this way, the presenter should speak loudly and make an extra effort to enunciate each word clearly. It helps to slow your rate in the beginning of the presentation to allow the audience to adapt to your accent.(10)

General Behavior

There are several common problems that can detract from the overall effectiveness of a presentation. One is to use the lectern as a crutch, staying rooted to the spot for the entire presentation. Similarly, movement may be restricted by various gadgets in and around the lectern such as a microphone around the neck, slide changer, or a light pointer. Many speakers also tend to rely excessively on notes or spend prolonged periods concentrating on a visual with their backs turned to the audience, virtually breaking off any effective contact. Remember that the lectern and any other presentation tools are there only to enhance a presentation. Whenever possible, a speaker should move away from the lectern a little to make more audience contact, placing the slide changer and pointer back on the lectern when not in use.

If the microphone is not fixed on the lectern, a speaker can move around much more and maintain better contact with the audience. While moving about, a speaker should try not to carry notes, as they become restrictive and prevent the use of hand movements for emphasis.

The laser pointer is frequently one of the biggest distractions in a presentation. Speakers often do not point accurately to a specific item on the screen and run the pointer across the screen in repetitive motions. Even worse, the pointer is at times inadvertently turned toward walls of the room or toward the unsuspecting audience. Practice is the best way to ensure the pointer is used effectively to point specifically to the desired item on the screen. The pointer should always be turned off when not in use.

All of these tips are part of creating the right environment for a receptive, responsive audience. Audience involvement, with the use of questions, feedback, and activity by the individuals, is highly recommended for successful presentations.(4) Maximize this involvement through positive reinforcement, acknowledging correct responses or good questions from the audience. Avoid reacting to wrong answers with negative nonverbal or verbal behavior.(10) Be aware of the messages the audience is sending by observing their behavior and reactions to the presentation.

When Things Go Wrong

Despite intense preparation and experience, things will occasionally go wrong, generally at the worst possible moment. There is only one way to handle this situation. Keep calm. The ability to handle these crises separates the true professional communicator from the amateur. If a slide is not advancing on the computer or the CD audio isn't working, ask the projectionist or someone who knows how to deal with the problem to help. Meanwhile, use the time to encourage the audience to ask questions or to further clarify a point that does not require the visual. If the problem can only be handled by leaving the front of the room, give the audience a task in the interim, but keep them focused on the topic. Letting the audience talk amongst themselves or taking a break will require additional time to get their attention once more. Always be prepared to give the presentation without the audiovisual support, in case this becomes necessary.

Microphones often malfunction. Banging them out of frustration only makes matters worse.

Sometimes problems cannot be corrected. To make the best of a bad situation, well prepared speakers always have a backup plan. They never show their frustration to the audience. When things are really going wrong, they know it is the perfect time for a long pause and a great smile.

Special Situations

The basic principles and techniques for effective presentations outlined in this chapter are applicable to any situation in which a surgeon is required to give a presentation. However, there are a few additional tips for some special situations.

SCIENTIFIC CONFERENCES

Scientific conferences are generally of great significance to the surgeon as a required path to achieve recognition and academic credibility. The conference itself may be very prestigious, but the audience may be difficult to identify for purposes of preparing the presentation. Some members of the audience may be unfamiliar with the surgeon's work; others may be experts in the area and may even be exceptionally critical. In addition, the time allowed for the presentation is relatively short. In most national meetings, 10 minutes are allowed for the presentation, and five minutes for the discussion. Consequently, the circumstances are unique and the stakes high. This might lead to heightened anxiety, which tends to adversely affect the presentation. Special steps will help to increase the likelihood of success.(14)

Careful preparation is critical. Begin by writing down in a few sentences what needs to be conveyed to the group. This will be based on the data available, and the results of analysis of these data. The speaker needs to be very selective about the amount of data presented. Presentation of excessive or ambiguous data, especially less relevant results, takes up precious time and usually results in a poorly delivered and rushed presentation.

The three parts of the presentation—introduction, body, and conclusion—must be carefully structured. Start with a brief introduction to the topic and personal work relating to it. Then go directly into the purpose of the research project. This opening segment should take about two minutes. The next three minutes should cover the methods used, with the following three minutes to cover results. The final two minutes are reserved for making succinctly presented conclusions.

Appropriate visual support must then be prepared. Limit your PowerPoint slides, if you use them, and make handouts especially for the occasion. Avoid the temptation to take graphs and charts directly from the data if they are too complicated. It is better to take complicated data and break them down into several simpler slides, with only portions of the data on each. During the discussion period, listen to the questions carefully. To avoid misunderstanding or misinterpretation, restate the question. Think for a few seconds, and then reply. Use simple, short answers; do not ramble on or go off on a tangent. The speaker should always remain in control and be polite, even when the questioner is in obvious disagreement or is trying to entrap the speaker.

JOURNAL CLUBS

Journal Clubs are a routine academic activity in many teaching programs. Generally, the group is small and the discussion involves a few selected articles from recent literature.

To enhance such presentations, it is critical for the leader of the discussion to have the journal articles distributed to the participants in advance. The speaker should become familiar with the articles to be discussed, writing on a separate sheet of paper the key features of the article and the items to be highlighted.

In order to enhance interaction between the participants, the group should be seated around a table, or the chairs should be placed in a U-shaped arrangement. The environment should be supportive to facilitate active participation.

Begin by briefly discussing the content of the article and adding personal comments. Use both nonverbal and verbal behaviors to make the presentation crisp, paying special attention to voice projection. In this situation, using notes or holding up the articles is acceptable. However, these materials should be set down regularly to allow for freer hand movements and regular eye contact. Finally, when asking for comments or answers to questions, encourage all the participants to look up and listen.

COMMUNITY FUNCTIONS

A community function is a situation in which the style is at least as an important a factor as content. It is important to capture and keep the attention of a diverse group which may include people who are not interested in the topic or are skeptical or have no concept of the issue to be discussed. The goal is to educate the group about the topic, not to prove how much the speaker may know.

When writing this type of presentation, plan on covering only a few key items. Use very simple sentences. Follow each medical term with a brief explanation in lay terms. Keep visuals simple, using more pictures than data. Avoid acronyms and abbreviations in the visuals, spelling out all medical words so the audience is not left guessing the correct spelling of the word or the terminology used.

Use the first few moments of the presentation to sweep audience members off their feet through effective verbal and nonverbal behavior and catchy statements. Include longer (> 3 second) pauses throughout the presentation, especially after introducing key concepts. Allow the audience to interrupt as often as necessary if they need further clarification and let everyone catch up before proceeding further. Even if no other visuals are used, it may be helpful to write down key words on a flip chart. Do not look disappointed or disgusted if a member of the audience is having a difficult time understanding a simple concept. Allow ample time at the end for questions.

After a strong closure, it is often helpful to give the audience a simple summary sheet, some literature, or an object which will serve as a reminder of the talk long after it is over.

SUMMARY

Presentation and communication skills are learned behavior. Appropriate training and repeated practice lead to polished presentations. Workshops that offer individualized attention are very helpful in improving presentation and communication skills, as well as bolstering self-confidence. Videotaping and critiquing presentations in a supportive environment and role modeling are other ways to effectively enhance such skills.(16-18)

The role of the surgeon as presenter is to convince and drive home clear messages with a lasting impact. The approach must be personalized with a clear focus on the various people that make up the audience. Addressing these individuals with appropriate verbal and nonverbal behavior is necessary to achieve the goals and objectives of an effective oral presentation.

Successful presentations are not spontaneous. They are the result of thorough preparation, sufficient practice, effective management of the environment, confident delivery incorporating positive behaviors, skill in dealing with unforeseen crises during the presentation, and the ability to adapt general communication principles to special occasions. These same communication techniques are applicable to any size group and can be tailored for addressing patients and their families as well as professionals, peers, trainees and the lay public. Surgeons, like politicians, are finding that good oral presentation skills can benefit their professional careers and reputations. With training, practice and experience, any surgeon can become a skilled communicator.

Use the Presentation Evaluation Form on page 115 to obtain feedback on crucial components of formal presentations. Speakers are encouraged to ask someone in the audience to return this form to them after a presentation so they can learn to improve their speaking behavior.

REFERENCES

1. Mitchell D, Goldsmith A, Green E, Slethaug M, Spekkens A. Preparing presentations: how to make yours a hit (Part 1). Dimensions in Health Service. 1988; 65(6):32-34.
2. Russell J, Hendricson WD, Herbert RJ. Effects of lecture information density on medical student achievement. J Med Education. 1984; 59:881-889.
3. Hammerschmidt DE. Don't crowd your slides! JAMA. 1984; 252:775-776.
4. Luria Sm, Neri DF and Jocobsen AR. The effects of set size on color matching using CRT displays. Human Factors and Ergonomic Society, Inc. 1986; 28:49-61.
5. Ward FE, Greene F and Martin W. Color discrimination as a function of saturation, field size and adaption level. Aviat Space Environ Med 1985; 56(3):251-3.
6. Neri DF, Luria SM and Kobus DA. The detection of various color combinations under different chromatic ambient illuminations. Aviat Space Environ Med. 1986; 57(6):555-60.
7. Workshop Manual, Effective Teaching: Improving your skills. The Medical College of Pennsylvania, Philadelphia; 1991.
8. Thompson WM, Mitchell RL, Halvorsen RA Jr, et al. Scientific presentations. What to do and what not to do. Invest Rad. 1987; 22(3):244-245.
9. Soderstrom RM. Effective medical communication. Current Problems in Obstetrics, Gynecology and Fertility. 1985; 8(11):32-47.
10. Smith TC. Making successful presentations. New York: John Wiley and Sons, Inc., 1984; 51-77.
11. Herbert WN. On improving the lecture. Obstet and Gyn. 1988; 72(6):937-939.
12. Paegle RD. Underutilization and misuse of audiovisual modes of communication by senior faculty. J Med Education. 1978; 53:727-733.
13. Van Liew HD. An initiation into teaching for graduate students. Am J Physiology. 1989; 257:S3-S5.
14. Irby D, DeMers J, Sher M, Matthews D. A model for the improvement of medical faculty teaching. J Med Education. 1976; 51:403-409.
15. Newble D, Cannon R. A Handbook for Medical Teachers, ed. 2. Lancaster, U.K.: MTP Press Ltd; 1987:21-29.
16. Foley R, Smilansky J, Bughman E, Sajid A. A departmental approach for improving lecture skills of medical teachers. J Med Education. 1976; 10:369-373.
17. Christensen JF, Levinson W, Colligan JL, Dunn PM, Jones SR, Morgenstern A. A one-day communication workshop for internal medicine residents. J Med Education. 1987; 62:687-690.
18. Sachdeva AK, Kelliher GJ. Use of a faculty development workshop to improve teaching skills. Innovations in Medical Education Exhibit Abstract Book. Association of American Medical Colleges; 1990:54.

SELECTED READINGS

1. Cooper GE, White MD, Lauber JK. Resource Management on the Flightdeck: Proceedings of a NASA/industry Workshop. (NASA CP-2120). Moffett Field, CA:NASA-Ames Research Center; 1980.
2. Healy GB, Barker J, Madonna G. Error Reduction Through Team Leadership: Applying Aviation's CRM Model in the OR. Bull Am Coll Surg. 2006; 91:10-15.
3. Helmreich RL, Ashleigh C and Wilhelm JA. The Evolution of Crew Resource Management Training in commercial Aviation. Int J of Aviation Psychology. 1999; 9:19-32.
5. McGreevy JM, Otten T, Poggi M, Robinson C, Castaneda D, Wade P., The Challenge of Changing Roles and Improving Surgical Care Now: Crew Resource Management Approach. Am Surgeon. 2006; 72:1082-1087.
4. Hurley D. Seven Lessons From Airline Safety: It's Not Just About the Pilot. Gen Surg News. 2006; 33:32-33.

Presentation Evaluation Form

To be completed by speaker before presentation

Purpose (circle) to inform to persuade to entertain

Residual message ______________________________

____

____

Speaker ______________________________

____

Content and Organization	**Appropriate**			**Needs Development**	
Introduction					
Get attention	1	2	3	4	5
Eye contact	1	2	3	4	5
Rate	1	2	3	4	5
Volume	1	2	3	4	5
Professional image	1	2	3	4	5
Development of Ideas					
Organization planned	1	2	3	4	5
Supporting materials clear	1	2	3	4	5
Rate	1	2	3	4	5
Volume	1	2	3	4	5
Eye Contact	1	2	3	4	5
Conclusion					
Economical	1	2	3	4	5
Volume	1	2	3	4	5
Eye contact	1	2	3	4	5
Delivery					
Language – Adapted to audience	1	2	3	4	5
Oral style (didn't read)	1	2	3	4	5
Meaningful movement (use of space)	1	2	3	4	5
Use of communicative gestures	1	2	3	4	5
Posture supports meaning (formal topic/formal posture)	1	2	3	4	5
Distinct (utterance) for this audience?	1	2	3	4	5
Adequate vocal variety (not monotone)	1	2	3	4	5
Fluency	1	2	3	4	5
Articulation	1	2	3	4	5
Overall Evaluation					
Did speaker achieve purpose?	1	2	3	4	5
Was residual message clear?	1	2	3	4	5

Next time focus more upon: ______________________________

____

____

Case Presentations: Objective and Subjective

Thomas TA Parrino, MD;
Deborah Peltier, MD

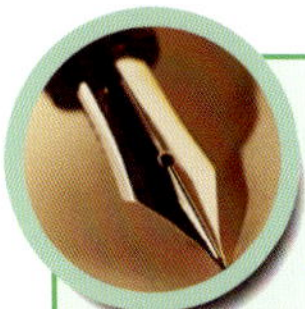

"You remember the patient in Room 202 with the fever of 105 degrees and the macular rash? Well I just did a spinal tap, and the fluid was very cloudy. I have sent the fluid to the lab for Gram stain, cell count, and chemistries, but meanwhile I want to get some antibiotics started. What should I order?"

"Let's see. This is community-acquired meningitis in a healthy young college student, right? Sounds most likely to me to be meningococcal meningitis. In this age group, Strep pneumonia and H. flu would be much less likely. These patients can die within hours of becoming symptomatic. The best thing to do right now is to start ceftriaxone and vancomycin until we see the Gram stain and get the cultures back. We can add or change antibiotics once we get the lab results, but that's the safest thing to do at the moment."

"OK, I'll call the pharmacy, write the orders and run over to the lab."

Although written records are considered the basis for assessment of the quality of clinical care, important clinical information is also exchanged in the hallways, on the telephone, and in conference rooms between two or more clinicians. The basic means for transferring verbal information is the case presentation, a structured method for organizing the critical pieces of patient data that are essential for clinical decision making.

The case presentation is an important communication tool in clinical medicine for transmitting information to expedite patient management, and to assess the clinical knowledge and skills of fellow physicians and trainees. These situations play themselves out every day in scenarios familiar to all clinicians. For example, the case presentation serves as the practical foundation for most basic patient management decisions, as in the opening scenario. It has evolved into a highly stylized form of communication. In most parts of the world, surgeons transmit clinical information in essentially the same style and in the same order to provide both a brief recapitulation of the patient's case and the therapeutic options.

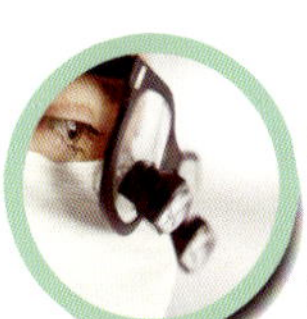

It's not what you say, but **HOW** you say it. In addition to using the case presentation for patient-management decisions, clinicians use case presentations in the evaluation of clinical performance. In this next example, the eight faculty members of the Clinical Competence Committee for an internal medicine training program are discussing the evaluation of Mary Smith, an intern just completing her rotation in the Critical Care Unit.

Dr. Wood: "Mary worked hard. She came in early, and she stayed late every day to make sure her patients were well managed. She was certainly a hard worker on this rotation. The only thing that concerns me is that she didn't seem to know her stuff. When she would present a case to me, I was never confident that she was on top of what was happening. Even though her records were impeccably kept, she never seemed to have the facts at the tip of her tongue, the way Sara Jones did. I'm not sure she's ready to be a junior resident. She certainly does try hard, though."

Dr. Bailey: "How often did you have a chance to work with Mary this month?"

Dr. Wood: "Well, let's see... We've had attending rounds three times a week for the last four weeks. That's 12 meetings so far. Mary has presented her admissions every four days, so that means she's presented about six cases to me informally, and two or three formally at rounds."

Dr. Bailey: "So you're basing most of your evaluation on these case presentations?"

Dr. Wood: "I never really thought about it but, yes, you may be right. I guess I rely on her case presentations, the reports of her junior resident, her medical records, and my own informal observations. On the basis of that, I would not put her in the top group of this year's crop of interns."

Dr. Bailey: "Of those things, what's most important?"

Dr. Wood: Clearly, I think the most important factor is my own gut instinct about what she knows. I just don't think she has it all figured out yet and it shows when she presents cases on rounds."

As both examples illustrate, the ability to make effective case presentations is crucial to transmitting critical information and demonstrating and evaluating clinical competence.

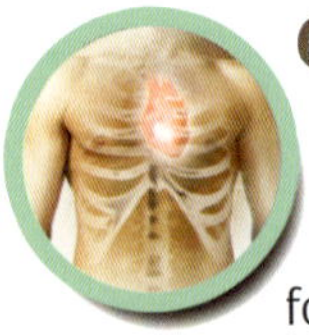

CASE PRESENTATIONS: JUST THE FACTS, PLEASE!

There are important parallels between the oral case presentation and the written medical record. Both require forethought and organization. The case presentation format is based on a set of established conventions. These conventions serve to standardize the way surgeons communicate.

There are seven basic elements to the standardized case presentation: the chief complaint, history of present illness, past medical history, review of systems, physical examination, assessment and plan.

Step One: Chief Complaint

The "headline" that directs attention to more detailed information to follow should indicate how sick the patient is.

Example:

"A 30-year-old gentleman walked into the clinic with a history of three days of mild diffuse abdominal pain."

Step Two: History Presentation Illness (HPI)

The HPI should include necessary elements for the listener to be able to draw a conclusion: location of the symptom, quality, severity, duration, timing, context, modifying factors, and associated signs and symptoms.

There are several ways to organize the presentation of the HPI.

Temporal Sequence:

"Two months ago Mr. Swanson began drinking heavily after losing his job. About three weeks ago he noticed mild abdominal pain, which gradually worsened. Two weeks ago he stopped his 8 to 12 daily beers and started taking antacids since he thought he had an ulcer. He continued to be sore in the mid and upper abdomen; his appetite has decreased. He developed mild intermittent nausea and 4 to 5 loose stools daily a week ago. He denied any vomiting until today.

During last night, about 16 hours before admission, he gradually developed constant mid-abdominal bloating pressure which started mild and increased to 6/10 by morning. He has no appetite; antacids have not helped. His pain began intensifying about three hours prior to admission and he vomited about one hour prior to admission with intense pain in mid-epigastric area."

Newspaper Style (temporal data in reverse order):

Mr. Swanson presented to the ER with intense abdominal pain and vomiting about an hour before admission.

He had been experiencing constant mid-abdominal bloating and pressure since last night. He had first noted mid-abdominal discomfort about three weeks ago with nausea and diarrhea for the past week."

Physiological Sequence:

"Mr. Swanson has been drinking heavily and eating little over the past 2 months; he has lost 20 lbs and has had 4-8 loose stools daily. In addition, he has had one day of severe unremitting upper abdominal pain, with nausea and vomiting; his wife brought him to the emergency room this morning as he is barely able to stand."

Anatomic Sequence:

"Initially Mr. Swanson's postoperative abdominal pain was mild, diffuse and hard to characterize. The day of admission the patient reported that the pain had localized to the midepigastrum and radiated to his right shoulder, and was worse with breathing."

Step Three: Past Medical History/Social History/Family History

Include current medications, allergies, and any medical or surgical information that may affect the diagnosis of the acute problem or proposed treatment.

(30-year-old Mr. Jones has presented with a suspected ruptured appendix and will need antibiotics.)

"Past medical history includes no medications and no prior serious medical problems or surgeries, but the patient has a penicillin allergy characterized by hives. He does not drink but says he has a family history of early heart attacks, as in his 35-year-old brother."

Step Four: Review of Symptoms

Include pertinent positives and negatives to strengthen the case for the diagnosis and to avoid missing important health information.

"Mr. Jones with the probable appendicitis had denied any medical problems, but on review of systems, he acknowledged easy bruising and heavy bleeding with a dental procedure three months ago."

Step Five: Physical Examination

Data from the physical exam is very important in supporting a diagnosis or in revealing a new problem.

"A 40-year-old, facing elective surgery for umbilical hernia repair, is a smoker and is chronically short of breath. Physical exam reveals pre-tibial 2+ edema and an S3 gallop which suggest heart failure and require further evaluation."

Step Six: Summary Statement

The summary statement recapitulates the most important aspects of the case, is one or two sentences, and includes NO new information.

Example:

"40-year-old smoker for elective umbilical hernia repair has new findings suggestive of CHF."

Step Seven: Decision Making: So What Are You Going to Do?

Use information from history, relevant past medical/social/family history, review of systems, physical exam and labs—in the generation of an assessment and plan.

"Mr. Swanson's history of alcohol ingestion, anorexia, weight loss, diarrhea, and his new severe abdominal pain, nausea and vomiting all suggest alcoholic pancreatitis, maybe acute on chronic. His marked elevation of lipase and amylase supports this, but his elevated wbc with marked left shift is concerning for possible infection, possibly an abscess. His IV is in, NG tube is in, and he is on his way to CT now and we will meet him there for further evaluation after the study."

LEVELS OF MEDICAL DECISION MAKING

While all elements of the patient's current condition and past history may be relevant to formulating a plan and making decisions, the presenter may choose to use shorthand to represent several elements:

> "Previously healthy 30-year-old with a negative social and family history."

Some patients will present with a focused problem that does not require complex interaction of many elements of the history:

> "This 24-year-old otherwise healthy female presents with a small caliber gun shot wound to the right hemothorax."

On the other hand, some patients require multiple laboratory and x-ray tests and repeat physical exams before the problem can be clearly identified and a treatment plan formulated. Many payers (insurance and Medicare) have recognized this by varying payment based on predetermined levels of decision making complexity. The scoring of this level is based in turn on the documentation in the record of the history and physical required to identify the patient's problem and plan an intervention. These elements will determine not only the quality of your communication during a presentation, but the reimbursement you receive once you enter practice. The history and physical must be as detailed and comprehensive as possible to identify the problem and plan the treatment.

CIRCUMSTANCES DETERMINE THE PRESENTATION TYPE

The decision about which type of presentation format to use depends mainly on the circumstances. In the Emergency Department setting, a brief summary of key information is all that is required to initiate urgent treatment. In the institutional outpatient setting, a more lengthy presentation sets the stage for a teaching exercise.

Billings and Stoeckle(1) in medicine case presentations divide case presentation formats into three basic types:

1. The "full" presentation includes all the information from the past medical history, review of systems, and physical examination. "Full" presentations can take up to 20 minutes.
2. The "brief" presentation omits noncontributory data from the past medical history, review of systems, and physical examination. "Brief" presentations should take about three minutes.
3. The "bullet" presentation presents only the most important information in one to three sentences. The "bullet" takes less than a minute.

An evaluation form designed for the outpatient setting is provided here. This can be used to score both formal and informal patient presentations and, with some modifications, can be adapted to the M&M conference presentation. Note that the term 'competent' is used here to indicate achievement of faculty skill level and not average.

OUTPATIENT COMMUNICATION SKILLS EVALUATION FORM

Student/Resident's name: ______________________ Date: __________

Preceptor's name: ______________________________

Seven Steps

	Needs work	Still developing	Average	Slightly above average	Competent	N/A
Step One **Chief Complaint (CC)**						
"The headline"						
Indicates "How sick is this patient?"						
Step Two **History Present Illness (HPI)**						
Includes relevant characteristics: location, quality, severity, duration, timing, context, modifying factors, and associated signs and symptoms						
Step Three **Past, Family and/or Social History (PFSH)**						
Includes relevant data						
Step Four **Review of Symptoms**						
Pertinent positives first, then pertinent negatives						
Step Five **Objective: Physical Exam and Labs**						
Includes general appearance, vital signs						
Includes relevant physical exam						
Relevant current tests or labs with trends						
Step Six **Summary Statement**						
Recapitulates important information						
Step Seven **Decision Making**						
Assessment						
Plan						
Overall: Use of time and organization						
Comments:						

PRESENTATION FORMAT

How does a surgeon determine which is the most appropriate presentation format for different clinical situations? Below are some general guidelines that may be helpful.

Attending Rounds

Attending rounds are a teaching exercise. For medical students and residents presenting during attending rounds, the "full" (2-3 minute) case presentation is most appropriate. The supervisor needs to hear about all of the medical issues concerning the patients under the care of the team.

Morning Work Rounds

Morning work rounds are usually conducted by the resident in charge of the service. The purpose is to acquaint all team members with the most important medical problems and plans for each patient. The patient care team must know about critical physical findings and changes in clinical status. Lengthy descriptions of unrelated medical problems would be counterproductive. Here the "brief" (3-minute) case presentation is clearly preferable.

Sign-out Rounds

During sign-out rounds, house officers usually sign-out their cases to covering staff at the end of the day. A departing resident might present eight or ten cases to the on-call team. In such cases, only the most important information should be reviewed. The "bullet" (1-minute) presentation is appropriate for such a situation.

The mandate of the 80-hour work week increased the number of sign-outs on each patient, thus increasing the possibility of medical errors. Some systems use electronic sign-outs (hand-offs), but most use face-to-face meetings in call rooms or hallway settings. Unfortunately, the electronic sign-out tempts a resident to transfer too much information rather than focus on the important bullets. Face-to-face allows the listener to ask questions and seek further explanation and for the speaker to read the nonverbal signals of the listener for understanding and confidence levels.

Due to the increase in frequency of hand-offs and the recognized potential for serious outcomes from errors occurring during this process, the Joint Commission on Accreditation of Healthcare Organizations (JCAHO) has recommended a tool for the hand-off procedure to improve communication and reduce error. The tool, SBAR, allows the provider and the receiver of information to agree on what and how information will be communicated. SBAR stands for Situation (What is going on with the patient?), Background (What is the clinical background?), Assessment (What is the current situation?) and Recommendation (What should be done?). This tool has been developed to reduce communication failure and the resulting patient harm resulting from communication errors during the physician to physician, physician to nurse and nurse to nurse hand-off. A 2003 study by JCAHO(7) that found 60 percent of 2,034 medical errors which resulted in 915 deaths had, as the root cause, a communication

60 percent of 2,034 medical errors which resulted in 915 deaths had as the root cause a communication breakdown.

breakdown, adds additional urgency to the message of using a standardized communication tool to reduce these errors. Regardless of the format of information transfer, critical elements include data on the patient's condition, expectations or plans, assessment of the patient and an agreement between the sender and receiver of the information as to the format of the information being shared. The goal of the standardized format is not only transfer of patient responsibility, but a reduction in communication error and the resulting potential for patient harm. Specific examples of presentations designed for different situations are provided in the following pages.

No matter how interesting a patient's history may be, make sure you boil things down and concentrate on what's important.

TAKE I

> "John Mahoney, is a 70-year-old retired U.S. Marine who has been experiencing increasing constipation and hematochezia for 6 to 8 weeks. His wife Mary finally prevailed on him to come to the clinic today after John spent a third straight night in the bathroom attempting to move his bowels. She became even more concerned when he reported seeing blood with the scanty amounts of stool in the toilet bowl. Embarrassed and uncomfortable about discussing this with a young medical student (and, perhaps, hoping that this whole problem will just go away), John finds an enthusiastic audience when he shares his medical history from his wartime experience in Vietnam."

It's often tempting to try to impress the team with the detailed research you have done on a complex and interesting subject, but that's not the name of the game in a busy surgical clinic. The goal is to assemble the most important facts and make sure you present them clearly, so that proper decisions can follow.

TAKE II

> "This 70-year-old man came in today with abdominal pain. He is a Vietnam veteran and had many medical problems while in Southeast Asia. He had falciparum malaria, typhoid, and dengue fever. He says his belly pain reminds him of when they treated him for typhoid. I looked up typhoid fever and, sure enough, typhoid can cause acute abdominal pain. So can malaria. I found out that falciparum malaria can be complicated by a condition known as blackwater fever, where there can be tissue infarction and organ failure, such as kidney failure, as a result. With dengue fever, the patient can have intense muscular pain that can mimic an abdominal crisis..." (The student goes on to discuss the pathophysiology of dengue fever.)

We know that normal human beings tend to lose interest in oral presentations after about three minutes. This means that we need to pretend we are journalists, writing stories for the newspaper or the evening news, presenting headlines first, key details, and then going back over the interesting sidelights only after the critical message has been delivered.

In real estate, the mantra is "location, location, location." In a case presentation, it's "prioritize, prioritize, prioritize."

TAKE III

"This 70-year-old ex-Marine was brought to the clinic against his protestations by his devoted wife. His main problem seems to be increasingly severe constipation occurring over about six weeks, with the appearance of bright red blood in the toilet bowl over the past couple of days. When I talked with the patient, he seemed uncomfortable in discussing this, and wanted to talk about his wartime medical history. I found his wife in the waiting room, and she gave me the real story. He has a very interesting past medical history, not really contributory to the present problem. I can tell you more about that later. Right now, I think the main problem may be lower intestinal obstruction, perhaps secondary to colorectal cancer."

Emergency Department

In Emergency Department Presentations brevity is most important. A new patient may have many clinical problems, but only one which requires emergency attention. The "bullet" presentation is the most appropriate format in an urgent situation.

"Doctor Franklin, I'm Alex Johnson, the new student on the Red Team."

(The student extends the right hand for a firm handshake.)

"The trauma team is just finishing up the primary and secondary survey, and Joe Simkin asked me to present this trauma case to you."

"Ok, go ahead."

"Thank you. The patient is a 22-year-old male with no known medical history who was the unrestrained, presumably intoxicated driver of an automobile involved in a witnessed, single vehicle rollover, driving at highway speed. The local EMTs arrived about 15 minutes after the accident and found him responsive and complaining of chest pain and with alcohol on his breath. They called for air rescue and when the helicopter team arrived about 20 minutes later, he had been extricated, had a collar on, and was on a backboard. His vital signs were a blood pressure of 90/60, a pulse of 120, respirations of 30, and his saturations were in the 80's. The copter crew intubated him and arrived here about 15 minutes later."

"What happened in the helicopter?"

"His saturations continued to be low. They report he had no breath sounds on the left, so they put in a Heimlich valve."

"What else could have resulted in low saturations with no breath sounds?"

"A hemothorax?"

"Yes, what else?"

"I'm not sure."

"OK, tell me more."

"After the tube was placed, his saturations improved but his blood pressure was still low, in the 90's. He was receiving his third liter of lactated Ringers, so they decided to give him O negative, un-crossmatched blood.

By the time of arrival here, his systolic was 110, his pulse in the 90's and his saturation 100% on an FIO2 of 100%."

"How many units of blood?"

"I think they said one."

"OK, what have we found here?"

"Well, right now he is sedated and intubated. He has decreased breath sounds on the left. His heart sounds are normal. His abdomen is distended and he has no bowel sounds. His extremities are cool, but he does have palpable pulses. His pelvis is stable. They just finished his chest and pelvis films and Joe is doing the FAST scan.

My preliminary assessment is that he has a left pneumothorax that needs a chest tube and that he could have hemorrhage into his abdomen, possibly a ruptured spleen. He is still in shock and he needs more intravascular volume. So, I would place a left chest tube in the 5th intercostal space, in the mid axillary line. If his FAST scan is positive for blood, I think he needs to go straight to the operating room. If the FAST scan is negative, then I would obtain a chest, abdomen, and pelvis CT scan. In the meantime, I would continue to run isotonic crystalloid and blood as quickly as possible."

HOW TO BILL FOR THESE EFFORTS?

The same data used in presentation and write ups will be critical for coding and billing. The following illustrates what is essential for different levels of reimbursement when seeing a new patient.

These efforts address the competencies of communication skills, patient care, and practicing medicine in a complex system.

*Caution: For a given ICD-9 code **all** of the requirements must be present and documented in the medical record, **not** just a single component.*

ICD Coding

ICD CODE	History Types	Examination Types	Level of Decision Making
99201	Problem focused history	Problem focused examination	Straight forward decision making
99202	Expanded problem focused history	Expanded problem focused examination	Straight forward decision making
99203	Detailed history	Detailed examination	Low complexity decision making
99204	Comprehensive history	Comprehensive examination	Moderate complexity decision making
99205	Comprehensive history	Comprehensive examination	High complexity

Billing depends on three factors: history type, examination type and level of decision making.

The History Type table below provides a definition of the different levels of documentation required for HPI, ROS, past history, family history and social history, as well as the elements of the history of present illness.

The ICD Coding table (page 126) provides definitions of each of four types of decision making that are used to define the billing codes.

WHAT DETERMINES HISTORY TYPE?

All require chief complaint +

History Type			
History of present Illness (HPI)	**Review of System (ROS)**	**Past, Family and/or Social History**	**Type of History**
Brief: 1-3 elements			Problem focused
Brief: 1-3 elements	Problem pertinent		Expanded problem focused
Extended: 4 or more elements	Extended	Pertinent	Detailed
Extended: 4 or more elements	Complete	Complete	Comprehensive

These are the elements of History of Present Illness (HPI)

- Location
- Quality
- Severity
- Duration
- Timing
- Context
- Modifying factors
- Associated signs and symptoms.

"The less time you have with patients, the more important communication becomes."

PA Rowland

Detailed definitions of the types of physical examination noted in the ICD Coding table are provided here.

Types of Physical Exam

- Problem focused — a limited examination of the affected body area or organ system.
- Expanded problem focused — a limited examination of the affected body area or organ system and other symptomatic or related organ system(s).
- Detailed — an extended examination of the affected body area(s) and other symptomatic or related organ system(s).
- Comprehensive — a general multi-system examination or complete examination of a single organ system.

Different codes are used when patients are evaluated in the inpatient setting.

For the ICD 9 code that is assigned, all of the components must be present and documented in the medical record, not just one component. The definitions of the elements are the same as noted above for the outpatient setting.

- 99221
  - A detailed or comprehensive history
  - A detailed or comprehensive examination
  - Medical decision making that is straightforward or of low complexity
- 99222
  - A comprehensive history
  - A comprehensive examination
  - Medical decision making of moderate complexity
- 99223
  - A comprehensive history
  - A comprehensive examination
  - Medical decision making of high complexity

Demonstrating Clinical Knowledge and Skill

The case presentation is a major determinant of how house officers and medical students are evaluated.

CONCLUSIONS

Presenting cases is a pivotal skill. Surgeons must convey information concisely and accurately in order to organize proper strategies for diagnosis and treatment.

Case presentations are important learning devices. Preparing full presentations emphasizes attention to clinical detail. Preparing brief presentations emphasizes clinical judgment. What is really important? What should be left out?

Case presentations are important for the demonstration of clinical knowledge and skill by students and house officers. In many situations, case presentations are the basis for evaluation of clinical knowledge. A quote from a popular handbook for medical students says:

"A good case presentation makes you look good."

The most important part of a case presentation is the preparation—the *reading, thinking, and questioning* that go into it. The result is a practical and essential tool in formulating patient-management decisions.

Finally, due to changes in graduate medical education, the use of patient hand-offs and the resulting need for patient presentations has dramatically increased. At the same time, studies of adverse patient outcomes identify communication errors as the leading cause of death and injury. These findings have led to the recommendation by JCAHO of the adoption of a standard format (SBAR) for transfer of patient information during the hand-off.

REFERENCES

1. Billings JA and Stoeckle JD. The Clinical Encounter, 2nd ed. St.Louis: Mosby; 1999; 294-303.
2. Parrino TA, Villanueva AG. The principles and practice of morning report. JAMA. 1986; 256:730-3.
3. Parrino TA. Editorial: The Social Transformation of Medical Morning Report. J Gen Intern Med. 1997; 12:322-3.
4. Parrino TA, Mitchell R. Diagnosis as a skill: A clinical perspective. Persp Bio and Med. 1989 Fall; 18-44.
5. Harrell RA, Firestein GS. The Effective Scutboy: A Survival Guide for Medical Students, 3rd Ed. Norwalk (CT): Appleton & Lange. 1988; 29-31.
6. Woods MS. How Communication Complicates the Patient Safety Movement. Patient Safety & Quality Healthcare. 2006 May/June. Available from http://www.psqh.com/mayjun06/dun.html. Accessed 10/2/07.
7. Dagmanra Scalise [researcher], Clinical Communication and Patient Safety. Citing Joint Commission on Accreditation of Healthcare Organizations, 2006; H&HN research.

Oral Examinations: A Survival Guide

Nicholas PW Coe, MD, FACS;
Pamela A. Rowland, PhD;
Kenneth W. Burchard, MD, FACS

The two seasoned surgeons stood when they heard the knock on the door of their hotel room in Chicago. One in a dark navy wool suit, tie knotted with the appropriate dimple against a crisp white shirt. The other in a conservative, 3-button charcoal suit. When the black linen pant suit opened the door, she asked, "Room Two?" She stood like a petite statute wearing a tight lavender blouse, open zippered jacket, clutching a small black purse under her right arm, obviously uncomfortable in two inch leather heels. Her hair simply parted to the side, fell to her shoulders in loopy curls, all but concealing one eye.

The examiner smiled briefly. "Doctor Carmel?" he extended his hand. "I'm Doctor Schwartz." "Doctor Schwartz?" Her hand darted out like a small bird. "Oh I.....dear. I read ....um..."

The process of becoming a medical practitioner is associated with several methods of evaluation, including formalized tests (i.e. standardized multiple choice exams) and more subjective assessment tools (i.e. ward evaluations, oral examinations). The greatest amount of time scheduled with test taking, of whatever type, is that spent in medical school. However, during residency, testing of the less formal type may be a daily, ongoing experience as the residents' problem solving skills are challenged by the faculty. Subsequent graduation from residency does not bring respite from various types of examinations, both formalized and more subjective.

All disciplines require examinations to grant board certification. The process may be different across specialties, but a board examination awaits all newly graduated residents entering practice. Even that hurdle is not the end of the road. Many boards now have or soon will announce recertification requirements. While the details may differ by specialty, the fact exists that physicians will face some form of testing throughout their professional lives.

As a method of examination, the oral examination appears to be associated with many myths, old wives tales, and preconceived ideas. Oral examinations also seem to engender more fear, dread, and aberrant behavior than other evaluation tools.

The purpose of this chapter is to outline the features unique to the oral examination as an evaluation tool as well as the variables which will influence performance ranking. In addition, a process for preparing for an oral examination is provided, as well as helpful hints for developing a valid and reliable test.

While this chapter is focused on the oral examination, the skills which foster a good performance during this test are skills that can be generalized to other verbal encounters such as bedside case presentations, lectures, discussions with family members, etc. Imagine the response of medical faculty, nurses, and other health care professionals if the examinee (Dr. Carmel) described above had shown up for morning ICU rounds looking and behaving as she did for the oral examination.

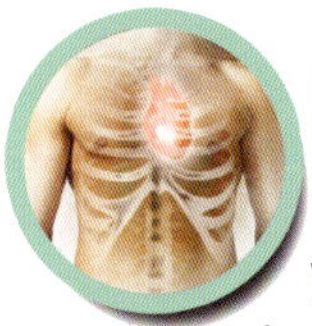

HISTORY OF ORAL EXAMINATION

Oral "examinations" have been used for thousands of years. Twenty-five hundred years ago, Socrates taught by asking questions and urging his students to examine their responses to better understand the reasoning therein. Socratic dialogue is, in effect, an extended oral examination seeking to plumb the depths of the thought processes of the discussants. Teaching reasoning by question and answer techniques has continued to be propounded by many educators and philosophers over the subsequent centuries. The history and theory of teaching and testing such deductive reasoning is succinctly reviewed by Baron and Sternberg.(1)

Recently, the technique of teaching by iterative hypothesis testing has been advocated.(2) For medical trainees, iterative hypothesis testing often requires the learner to form a diagnostic hypothesis from initial presenting data. As a result of this examination of facts, further data are gathered and the initial hypothesis refined. This process proceeds with increasing definition of the diagnosis until a final decision is reached. In other words, such iterative hypothesis testing is Socratic dialogue applied to medicine.

Oral examinations are ideally suited to evaluate this reasoning process and to discover why directions were chosen and choices made.

Oral examinations in conjunction with written examinations have been the mainstay for graduation requirements from European medical schools for decades. In the United States, some disciplines, notably internal medicine and pediatrics, have moved away from oral exams to concentrate exclusively on multiple choice written exams. Nevertheless, a majority of specialty boards, including surgery and most surgical specialties, anesthesia, obstetrics and gynecology, emergency medicine, psychiatry, neurology, and radiology still require an oral examination in the certification process.(3)

Also, many third year medical school rotations use an oral examination as part of the formal evaluation at the end of the clerkship.

What Does the Oral Examination Measure?

Arguably the best answer to this question is to determine which variables of performance influence the score or grade achieved by the examinee. Another method is to assess the validity of the test. Test validity is a measure of the examination's ability to properly rank the performance variables tested. This usually requires comparing an examinee's performance on the test with other measures of this achievement.

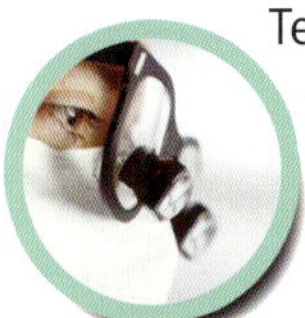

The determinants of a good score on the oral examination have varied in keeping with the structure or format of the examination process. For instance, earlier this century oral examinations for medical students were often recall in structure and, therefore, little more than a verbal version of a fill in the blank written examination. (4-6) Curiously, as an assessment of validity, this format did not correlate well with written tests and other measures of student performance. (4-6)

By the late 1960's, the oral examination evolved into more of an evaluation of problem solving and communication skills and less a test of recall. Using this emphasis, oral examinations were found to correlate well with overall clinical ranking. (7-9)

In the 1990's, continuing attention to the structure of an oral examination (i.e. programmed cases) and training of examiners has resulted in further documentation that examinees who perform well on this test also score well using other clinical performance measures. (10-12)

In 1992, more detailed information about the factors that influence performance scores of the oral examination was reported. In this study, actors representing surgical residents were examined with three performance variables (the content of their responses, their verbal style, and their dress) purposely adjusted. The examinations were videotaped and scored by surgeons unaware of the adjusted variables. All three of these factors significantly influenced the performance scores. Residents who had good problem solving skills, had good verbal communication skills, and were dressed in a professional manner achieved the highest scores. Residents with poor problem solving skills could achieve significantly higher ranking if they exhibited good verbal communication skills and were dressed well. (3)

This and a similar study (13) emphasize that the oral examination measures at least three variables that relate to good clinical performance—problem solving, communication, and professional image. Since oral examination scores have repeatedly been demonstrated to correlate well with other measures of clinical ranking, the logical conclusion is that the factors which influence oral examination performance are valid and worthy of assessment and, when necessary, remediation.

HOW TO PREPARE FOR AN ORAL EXAMINATION

Oral examinations are alarming to many, terrifying to some and paralyzing to a few. To say the least, an examination of the last group of candidates would be unsatisfactory. Therefore, it is appropriate for both candidate and examiner to strive to eliminate the element of fear from the examination.

The first strategy is for both to recognize the fear engendered. On the examinee's part it is to transcend terror and on the examiner's to conduct the examination in a way that relaxes the examinee and allows efficient and useful evaluation of the process of patient management.

The examinee can probably best prepare by remembering that the oral examination is about patient management. Assuming that candidates have the requisite knowledge to pass the examination, they should begin by following the course the examiner charts for the patient. Since verbal and nonverbal (i.e. professional image) communication skills do influence performance ranking, some hints about these skills are listed on the following pages, in no particular order of importance.

Verbal

1. **Be succinct, but be complete**. After the examiner has given the stem of the question, a simple way to begin the answer is to ask for a complete history and physical. The examiner then has the option of either asking what particular details the candidate is concerned with or simply giving the brief outline necessary for the candidate to continue with the question. However, if the situation presented is an emergency or trauma scenario, the candidate should stabilize the patient first (attend to the ABC's of resuscitation) and ask detailed questions later.

2. **Clear speech**. Speak clearly and deliberately. Don't rattle off an answer too fast or, conversely, drag out thoughts. Avoid habit phrases such as:

   "you know,"

   "like,"

   "so forth,"

   "probably,"

   "some people would," or

   "the literature says..."

   Incidentally, a candidate who uses "the literature says..." should know that research by heart. An example of a poor presentation might be:

   "Well, like, I'd probably, give some, like, Lactated Ringer's, but, well, the literature, um, er, should I use normal saline?"

   Most people would agree that this answer does not indicate a clear, reasoned thought process.

3. **Let the examiner guide the question.** The examiner is, in a sense, the patient. It follows, therefore, that the candidate should not argue with the examiner or interrupt when information is being given. It should also be self-evident that arguing or interrupting under these circumstances will not impress any examiners.

4. **Mention thought processes but don't recapitulate**. It is acceptable to say, for example:

   "My principle diagnosis would be diverticulitis, but I am also concerned about colon cancer..."

   What is not acceptable is to repeat verbatim the information the examiner has already given. This wastes time, bores the examiner and gains no points for the examinee.

   "Well, the woman is 54...and she has no history of colon cancer in her family...no family history...no previous significant problems...hmmm..."

5. **Raise points and don't be afraid to ask questions**. Many examinees are afraid to ask a question for fear that the examiner will then pounce on that point and propel them down the "pimping" path. For instance, in dealing with a patient with a peptic ulcer the

examinee may ask for a serum gastrin. The fear is the examiner will then ask for the amino acid sequence for big gastrin. The only cure for this behavior is examiner education. A suggested response would be to simply give the gastrin value and give the examiner credit for asking an appropriate question. When asked for Bilroth's mother's maiden name or the action of Bombesin on the reticular activating system, try saying,

"I'm sorry, I don't know. Could you please tell me how the patient is progressing and the results of the lab studies I requested."

The addition of "Sir" or "Ma'am" is at the candidate's discretion.

6. **Don't be afraid to say "I don't know."** There are times when the question will simply be beyond the candidate's knowledge (excluding "pimp" questions). Attempting to fool the examiner will usually result in abject failure. It is far better to admit a knowledge gap and move on. It is hoped the candidate will be able to impress the examiner in subsequent questions to such an extent that the point of ignorance is overshadowed or forgotten.

7. **Answer the question**. Some candidates use a politician's strategy and avoid giving an answer to a question they don't know by answering a question that wasn't asked. For instance:

   "How would you treat acute cholecystitis?"

   "I could give intravenous fluids and antibiotics."

   "Good. Which antibiotic?"

   "An alternative would be to operate on the patient." The examiner pauses, puzzled. "When?" he asks, hopefully.

   "I also think the intravenous is important. And a nasogastric tube," the resident offers.

   "Why?" The examiner groans, resignedly.

   "I'd also like to get some more tests to make sure the patient hasn't got a perforated ulcer."

   Although the answers were correct in themselves, they didn't answer the examiner's questions. This technique is very obvious and irritating to an examiner who is conscientiously trying to discover what the candidate knows.

8. **Avoid long pauses**. It is natural to want to stop and think about the question; however, there is only so much time during the examination and the examiner only grades on what you say. A few moments (2-3 seconds) for reflection are acceptable, but long pauses (>4 seconds) and awkward silences will not help.

   For instance, when reviewing a recent videotaped oral examination, the candidate asked if the tape was broken, because nothing seemed to be happening. In fact, however, the prolonged pauses were his and not the fault of the machine. He was taking so long to think about his answers and agonizing over what possible trick questions could be in store for him that he entered a state which resembled suspended animation. This was highlighted on the videotape.

9. **Don't prejudge the outcome**. Many oral examination formats incorporate several examination sessions with different examiners. Candidates often finish one examination feeling they have done badly and then proceed to the next room with the assumption that they will do equally badly. Clearly, this is not necessarily so.

   Each examination is completely independent of the others. If candidates believe they gave a disappointing performance in one, the next examination offers a golden opportunity to remedy that situation. Candidates should take a deep breath and proceed to the next room as if it were the first. It is also useful to remember that the examiner will not necessarily recognize all the areas of ignorance that the candidate may have realized. Sometimes a candidate sets too high a personal standard. The answer given may have been perfectly acceptable to the examiner, even if the candidate felt it was unacceptable.

10. **Mental blocks.** Mental blocks are common in oral examinations. A good examiner will understand how a candidate may stumble from time to time and will grant credit for something the candidate clearly knows, but cannot enunciate. Candidates will do more harm than good castigating themselves for blocking on a name or a point when, in fact, the examiner can see that the decision process was clear and the block was an irrelevant artifact of the examination process.

11. **Don't be alarmed if the examiner terminates the question.** This means neither that the candidate is doing abysmally badly nor wonderfully well. The examiner may simply want to get on to another subject. The more that can be learned about different areas of knowledge, the more comfortable that examiner will be in giving the final grade.

12. **Don't ask if the answer was correct.** This is inappropriate at any time during an oral examination. The oral examination is almost exclusively a summative evaluation and feedback will be given at a later time. Therefore, it is also inappropriate to ask questions such as,

    "Should I have done...?" Or, upon exiting the examination room, "How did I do?"

If you fail your first room, think like a quarterback!!

As is often said, quarterbacks have to have bad memories. Forget the first room and start fresh in rooms 2 & 3. You can fail one room and still pass.

13. **Don't try to find out what is being asked.** Anxious candidates often try ahead of time to learn what questions are being asked. Candidates sometimes ask for copies of potential examination questions or try to intercept other candidates as they leave the room the examinee is about to enter. The hope is to gain an edge by learning what the examiners are asking. The inherent flexibility of the oral examination renders this technique

If verbal and nonverbal behaviors conflict, the examiner believes the nonverbal.

relatively useless and has great potential for harm. Imagine a candidate who learns that a certain room is asking about upper GI bleeding from a peptic ulcer. The candidate will then fixate on that problem and proceeds to answer that question without paying adequate attention to the examiner, who has meanwhile grown bored (they are, after all, only human) with peptic ulcers and has decided to shift the questioning to bleeding varices. Even in strictly standardized oral exams where examiners are asked to keep the questions as nearly the same for each candidate as possible, an examiner recognizing that a candidate is answering well may change the "patient's" course. Unless the candidate is alert and willing to listen, the result will be disastrous.

The best preparation is to know the subject. Any candidate could write a question item. An oral examination is not a guessing game, but a testing modality designed to evaluate how the candidate thinks. That capability cannot be gleaned from the previous candidate or knowing the questions ahead of time.

14. **Don't be paranoid.** A common reaction to the fear of an oral examination is to think the examiner is out to trick the candidate. Nothing could (or should) be further from the truth. The examiner wants to know how the candidate reasons within a framework of expected knowledge. The suspicion that the examiner is after zebras (obscure diagnoses) hinders good answers and defeats the purpose of the examination. It is a common occurrence to see a candidate begin to answer, stop, wondering if the answer could really be that simple, and then dive off towards an obscure, irrelevant and highly unlikely diagnosis and management plan. Have faith in the examiner and remember: "Common things occur commonly!"

If you are in a fellowship, you may need to refresh your general surgery knowledge:

- **Attend general surgery grand rounds**
- **Attend breast tumor board**
- **Review or retake an ATLS course**
- **Review a current text; use uptodate.com**
- **Arrange for practice sessions with someone who will be tough on you**

15. **Practice.** Probably the most useful way to prepare for an oral examination is to practice aloud. Either practice alone, such as by answering imaginary questions in front of a mirror, or simply envision during rounds how to manage the patient being discussed. It is also worthwhile running through practice questions with a friend or colleague, asking each other questions and grading each other on the answers. It may be possible to ask a senior resident to provide more intensive questioning.

A good training program will make faculty members available to give students and residents practice sessions. If not, ask if a consultant can be obtained. These exercises will familiarize examinees with the process and what is expected of them. It may be helpful to review some of the points mentioned above to help make the examination fair and useful. Such training sessions train both the examinee and examiner.

Nonverbal Skills

Nonverbal signals deliver some of the most powerful messages, whether in an oral examination or in life in general. When verbal signals say one thing and nonverbal signals send a different message, people tend to believe the nonverbal. Remember that examiners are only human. However hard they try to ignore nonverbal signals, they may not always be successful. A candidate may not be aware of sending nonverbal signals just as the examiner may not be conscious of registering those signals. Candidates should evaluate their own nonverbal habits based on some of the following criteria.

1. **Dress**. Appearing for an oral examination in casual attire with eye-catching jewelry will give a poorer impression than conservative, professional dress (see example at the beginning of this chapter). For students, the white, clinical clerk jacket is acceptable in place of a sports jacket or blazer if it is clean, pressed and not adorned by excessive paraphernalia (pens, manuals, eye charts, etc.) For women, a white, simple blouse with a dark skirt, natural colored stockings and closed-toe shoes is "professional." For men, a white shirt, conservative tie, dark pants and socks, and leather shoes are acceptable. A business suit is more appropriate for either men or women residents for board examinations. Hair should always be neat and off the face.
2. **Eye Contact**. Eye contact means maintaining a steady, courteous look in the examiner's eye, not a fixed stare or a battle of wills. A shifty-eyed candidate or one who concentrates more on the window and activity outside or the ceiling appears weak to the examiners. It creates a poorer impression, both of knowledge and thought processes, than candidates who appear to be paying attention by looking at the examiner.
3. **Distractions**. Try to avoid scratching, picking, twitching, sniffing or otherwise distracting the examiner's attention. Potentially, this may result in the examiner not hearing an appropriate answer because of the distraction. A very common, often unconscious, response to stress is the "bouncing leg" that results from crossing one leg over the other, or nervous candidates who proceed unconsciously to bounce the foot up and down like a jackhammer.

   It should also be pointed out that bringing food or beverages into an examination is unacceptable.
4. **Taking Notes**. Generally speaking, keeping a note pad and taking notes during the examination is distracting, wastes time and is of very little value.
5. **Defensive Posturing**. There are several forms of defensive posturing that tend to set up barriers to effective communication. Some are formed from habit, while others are simply nervous reactions to stress. Avoid placing a hand over the mouth while answering. Not only might the examiner not be able to hear what is being said, but this maneuver also sends a clear signal of uncertainty. Candidates may find that folding their arms across the chest may be a comfortable, relaxed way to sit, but it can be another barrier between the candidate and the examiner. Women must be careful of crossing their legs above the knee when wearing certain skirts. Slouching may also send negative messages to the examiners.

WHAT CAN THE EXAMINEE LEARN?

1. **Recognize Knowledge Gaps**. Candidates invariably recognize more gaps in their knowledge than the examiners will. Almost everyone who has taken an oral examination remembers the experience for years to come. These areas of ignorance can be promptly remedied in the aftermath of the examination.

2. **Recognize Stress Responses**. Stress brings out many inappropriate verbal and nonverbal responses. Mumbling, covering the mouth, freezing and other defensive maneuvers are frequently observed. It is a common experience to see a student or resident, who the examiner knows is bright and capable, turn into a sullen, defensive, uncommunicative antagonist.

   It is not too great a leap of faith to suggest that an inappropriate response to stress in an oral examination may be manifested by a similar response to stress in clinical or personal life. The oral examination represents a test in a controlled environment conducted by trained educators. Observation of an inappropriate stress response is ideally followed by counseling at an appropriate level of complexity. This may be as simple as describing which behaviors need to be changed and methods to increase positive change. At the other end of the spectrum, it may be necessary to have a formal behavioral or psychological evaluation for a major stress reaction.

   Although a candidate can learn from a stress response, there are ways to reduce the appearance of stress. It can be avoided or at least reduced by appropriate preparation, oral practice and education about the oral examination process. The purpose of the examination is not intended to engender and reveal stress reactions.

3. **Think Clearly.** Candidates must be able to think and reason clearly to successfully pass the examination. The oral examination tests the iterative hypothesis testing process. Practicing this technique will prepare a candidate for the oral examination or, conversely, practicing for the examination is excellent training for this most basic way of dealing with clinical decision making. This process offers a formal opportunity for a candidate's reasoning to be evaluated. A successful result confirms a candidate's capability; a negative outcome signals the need for work. It is surely better for students, residents and clinicians to discover their deficits in the artificial microcosm of the oral examination than in their real life practice.

IMPROVING AND PREPARING FOR THE ORAL EXAMINATION

What are the steps for preparing or improving existing oral examinations?

1. **Standardized Questions with a Formal Stem.** (i.e. the patient history and appropriate physical and laboratory studies). These and key or prompter words are very helpful in standardizing the examination and increasing reliability among examiners and examinees.

2. **Examiner Education.** The American Board of Surgery and other specialty boards give detailed instructions to the examiners. Such formal training may be impractical for residency training programs and medical school faculty. However, if examiners are given a standardized scoring sheet, inter-rater reliability is high, especially for ranking the good performance, and may not be greatly influenced by the experience of the examiner. (14-16)

3. **One Versus Two Examiners.** Some authors have suggested that one examiner is less threatening to candidates and, therefore, preferable. Others believe that having two examiners gives some internal reliability and helps prevent adverse interpersonal exchanges between the examiners and candidates.

   In general, having two examiners is also less tiring to the examiners and, therefore, perhaps leads to a more valid and reliable examination. It should be remembered that examiners often work for several hours at a time, whereas the examinee completes the examination in less time.

4. **Review Courses.**

   For content issues: Knowledge base trumps everything else. However, do not assume you can learn five years of general surgery in the few days before the examination, as some commercial courses promise.

   Southeastern Surgical Congress and Southwestern Surgical Congress have jointly sponsored a surgery review course in the fall.

   Website: www.sesc.org

   Telephone: USA 1-800-558-8958 Bobbie Moore

   USA 630-986-5811 Christa Hanzlik

   To review nuts and bolts of specific procedures that you don't often perform, go to www.cine-med.com.

   For communication skills: Clinical Performance and Oral Examination in Surgery has over 20 years of solid data to support its methods for analyzing and correcting each individual's weaknesses. These small courses offer individual attention. The nationally selected faculty are hand picked for their area of expertise and, unlike other review courses, are not paid for their participation.

   Website: www.oralboardreview.net

   Telephone: USA 207-662-2515 June Cameron

   USA 603-359-0824 Pamela Rowland, PhD

CONCLUSION

While an oral examination can be a stressful situation, learning to deal with that stress is beneficial. The oral examination process of iterative hypothesis testing requires a candidate to refine a diagnostic hypothesis progressively based on the initial and subsequent data. It, therefore, tests a candidate's knowledge, but more importantly evaluates the candidate's thought processes. Along with other forms of testing such as written exams, actual patient evaluations, objective structured clinical exams, stimulated recall exams, and interactive computer-based patient simulations, the oral examination can help provide a comprehensive evaluation of the candidate's abilities to deal with a wide spectrum of situations.

Reaction time latency is 2-3 seconds

Preparation for an oral examination should include a careful look at the candidate's verbal and nonverbal communication skills. Mastering these skills will not only serve to boost the candidate's confidence during the examination, but will be a valuable resource in practice. After successfully completing an oral examination, handling an angry, grieving relative, a combative patient or truculent faculty member may seem simple in comparison.

Fairness: Candidates who fail and retake the certifying examination, will never see the same examiners in future examinations.

REFERENCES

1. Baron JB, Sternberg RJ. Teaching thinking skills: theory and practice. W.H.Freeman. 1987.
2. Kassirer JP. Teaching clinical medicine by iterative hypothesis testing. N Eng J of Med. 1983; 309:921.
3. Coe NP, Rowland-Morin PA, Burchard KW, et. al. Factors affecting the evaluation of the oral examination. Curr Surg. 1992; 459-464.
4. Barnes EJ and Pressey SL. The reliability and validity of oral examinations. School and Society. 1929; 30:719-722.
5. Evans LR, Ingersoll RW, Smith EJ. The reliability, validity and taxonomic structure of the oral examination. J Med Educ. 1966; 41:651-657.
6. McGuire CH. The oral examination as a measure of professional competence. J Med Educ. 1966; 41:267-274.
7. Colton T, Peterson OL. An assay of medical students' abilities by oral examination. J Med Educ. 1966; 42:1005-1014.
8. Levine HG, McGuire CH. The validity and reliability of oral examinations in assessing cognitive skills in medicine. J Educ Measure. 1970; 7:63-74.
9. Quattlebaum TG, Darden PM, Sperry JB. In-training examinations as predictors of resident clinical performance. Pediatrics 1989; 84:165-172.
10. Anastakis DJ, Cohen R, Reznick RK. The structured oral examination as a method for assessing surgical residents. Am J Surg. 1991; 162:67-70.
11. Hassett J, Luchette F, Doerr R, et al. Utility of an oral examination in a surgical clerkship. Am J Surg. 1992; 164:372-376.
12. Wade TP, Andrus CH, Kaminishi DL. Evaluations of surgery resident performance correlate with success in board examinations. Surgery. 1993; 113:644-648.
13. Rowland-Morin PA, Burchard KW, Garb JL, et al. Influence of effective communication by surgery students on their oral examination scores. J Acad Med. 1991; 66:169-171.
14. Burchard KW, Rowland-Morin PA, Coe NP, Garb JL. A Surgery oral examination: inter-rater agreement and the influence of rater characteristics. Acad Med. 1995; 70(11):91-93.
15. Kelley PR, Matthews JH, Schumacher CF. Analysis of the oral examination of the American Board of Anesthesiology. J Med Ed. 1971; 46:982-988.
16. Schwiebert P, Davis A. Increasing inter-rater agreement on a family medicine clerkship oral examination - a pilot study. Family Med. 1993; 25:182-185.

Oral Examination Practice Questions Area One

This will include questions in the following areas:

Stomach

Esophagus

Biliary

Pancreas

Lung/Thoracic

Head & Neck

Spleen

Small Bowel

Pediatric Surgery

CASE #1 - Stomach - Perforated Ulcer

A 65-year-old white male is admitted with a six-hour history of progressively increasing epigastric and then diffuse abdominal pain. He has COPD and three days ago received prednisone, 30 mg/day, for an exacerbation. His only other medication is famotidine twice a day. On examination his T-100°F, BP-110/60, P-120. He is lying still with a mildly distended abdomen. There are no bowel sounds. There is tenderness to percussion throughout with involuntary guarding in all regions. His laboratory data are: HCT 50, WBC 15,000, Na 137, K-3, CL-109, $C0_2$-22, BUN-32, creatinine-1.2, and glucose-135.

Prompter words:

- Free air
- Volume resuscitation
- Antibiotics – Candida likely
- Graham patch
- Definitive operation

CASE #2 - Acute Cholecystitis

A 60-year-old non-insulin dependent diabetic woman comes to the Emergency Department because of 2 days of upper abdominal pain. When the pain started it was similar to other episodes she has had over several years and is different from the pain she had with her "heart attack" last year (she is confident of that). After an hour or so, the pain became more constant, and has been associated with nausea with one episode of vomiting. The pain radiates to her back. She tried her sublingual nitroglycerin and it did not help the pain.

On examination, she is lying still but does not appear toxic. P-80 (reg), BP-150/90, temp 37.7°C. She has no abdominal scars or masses. Bowel sounds are present. She has percussion tenderness and involuntary guarding in the epigastrium and RUQ. HCT-42; WBC-14k; lytes - WNL; BUN-25; Creat 1.1; glucose-200.

Prompter words:

Diagnosis:

- Ultrasound findings/reliability
- HIDA scans/clinical
- EKG
- Bloods (amylase/LFT's Bili - 2.3)
- Colic vs. acute cholecystitis

Treatment:

- Antibiotic - choice
- Timing of operation ("golden period")
- Open or laparoscopic or tube
- Cholangiography
- Medical treatment (natural history/complication)

Variations:

1. Patient watched and treated with antibiotics
    - Fails to improve
    - Worsens
2. Patient operated upon laparoscopically
    - Dense adhesions - taken down, GB difficult to grab, etc.
    - When to do cholangiogram
    - When to convert to open
    - Drain vs. no drain
    - Role of cholecystostomy (even open, cholecystectomy too hard)
3. Patient also alcoholic - question of liver disease

    Post-op Complication:

    - Pancreatitis/abscess/CBO injury

Oral Examination Practice Questions Area Two

This will include questions in the following areas:

Trauma - Blunt

Trauma - Penetrating

Burns

Evaluation of Shock

Pulmonary Embolus

Organ Failure

Metabolic Derangements/Nutrition

Coagulation

Gastric Outlet Obstruction

CASE #1 - Critical Care - Multiple Trauma Priorities: Chest

(including cardiac, aorta, pulmonary contusion abdomen [pancreas, duodenum]

An 18-year-old white male is seen at the Level I Trauma Center following a two-car motor vehicle accident. He was the driver of one of the cars. EMTs report that it took 15 minutes to extricate him from his automobile; the steering wheel was broken. On examination, BP-110/60, P-100. He is alert complaining of severe anterior chest and epigastric pain.

Prompter words:

- ABCs
- Chest x-ray
- Cardiogram
- Arterial blood gases
- Cardiac contusion
- Cardiac tamponade
- Cardiac rupture (atrio-caval avulsion)
- Pulmonary contusion
- Aortic transection
- Peritoneal lavage
- Serum amylase
- Retroperitoneal area
- Gastrografin study
- Pancreatic trauma (head) management
- Duodenal trauma management

CASE #2 - Trauma - Pelvic

A robust 38-year-old male is brought to the ER 15 minutes after being crushed by a dump truck rolling over his lower abdomen and hips. He is awake, alert, and diaphoretic. His BP is 90/50, P-120, respiration-22, and temp-35.5˚C. There are ecchymoses and tire tracks from the iliac crests to the mid-thigh.

Prompter words:

- Resuscitation
- Examination of pelvic stability
- Urinary tract/ perineum – blood at meatus
- Rectal - +/- blood/bony fragments
- Pulses
- Neurologic function
- Continued volume need
- Peritoneal lavage vs. CT
- Pelvic hematoma
- Indications for pelvic stabilization
- Indications for arteriography

Oral Examination Practice Questions Area Three

This will include questions in the following areas:

Breast

Endocrine

Venous Disease/Leg Ulcer

Vascular

Colon & Anus

Appendix/I.B.D.

Ovarian CA

Skin & Soft Tissue

CASE #1 - Inflammatory Carcinoma of the Breast

A 39-year-old nurse presents to her family practitioner with a two- month history of right breast enlargement and a reddish, purple hue to the breast. There is no family history of a breast carcinoma. A mammogram did not reveal any mass; however, it did reveal skin thickening over the upper outer quadrant of the breast. She is sent to you for surgical evaluation.

Physical examination reveals a somewhat tender right breast with obvious erythema, peau d' orange, and ridging. The breast is somewhat tender. There is no nipple discharge or puckering of the skin. Evaluation of the axilla reveals 2 to 3 somewhat enlarged lymph nodes that are only mildly tender. You proceed with your work-up.

Prompter words:

- Evaluation of erythematous, non-tender breast
- The role of needle aspiration
- The role of biopsy
- The role of antibiotic trial
- Histopathologic criteria for inflammatory carcinoma of the breast
- Surgical and non-surgical therapy options
- The role of ER and PR receptors
- The role of radiation therapy and combined modality therapy

CASE #2 - Endocrine - Parathyroid Adenoma

A 62-year-old white female is referred to you for evaluation of a persistently elevated serum calcium (12.5) of two months duration. She reports some generalized weakness and a five-pound weight loss during this two-month period.

Prompter Words:

- "Bones, stones, moans and groans"
  (Bone resorption, nephrolithiasis, nephrocalcinosis, pancreatitis, peptic ulcer, altered mental status)
- Work-up
- Parathormone levels – intact v. C-terminal
- Milk-alkali syndrome
- Sarcoidosis
- Myeloma
- Breast cancer
- PTHrP regarding differential diagnosis
- MEN syndromes
- Operative approach: collar vs. lateral approach, intraoperative PTH
- Number of glands resected
- Postoperative complications – hypocalcemia, recurrent nerve damage

Letters from American Board of Surgery (ABS)

There are two letters provided after the certifying examination by the executive director of the ABS. Most bring good news and let candidates know that they have successfully completed the certifying examination; a certain percentage contain disappointing news. If your letter brings bad news:

Request a letter from the ABS (within 30 days of the examination) outlining the reasons for failure.

Although this may be difficult to do at this time, it may be helpful. What you read may not be consistent with what you think happened. Often candidates will say, "That's NOT what I said." However, what matters is what the examiners heard. It's all about your ability to communicate.

This is an example of what you may learn:

Dear Dr. Washington:

I have your letter of August 01 in which you request a critique of the Certifying Examination which you took on July 14, 2007 in Dallas, TX. I can give you a broad outline of the results. As an overview, while it was clear that you had some strengths, it was also clear that you had sufficient areas of weakness such that the majority of your examiners felt that you had not performed in a manner commensurate with that of a certifiable surgeon.

This letter will outline your performance in each room, identifying the questions asked and the examiner's evaluation of your performance on each question.

During your first interview, you were given a patient with small bowel fistula. Your response was considered unsatisfactory, especially with respect to your failure to recognize the problem despite postoperative bilious drainage from the wound, with respect to your failure to evaluate for a possible associated intrabdominal process, with respect to your failure to protect the skin in the region of the fistulous opening, and with respect to your understanding for the indications and duration of non-operative therapy. You were given a patient requiring a laparoscopic cholecystectomy. Your response was considered satisfactory, although your examiners did express some concern about your understanding of the options in management for a leak from a cystic duct stump. You were given a patient with a hiatal hernia and reflux. Your response was also considered satisfactory, but again your examiners did express concern about your ability to evaluate and treat a slipped Nissen fundoplication. You were given a patient with liver metastases. Your response was considered satisfactory, although the examiners noted that you did not initially biopsy the lesion and were reluctant to carry out a synchronous resection.

During your second interview, you were given a patient with ARDS. Your response was considered satisfactory, although the examiners noted that your knowledge in the area lacked some depth. You were given a patient with a duodenal hematoma. Your response was considered less than satisfactory, especially with respect to the technical details of the operative management.

You were given a patient with septic shock. Your response was considered unsatisfactory, especially with respect to inadequate fluid resuscitation, with respect to selection of antibiotics, and with respect to an unorganized approach to evaluating the differential diagnoses.

During your third interview, you were given a patient with a perforated sigmoid colon. Your response was considered less than satisfactory, especially with respect to lack of consideration of a perforated malignancy rather than diverticulitis, with respect to not obtaining a biopsy of the mass, and with respect to the operative management of abdominal wall adherence. You were given a patient with Stage III breast cancer. Your response was considered less than satisfactory, especially with respect to the role of preoperative chemotherapy.

Permit me to offer you two pieces of advice which I sincerely hope you will take. First, do not dwell on the results of this examination; what's past is past. Second, and in that connection, I would encourage you to "practice" taking oral examinations in preparation for your next attempt. This means that you should ask a colleague, preferably a Board Certified general surgeon, to question you for two or three hours every week for the next several months. Your questioner should probe deeply enough into your answer to make certain that you have adequate information and then critique your answers with regard to promptness, clarity, logic, and evidence of problem-solving ability. If you can follow this course, your next oral examination should be less stressful and hopefully will have a different outcome.

Sincerely,

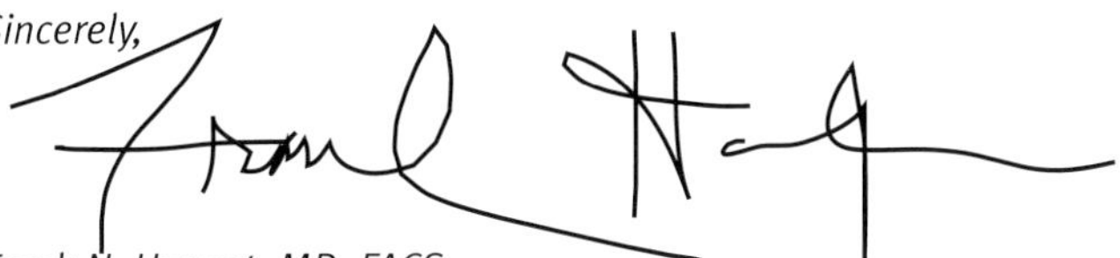

Frank N. Honest, MD, FACS

Executive Director

Critical Care: The Unknown

Kenneth W. Burchard, MD, FACS

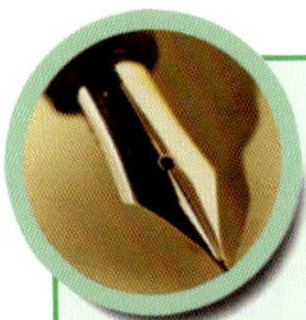

"Mrs. Allinson, I'm Doctor Frank. Your son has been badly injured."

"What do you mean?" Mrs Allinson gasped.

"He has suffered major intra-abdominal injuries and lost a lot of blood. His blood pressure was very low many times. He is also unconscious and appears to have a bruised brain. His left leg has many fractures as well as loss of muscle and skin. He may need an amputation. His life is in severe danger."

"They told me he was all right in the ambulance. Now you tell me he might die?"

"He's requiring many life support systems at present; a respirator, inotropes. He may not make it through the night."

"Are you an expert in this? You don't know my son. He's strong, he'll pull through anything. I have to call my doctor and find out who can take the best care of him."

Despite depictions of critical care units on television and in the movies, few family members and friends of the critically ill are familiar with modern critical care facilities either from an environmental or medical therapy standpoint. Usually, patients are admitted to intensive care units (ICU) because of severe illness, trauma, or after major surgery. The family and friends of these patients rarely arrive immediately in the ICU with the patient. Therefore, the physician meets the loved ones in a waiting room or lobby to prepare them for the critical care unit experience and to present realistic outcome expectations. Failure to perform this task properly early in the encounter sets the stage for anger and confrontations regarding further medical care decisions. Preparing a family may be difficult, especially when the critically ill person was previously healthy and vigorous (for instance, a young trauma victim). However, it is better to be realistic initially than to be faced later with the aftermath of a rosy prediction which did not come true.

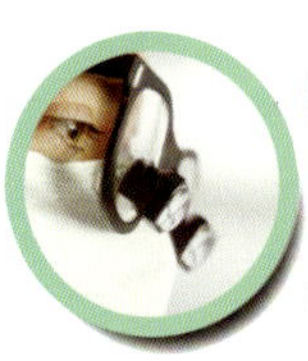

NEEDS OF THE FAMILY

Most studies about the concerns of families of critically ill patients have appeared in nursing literature and catalogue the most common "needs." (1-5)

Most Common Needs of Families of Critically Ill Patients

(In descending frequency)

1. Honest answers to questions
2. Knowledge of specific facts of the illness
3. Knowledge of prognosis
4. Notification of major changes in patient's condition

5. Daily information
6. Information that is understandable
7. Some sense that the hospital personnel care
8. Have hope
9. Know what and why particular care is being provided
10. Reassurance that best possible care is being provided
11. See patient frequently
12. Understand the medical treatment given
13. Talk with the physician.

Note that speaking specifically to the physician is *not* the highest priority. In fact, some of this information can be provided by the nursing staff. However, it is crucial that physicians in the critical care environment anticipate the priorities of family members, attend to these needs, and provide the health care team, which may include other physicians, with consistent guidelines for communicating with the family.

In communicating with the families of critically ill patients, the most common needs are for honesty, realistic predictions of outcome, and clear descriptions of disease.

Honesty

> "...at about this time they began to speak the truth to each other. The truth, he thought, has never been of any real value to any human being - - it is a symbol for mathematicians and philosophers to pursue. In human relations, kindness and lies are worth a thousand truths."(6)

A requirement of honesty implies that physicians and other health care personnel are truthful during discussions with the family about the patient's illness. Since absolute *truth* is an abstraction and possibly never fully attained, *truthfulness* becomes the practical goal.(7) Much has been written about the concept of truth, but little of it has been written in the context of medical practice. In fact, lying, especially the use of "white lies" that are not intended to do harm, has been considered essential to protect patients.

The utility of such white lies has been questioned, particularly for dying patients who, when denied clear prognostic information, are inhibited from acknowledging fears and concerns, as well as discussing them with family members and health care professionals.(8)

However, truthfulness can be brutal and cruel. Rather than

WHITE LIES

1. **WHITE LIE:** "We are worried that there may be some infection in the belly after the operation."

   TRUTH: A leaking colonic anastomosis is suspected.

2. **WHITE LIE:** "His heart is responding to the medicines which make it pump harder."

   TRUTH: If he were doing well, he shouldn't need inotropes.

3. **WHITE LIE:** "If his kidneys fail we can always use dialysis to replace kidney function and keep him going."

   TRUTH: Acute renal failure is associated with a 50% chance of dying.

tell a family member that a patient is certain to die, is it untruthful to state that the survival of a family member is unlikely? During the initial conversation about a critically ill patient, should a physician state categorically that a family member will be dead within a few hours or days? The following example points out the problems that can occur by not telling the truth initially.

A seventy-five year old woman is operated on for a large thyroid malignancy which required a partial sternotomy for removal. The patient's preoperative history indicated severe pulmonary dysfunction, with dyspnea at rest, an FEV1 of 700ml, and room air PaO_2-55, $PaCO_2$-50. Despite knowledge of this severe degree of pulmonary dysfunction, the operating surgeon predicted that the patient would need a ventilator only overnight and be ready for hospital discharge in about seven days.

The patient's respiratory mechanics did not allow immediate extubation and the patient's course was complicated by a wound infection and pneumonia. Her illness was of such severity that the ICU staff and the attending surgeon discussed with an ethicist the possibility of withdrawing ventilator assistance. These discussions did not include the patient's husband, who was repeatedly told by the operating surgeon that his wife was responding to therapy and that only small hurdles needed to be surmounted. As a result, the husband did not appear to have a realistic sense of the degree of his wife's illness and the prolonged ICU course that would be required for potential recovery. He echoed the stance the operating surgeon presented to him, not the ICU staff. He seemed perplexed that his wife was not progressing more quickly and questioned the quality of care provided in the ICU. Eventually the patient did recover, but only after three weeks of ICU management and two more weeks on the regular floor.

The discussion with the ethicist demonstrated that the operating surgeon did have a realistic appraisal of his patient's degree of illness and potential for persistent ventilator requirements. However, he did not relay this to the family. While this led to tension between the ICU staff and the family, there was apparently little questioning of the attending surgeon's care by the husband.

Regardless of the capability of a physician to predict the future accurately and therefore "tell the truth," such frankness can adversely affect family necessities. Most families wish to have some hope and to feel that the best possible care is being provided. Families may believe that if there is no hope, there is little reason to provide top quality care. Therefore, both of these needs may not be met by "the truth." However, this does not imply that false hope and maximum medical therapy for every patient is warranted. Instead, a middle ground, which is realistic yet supportive, is most appropriate.

How does a family discern if the health care team is honest? Possible methods include nonverbal communication, consistency, and eventual patient outcome.

Methods For Discerning Honesty

1. Do the nonverbal behaviors support or conflict with verbal behaviors?
2. Am I getting a consistent message?
3. What is the final patient outcome?

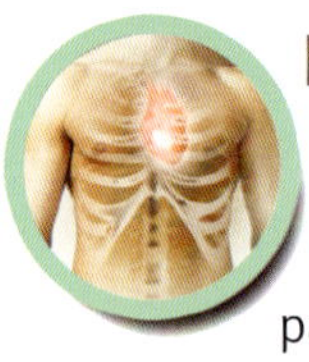

FIRST IMPRESSIONS

First impressions are important and communication at the time of a first meeting should convey both verbal and nonverbal messages of caring and warmth for both the patient and family members.

Do's And Don'ts For Nonverbal Communication

DO:	DON'T:
If standing, stand nearby.	Don't be distanced.
Make eye contact at same level.	Don't sit behind a desk.
Be patient.	Don't stand over patient or family members.
Wait for an acknowledged end to the conversation.	Don't fidget, tap feet, or run away.
	Don't walk away.

NONVERBAL COMMUNICATION

Nonverbal communication means messages that are conveyed without words by such methods as body movements, facial and eye activities, touching, dress and smell.(9) Impressions are largely based on nonverbal communication. When verbal and nonverbal messages conflict, Americans will tend to believe the nonverbal message. Studies are inconclusive about an individual's ability to discern who is actually telling the truth simply by assessing nonverbal clues. However, a conclusion that a member of the health care team is lying will require much effort to overcome even when false.

Avoid appearing aloof and distanced from the family because of a barrier like a desk. Make eye contact at the same level. Avoid standing over a family member. Sit down! Even when pressed to move on to other responsibilities, avoid appearing eager to leave. If you sit, the family will feel as if you spent more time with them than if you stand. Psychological time is usually longer than real time. Don't fidget, don't resort to foot tapping or other exhibitions of impatience, and don't run away. Wait for the family to acknowledge understanding and willingness to end the communication. This will be evident in their silence or other nonverbal communications such as nodding the head or extending a hand for a "thank you" hand shake.

CONSISTENCY IN MEDICAL STAFF

Any physician (attending, resident, and medical student) who communicates with a family should inform the other medical staff as to what the family has been told. This should include any plans that were outlined, so that the message can be reinforced. Appropriate entries of the content of such discussions can be entered in the patient's medical record. With careful attention to this process, the critical care staff can avoid providing discordant information. When a physician is unaware of a change in the patient's condition, it is better to be honest rather than trying to cover up the fact that the physician had not yet seen the patient that day.

EVENTUAL PATIENT OUTCOME

In the end, the patient's final outcome will be the truest test of honesty.

Honesty is more likely to be questioned when the patient does worse than predicted, than when the patient does better.
KW Burchard

Therefore, it is best to err on the side of pessimism without being brutal, than to err on the side of optimism when unwarranted. Most physicians need little assistance recognizing the critically ill patient who is likely to have a poor outcome. Prognostication can be supported by several numerical scoring systems such as the Multiorgan Dysfunction Score, APACHE, and Injury Severity Score.(10) However, since individual patients may not fit a particular predicted pattern derived from large numbers, it is better to use more general descriptions such as:

"a 50:50 chance of surviving,"

"most likely will be paralyzed," and

"may be in the hospital for several weeks."

In the example of the woman with pulmonary and respiratory complications, the operating surgeon would have better prepared the family if he had explained before the surgery that the patient's underlying lung disease would potentially make the postoperative care difficult. This could then be re-emphasized in the first postoperative conversation. If the patient did well, the patient and family would be pleased that an adverse outcome did not occur. If it did occur, as was the case, they would have been well prepared. An unexpected adverse outcome will lead to concerns about the quality of care provided by the physicians, other ICU staff, or both.

The inconsistency between predictions of the ICU staff and the operating surgeon in the above case evoked questions about the quality of ICU care.

TERMINOLOGY

Difficulties using lay language to explain disease and treatment are accentuated in the critical care environment with its attendant plethora of equipment, personnel, and laboratory tests.

Medical Translations

NOTE: Both terms used together works best

Physician Speak...	Non-physician Speak...
"electrolytes"	"blood chemicals"
"malignancy"	"cancer"
"differential diagnosis"	"what could be the problem"
"needs support"	"airways, breathing machine, feeding tubes, kidney machine"
"hypoperfusion"	"decreased blood flow"
"hypoxia"	"too little oxygen"
"benign"	"is not cancer"
"sepsis"	"severe infection"
"stable"	"neither sicker nor better"
"vertigo"	"dizziness"
"dysfunction"	"problem"
"referral"	"ask another doctor for another opinion"
"inhibitor"	"stops something from working"
"low intensity exercise"	"walking not running"
"prosthesis"	"body part that is made to replace a human part"
"adverse reaction"	"not good"
"tore ligament"	"sprained"
"perforation"	"hole"
"termination"	"stop"
"embolism"	"clot or lump of blood"
"impair"	"harm"
"indication"	"sign"
"cerebral hemorrhage"	"stroke"
"coronary thrombosis"	"heart attack"
"bacteria"	"germs"
"conversion"	"change"
"inadvertent"	"not planned"
"sensation"	"feeling"
"equivocal"	"not positive or negative"
"sutures"	"stitches"
"soluble"	"will disappear/dissolve over time"
"adequate"	"enough"
"progressive"	"continue to get worse or better"
"diagnosis"	"name for condition of problem"
"annually"	"every year"

Medical personnel may hide behind terminology intended to emphasize the complexity of illness, thus adding to the difficulties for nonprofessionals to understand and make conclusions. Some patients and their families are easily intimidated by medical jargon and willingly accept a dependent position with such statements as:

"You're the doctor, you know best."

"Whatever you think is right, we'll do."

Such conclusions by patients and family members inappropriately divests them of decision-making responsibilities and is another potential source of anger if the outcome is not favorable. A physician faced with this type of statement should presume that the explanation of the disease and/or treatment options was not well understood. An attempt to re-explain should be made with the intent of helping, not supplanting, the decision process. The physician should emphasize that the decision is still the patient's or the family's.

The lay public will likely understand such terminology as "breathing machine," "medicine to increase the blood pressure," or "a tube which will help us measure how the heart is doing" better than such terms as respirator, vasoconstrictor, and pulmonary artery catheter. By avoiding technical jargon and providing a caring, warm approach to the critical care environment, the physician can improve understanding and reduce intimidation.

COUNTERING HOSTILITY

Despite all such efforts, an occasional family member may exhibit hostility, usually with disbelief that his or her loved one is as ill as the critical care staff is describing. Such individuals will seek inconsistencies in medical staff statements to reinforce the notion that the medical staff is not quite sure of the disease process and/or treatment. It can be easier to accept incompetence in the medical staff than a life threatening or disabling disease in a loved one. Conflicts often arise about the necessity of uncomfortable tests or treatments or the use of pain medication and sedatives.

When such hostile interactions are recognized, one effective method for resolution is to have a discussion involving the family member, other family members, the physicians and the patient's nurse(s), as well as a "non-medical" professional, such as a member of the clergy or a person from risk management. With such an audience, it is difficult for the hostile family member to claim inconsistency. It also provides the health care team the opportunity to discern the level of understanding of the family member and to answer questions. Frequently, guidelines about acceptable family member behavior and subsequent communication channels can be agreed upon.

CONCLUSION

Critical care units require honest, consistent, and clearly understood communications to patients and patient family members from the entire health care team. As a primary role model for the health care team, it is incumbent on the critical care physician to become proficient in both verbal and nonverbal communication methods that will foster trust and decrease hostility or questioning of the quality of care.

REFERENCES

1. Forrester DA, Murphy PA, Price DM, Monaghan JF. Critical care family needs: Nurse-family member confederate pairs. Heart Lung. 1990; 19:655-661.
2. Meijs CA. Care of the Family of the ICU Patient. Crit Care Nurse. 1989; 9:42-44.
3. Hickey M. What are the needs of families of critically ill patients? A review of the literature since 1976. Heart Lung. 1990; 19:401-415.
4. Kirchoff KT, Song MK and Kehl K. Caring for the family of the critically ill patient. Crit Care Clin. 2004; 20(3): 453-66.
5. Vincent JL. Communication in the ICU. Intensive Care Med. 1997; 23(10):1093-8.
6. Greene G. The Heart of the Matter. New York: Viking Press; 1948.
7. Bok S. Lying: Moral Choice in Public and Private Life. New York: Vintage Books, 1979.
8. Kubler-Ross E. On Death and Dying. New York: Macmillan Co.; 1969.
9. DeVito JA, Hecht ML. The Nonverbal Communication Reader. Prospect Heights: Waveland Press; 1990.
10. Rocker G et al. Clinician predictions of intensive care unit mortality. Crit Care Med. 2004; 32(5): 1149-54.

Asking for Tissues and Organs: Balancing Needs

William P. Fiser, Jr. MD, FACS

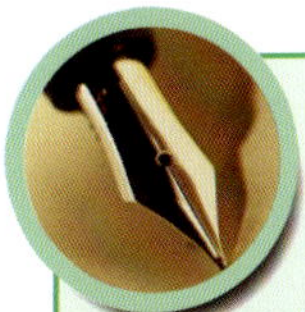

Four family members sat in silence in the ICU conference room. Three daughters and Mom. An empty tissue box sat between them and the resident on the table. One of the daughters wept with her chair turned partly away from the table. Mom faced the resident with an expectant expression.

"My attending should be here soon," the resident said. "We got a question for you."

The oldest daughter sat beside her mother. She removed half-glasses and asked, "Does it involve requesting our father's organs?"

"Kidneys," said the resident. "That's all we need."

"Need?" The weeping daughter twisted back and faced him. "Did you say 'need'?"

"Yeah, we have a list. There's always a shortage."

"So my husband has been declared officially dead?" the wife asked. She squeezed her daughter's hand. "When did this happen?"

The middle daughter stood. "Mom, no one said Dad's gone. They're just preparing us for the possibility."

Leaning back, the resident toyed with the stethoscope around his neck. "Actually, a neurologist is examining him as we speak. Not much doubt. He's brain dead, I'm sure."

The four women glanced around at each other. The oldest daughter stood with her sister. "Now just a moment! You're saying Dad's as good as dead? And this is the first we hear about it?"

The resident frowned. "Look, we've been trying to tell you for days that he's going to die. You're not listening. I told you his gases are lousy, he needs max pressors, got a new ST elevation." He folded his arms. "Didn't I tell you all this? Why waste a couple of good kidneys?"

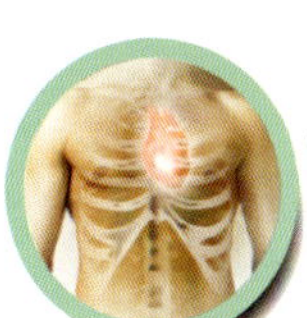

Although the majority of organ donor cases are from head trauma, the following example represents a significant and increasing percentage of donor cases.(1) A 58-year-old white male was admitted to a rural hospital with mental status changes. The patient deteriorated in the ER, became unresponsive, and required intubation with mechanical ventilation. Several hours later the patient was transported to a tertiary care center. The patient arrived in the emergency room unresponsive with a Glasgow Coma Scale (GCS) of 3 on no sedation. Because of the GCS <5 and mechanical ventilation, the patient met clinical triggers and the organ procurement organization (OPO) was notified.

A CT scan revealed a very large hemorrhage centered within the right basal ganglia which was likely a hypertensive bleed. There was an extensive midline shift to the left noted along with effacement compatible with herniation. The attending physician spoke with the family about the poor prognosis. The physician implemented catastrophic brain injury guidelines to keep the potential donor stable.

The OPO family services coordinator (FSC) arrived within one hour to meet with hospital staff to determine suitability for donation and begin family support if appropriate. A short team huddle with the health care team was held in which the physician explained that he had spoken with the family about the poor prognosis and was planning confirmatory brain death testing. The nurse and chaplain added that the wife and adult daughters did not comprehend the gravity of the situation and expected him to get better and go home. The FSC said that the patient was not in the donor registry. A plan was made to have a family discussion after results of an apnea test.

The physician was able to introduce the FSC to the family by explaining, "She is a part of our team who is here to help families who find themselves in circumstances similar to yours." The FSC began meeting family needs such as making phone calls and helping the family find their way around the hospital, but with no mention of donation.

The apnea test was performed and was consistent with brain death. The attending physician wrote a brain death note in the chart declaring the patient dead. A short team huddle was held to make a plan for the family discussions. The social worker made sure the family room was ready. The nurse, chaplain and FSC accompanied the family to the sitting room. The attending physician arrived and expressed sympathy, sat at eye level with the family and explained events that led up to the point of brain death. Brain death was clearly explained along with the confirmatory testing. Family questions and concerns were addressed by the physician with no mention of donation. When the family asked, "What happens next?" the physician explained, "These family representatives (FSC, chaplain, social worker, and nurse) will help you through the next steps and will give you the information you need." He expressed condolences again to the family and left. The family was escorted back to the bedside for grieving and their farewell to their loved one.

When the family was ready, a second family discussion was held to discuss end of life issues. With other team members present, organ and tissue donation was addressed by the FSC. Included in this discussion were decisions about selecting a funeral home and funeral services, and information was given to the family about donation. After all family questions and concerns were addressed, the family decided that they would like to consent for organ and tissue donation. They felt that their loved one would want to help others. A careful review of the patient's medical social history was completed for both organ and tissue donation. The patient was a nonsmoker in otherwise good health with recent onset of hypertension making him acceptable for tissue donation.

A second OPO team arrived on the scene and began managing the donor. The patient began receiving volume resuscitation while a central line was started. Baseline lab was sent including serology for HIV, HBV, HCV and EBV. Initial crystalloid fluids were switched to colloid. FFP was given for an INR >1.5 control. The patient remained hypotensive so dopamine was started. Hormonal resuscitation was given of steroids, insulin drip, and thyroid hormone. The blood pressure stabilized. After four hours of reperfusion, a cardiac ECHO was performed that showed good left ventricular function. Because of the age, a coronary arteriogram was performed, which showed normal coronary arteries. An oxygen challenge test was done and the patient had a FiO2 of 500 on 100% oxygen. Liver and kidney numbers were excellent. Serology came back negative.

A UNOS match run based on blood type which was A-positive was completed and electronic offers were made to transplant centers to place the heart, lungs, liver, kidneys and pancreas. All organs were placed except the pancreas which was declined because of age. An operating room time was scheduled and six organs were recovered and transplanted. After the organs were recovered, the corneas, bone and skin were recovered. The ligaments and saphenous vein were declined because of age.

The patient had a normal open casket funeral two days following the recovery. The OPO followed up with the family and invited them to participate in an aftercare program with support groups of donor families. In addition, the family was provided information about the organ recipients such as age, geographical location and success of transplant.

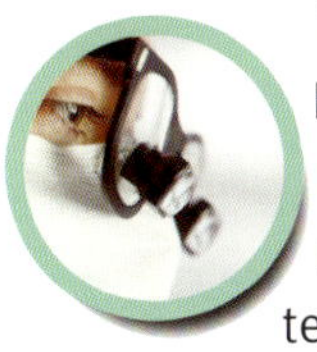

The above case scenario illustrates the principles of best practices identified by the HRSA-sponsored study of the highest performing Organ Procurement Organization (OPO) and donor hospitals.(2) The patient was rapidly evaluated and determined to meet **clinical triggers** resulting in an early referral to the OPO. Rapid brain death testing was performed; if the apnea test was not feasible, a nuclear medicine blood flow study would have been performed. An OPO coordinator who specializes in working with families came on site and met with the health care team to asses the situation. The OPO representative or **FSC**(3), with approval from the attending physician, began interacting with the family. The FSC was introduced as a member of the health care team that deals with families that find themselves in situations like theirs. The FSC did not bring up organ donation but provided support to the family and facilitated communication with the medical team. When the attending physician determined that the patient was brain dead, the **team** had a brief **huddle** before talking to the family to define their roles. The attending physician then took the FSC nurse into the family conference and gave the family the bad news which included a clear explanation of brain death. At this point, the attending physician left the FSC with the family and returned to his other patient responsibilities. The family, although they did not have any more questions for the attending, asked "What did Dr. Attending say?" and often the FSC parroted things the attending said to help the family grasp that a death had occurred. The FSC provided support from her background in grief counseling. The FSC worked with the family and when they had accepted the death, discussed the organ and tissue donation option **(decoupling)**(4-6) as one of the end of life decisions to be made along with things like funeral plans. The FSC emphasized the possibility of saving other lives from this tragedy and gave the family the information they needed to make an informed decision. The FSC used her skills and training to make an **appropriate request**. Some families are eager to donate and have already made this decision; some families are undecided and have to wrestle with the decision. It is obviously in this latter group that most improvements in donation rate can be made.

Once a family decides to donate organs and tissues, a lengthy medical social history must be performed. The history for tissue donation is even more extensive than organ donation because there are so many medical social contraindications to tissue donation. After the consent was signed, the FSC stayed with the family and continued to provide support while the procurement coordinators began managing the donor to improve organ function and began the lengthy process of placing organs. To maximize the number of transplantable organs, the donor must be resuscitated and stabilized to overcome damage that has occurred during brain death.(7)

BRAIN DEATH

In the process of brain death, most patients experience a period of hypertension associated with a sympathetic storm. It appears that this phase is particularly damaging to the heart and lungs, causing ischemia and activation of a generalized inflammatory response. After brain death is complete, the potential donor usually has vascular collapse and shock from hypovolemia and marked vasodilatation. Once they are volume loaded, treated with pressers and given hormonal resuscitation, the blood pressure and cardiac output can be restored, but it takes reperfusion time for the damaged organs to recover. It is amazing how much the heart and lungs can improve with good donor management. Organs that would have been unacceptable for transplant become usable with good management.

Communication with a family about organ and tissue donation at the time of death has many pitfalls and really should be avoided unless you have received additional training and have been certified by your organ procurement organization or tissue procurement organization as a designated requestor. This principle often is misunderstood and resented by physicians because they see it as a violation of the sacred doctor-patient relationship. Stating your support of donation when asked by the family is appropriate. When asked, giving information that you are certain is current is also appropriate. Donation is a rapidly changing field and misinformation is very detrimental to the process, so be careful. There are many myths that family members have about organ and tissue donation that are driven by fear. One of the most common myths is that the patient may receive worse care if they consent to donation because the doctors want to recover organs and tissue for transplantation. When a physician speaks with a family and requests donation, it can be seen as a conflict of interest and adds to the family's suspicion. These suspicions are irrational, but real to the families that harbor them. Also, the physician stating to the family, **"By law I have to introduce you to the OPO representative,"** undermines the request process.

Most organ donations only occur when the organs are still perfused just up until the time of recovery. This is primarily in situations where the patient is declared dead by brain death criteria. Another organ donation option is in patients who are going to have life support discontinued and is called donation after cardiac death (DCD).(8) This is the method by which organs were procured prior to the brain death laws being enacted and in some regions of the country still account for 10% of organ donors. There is a national movement to increase this type of donation. Tissue donation occurs after death and circulation ceases. Corneas can be recovered for up to six hours after death and other tissues can be recovered up to 12 hours after death, or even up to 24 hours if the body is refrigerated. Because there are many reasons potential donors are unacceptable for tissue donation, it is important not to raise the family's expectations regarding tissue donation until all these issues have been reviewed and the donor is found to be acceptable. One of the mistakes made by well meaning physicians is getting consent from the family for tissue donation, only to learn that their loved one is not an eligible donor. This can be devastating to a family that has managed their grief by wanting to make a gift to help other people.

Although the rules are constantly changing, a number of medical social history items will result in exclusion for tissue donation such as any history of drug abuse, homemade tattoos, incarceration or living outside the US for extended periods of time.

Exciting improvements are occurring in organ donation. Public opinion polls have shown that about 75 to 85% of the population is in favor of organ transplantation and organ donation.(9) One would think therefore that 75 to 85% of eligible donors would consent for organ donation. That has not previously been the case and for years the donation rate in eligible donors has been about 50%. There has been significant improvement recently, attributable to the HRSA-sponsored Organ Donation Breakthrough Collaborative (ODBC). The key lies with the 25 to 35% that say they favor organ transplantation and donation but do not make a gift when the opportunity presents itself. It has become apparent that this 35% take special handling to obtain consent.

DE-COUPLING

One method of approaching these potential donor families is called de-coupling. This concept was proposed in 1990 by KODA (Kentucky Organ Donor Affiliates), working with the University of Kentucky.(10) Simply stated, the discussion of death should be a separate conversation from the request for donation. Families cannot give consent for donation when they are still in the first stage of grief, identified by Kubler-Ross as denial (11) and have not accepted that death has occurred. Pushing for an answer to the request for donation in this stage of grieving will likely result in a refusal. No is the answer for everything in the stage of denial. A skilled requestor works with the family and requests donation when they are ready to discuss end of life decisions. Good consent rates can also be attributable to a good requestor. Some people just have more skill in connecting with the family and allowing them to understand the importance of saving someone else's life in their time of tragedy. The other method of talking to families is to plant the seed early. Although this is not the recommended method, a skilled requestor may be able to get high consent rates using this method.

HOUSTON LIFEGIFT

One of the high performing OPO's studied by the HRSA for best practices was Houston LifeGift. They utilize in-house coordinators at their larger hospitals to interact with potential donor families early in the process and to provide support to these families.(3) They do not mention organ donation until after death declaration unless the family asks a specific question. These coordinators provide appropriate requesting and their consent rates are exceptional in inner-city hospitals with diverse racial and ethnic groups. HRSA provided a grant to duplicate this approach in five hospitals in New York and California. The consent rate for organ donation increased over 22%, collectively, in these five hospitals, thus validating this approach.(12) This approach has met with quite a bit of resistance from some of the medical staff despite approval of the ethics committee and medical board of the respective hospitals. The physicians complain that patients are being deceived by not being told at introduction that the organ and tissue donation is driving this service provided by the FSC. This is despite the families being very pleased to have this additional service. Another interpretation of this interaction is that the FSC is managing information. In medical practice, information is managed all the time. For example, if a patient comes into the office with radiographs that show that they most likely have incurable cancer, most physicians don't inform the patient at that time of the grim outlook. Certainly it is appropriate to say this looks bad and more tests are necessary. Most physicians would not have a discussion of the cancer until they have confirmatory tests such as a biopsy and pathological examination. Likewise it is not appropriate to discuss brain death until there is a diagnosis of brain death. Discussing organ donation before a diagnosis of brain death is getting the cart before the horse, and implies that brain death has already been diagnosed. With that being said, it is appropriate to tell the family that things look bad and to prepare them for a bad outcome.

Up until 2004 and 2005, national organ donation rates had remained relatively flat and then they increased 10.6 and 5.9% respectively.(13) There were wide variations in the consent and donation rate in various hospitals and organ procurement organization's (OPO) service areas.(2) Former Secretary of Health, Tommy Thompson, directed HRSA to fund a best practices study to focus on the five high performing OPO's in the USA and territories. The concept was to identify the best practices and make them common practices. An Organ Donation Breakthrough Collaborative (ODBC) was organized by HRSA to bring together a number of key health care organizations including JCAHO and CMS as participants to discuss and implement these best practices. The ODBC also used the methodology of the Institute for Health Care Improvement including: Plan, Do, Study and Act cycles to evaluate changes. ODBC focused on data and measuring changes. To participate in the ODBC, individual hospitals executed contracts with HRSA requiring signatures of upper hospital management. The point was to make hospitals more responsible for their donation rates.

As organ transplantation has become more and more successful primarily due to the improvement in drugs and management of rejection, the demand for organs has grown exponentially. The waiting list continues to grow with more than 91,999 men, women and children currently awaiting life-saving transplants. Every 13 minutes another name is added to the national transplant waiting list. Seventeen people die each day from the lack of available organs for transplant.(14) Fortunately, the national organ donation rate is now growing for the first time and the successor to the ODBC, the Organ Transplant Breakthrough Collaborative (OTBC), has set a goal of no deaths on the waiting list through implementation of best practices identified in the ODBC and through better management of potential organ donors.

MISSION STATEMENT FOR THE ODBC

> "Commit to saving or enhancing thousands of lives a year by spreading known best practices to the nation's largest hospitals, to achieve organ donation rates of 75% or higher in these hospitals."
>
> *Former Secretary of Health, Tommy Thompson*

Principles of the ODBC:

1. Establish joint accountability for increasing the number of organ donors because donation will increase if OPO's and hospitals work together.
2. Unrelenting focus on change and improvement.
3. Rapid, early referral and linkage. Key OPO and/or hospital donation staff are linked rapidly and early to potential donor families.

4. Integrated donation process management. OPO and hospitals establish and manage an integrated donation process that clearly defines roles and responsibilities and provides feedback.
5. Aggressively pursue every donation opportunity.

   Every possibility for increased donation is maximized and routinely evaluated through:

   - quick deployment
   - reproaches
   - donor management
   - aggressive organ placement.
6. Establish strong culture of accountability for results.

   Analyze and schedule debriefings about results.
7. Set Goals

   Outcome Measures:

   75% conversion rate (organ donors/eligible organ donors)

   ZERO medical examiner/coroner denials

   Process measures:

   - 100% Referral rate
   - 100% timely notification rate
   - 100% appropriate requestor rate

High Leverage Changes of the Organ Donation Breakthrough Collaborative

- Advocate organ donation as the mission.
- Involve senior leadership to get results.
- Deploy a self-organizing OPO/hospital team.
- Practice early referral, rapid response.
- Master effective requesting.
- Implement donation after cardiac death.

Prior to the ODBC, request laws were passed and implemented by the CMS as a condition of participation. One requirement is that all hospitals must routinely refer all deaths. These were easy to measure and directly related to increases in tissue donors, but only indirectly related to increases in organ donors. It became clear that they were not the gold standard or even close to it for measuring hospital performance in organ donation. For organ donation, the referral of ventilated patients that may progress to brain death or donation must be timely for the process to work effectively.

- Referrals must be made on all imminent deaths and cardiac deaths

  Regardless of diagnosis and/or condition

  Call to be made in a "timely manner" (early!)

  Using a clinical trigger that creates a very systematic, automatic occurrence

The concept of clinical triggers is not reliant on obtaining permission from physicians to call in a referral of a potential organ donor. The most common clinical triggers are based on severe neurological injury with a Glasgow coma scale of five or lower and requiring mechanical ventilation. Each individual hospital can custom design their clinical trigger but, once in place, it makes referrals to the OPO more consistent and avoids missing potential donor referrals. While physicians lose control over when the referral is made, after these processes are in place, they have been well accepted.

Tracking data on conversion rates (organ donors/eligible donor) requires defining an eligible donor as any patient that meets brain death criteria whether declared brain dead or not. The definition of an organ donor for the ODBC is defined as any patient that has organs recovered for transplantation and at least one organ is transplanted. This data collection was started with the ODBC and has now been adopted by JCAHO for their survey of hospitals. All hospitals are now required to report their conversion rates. When JCAHO comes for a visit, they will ask for a report on your hospital conversion rate and what is being done to improve it.

Medical examiner denials have been a problem in certain geographical areas.(15) Tthe National Association of Medical Examiners (NAME) became very involved in the ODBC. Because of the involvement of senior leadership of this organization reaching out to its membership, marked improvement has been observed in the frequency of medical examiner denials. In Arkansas, there were usually five or more denials per year and this number has dropped to one for the past year, and this is a rural state with elected county coroners and prosecuting attorneys who may have little medical knowledge. It is actually the county coroners that give the release, but because of the proactive stance of the state medical examiner, denials have almost been eliminated. During the 2005 legislative session, a bill was passed and signed into law that requires the coroners to consult with the medical examiner, write a letter explaining any denial for organ donation to the OPO and attend the autopsy if they refuse release for donation. There are times when it is appropriate to limit the organs that can be recovered. We see this most frequently in child abuse cases. With modern forensics, organ donation should not prevent the collection of evidence in criminal cases. The OPO has willingly agreed to participate in the process and facilitate collection of evidence to preserve organ donation as an option. During the

Below are listed the process measures expected by JCAHO along with the observed rates reported at the time of the ODBC.

- **75-80% conversion rate *(Collaborative average 61%)***
- **100% referral rate *(Collaborative average 90%)***
- **100% timely notification rate *(Collaborative average 75%)***
- **100% appropriate requestor rate *(Collaborative average: 90%)***
- **ZERO medical examiner denials *(Most locations at zero)***

2007 legislative session in Arkansas, the new revised uniform anatomical gift act was passed and signed into law. It gives the state medical examiner authority over county coroners regarding organ and tissue donation.

DONATION AFTER CARDIAC DEATH (DCD)

On April 7-8, 2005, a national conference on organ donation after cardiac death (DCD) was convened in Philadelphia, PA, to address the increasing experience of DCD and to affirm the ethical propriety of transplanting organs from such donors.(8) The professional affiliation of participants included the American Medical Association (AMA), the Society of Critical Care Medicine (SCCM), the American Association of Critical Care Nurses (ACCN), the American Society of Anesthesiologists (ASA), the Joint Commission on the Accreditation of Hospital Organizations (JCAHO), the American Society of Transplant Surgeons (ASTS), the American Society of Transplantation (AST), the Association of Organ Procurement Organizations (AOPO), the Scientific Registry of Transplant Recipients (SRTR), Eurotransplant, the North American Transplant Coordinators Organization (NATCO), the National Association of Medical Examiners (NAME), the United Network for Organ Sharing (UNOS) contractor of the Organ Procurement Transplant Network (OPTN), the Division of Transplantation of the Department of Health and Human Services (DOT), Centers for Medicare and Medicaid Services (CMS), the National Kidney Foundation (NKF) and the World Health Organization (WHO). The neuroscience community was represented by renowned physicians from the Neurocritical Care Society. Distinguished bioethicists from the medical and lay community participated as well. They were broken into six working groups to address different questions with the report of their conclusion now published in American Journal of Transplantation. This is an overview of that report and is the most current thinking on DCD.

The Institute of Medicine (IOM), SCCM, and JCAHO have concluded that "DCD is an ethically proper approach of recovering organs from a deceased patient for the purpose of transplantation." (8,16-19) When the withdrawal of life support has been consensually decided by the attending physician and patient, or by the attending physician and family member or surrogate (particularly in the hospital setting of the intensive care unit), a routine opportunity for DCD should now be available to all families for consideration and to honor deceased donor wishes. The message derived from the conference was to convey a societal responsibility that regularly enables organ transplantation from deceased donors, determined to be dead either by circulatory or brain criteria. The ethical axiom of organ donation is to adhere to the dead donor rule: the retrieval of organs for transplantation should not cause the death of a donor.(20,21) The circulatory criterion of death (used in DCD) is employed when the donor does not fulfill brain death tests, ventilatory support has been withdrawn, and circulation and respiration cease. In clinical situations where death is expected: once respiration and circulation cease (irrespective of electrical cardiac activity), the period of observation necessary to determine that circulation will not recur spontaneously (autoresuscitation) may be only a few minutes. In analyzing current data on auto-resuscitation, the relevant event is cessation of circulation; it is not cessation of electrical activity. When life-sustaining therapy is withdrawn, based on the limited data available, spontaneous circulation does not return after two minutes of cessation of circulation. A survey of all OPOs conducted for the DCD conference determined that 92% (47) of all OPOs use a five-minute interval from asystole to the declaration of death, consistent with the IOM recommendations. Nevertheless, there are four OPOs that use an interval of two minutes (3 OPOs) and four minutes (1 OPO).(8) The Society of Critical Care Medicine (SCCM) concluded that "at least two minutes of observation is required, and more than five minutes is not recommended".(18)

> "This decision to withdraw or withhold treatments should be made on its own merit, with the patient's physician having established the futility of any further treatment, and not for the purpose of organ donation. Decisions regarding the suitability of a donor should be made by the OPO in consultation with the patient's health care providers. The administration of sedatives and opioids should be the same as that which is customary for all end-of-life care and should treat patient discomfort and/or the appearance of discomfort."(8) Evidence based clinical judgment should be used to assess whether cardiac death will likely occur within a time period allowing successful DCD. The University of Wisconsin has developed an algorithm for the assessment of the potential DCD donor.(22) A score is computed which is based upon the patients age, BMI, O2 saturation, method of intubation (endotracheal versus tracheostomy), level of spontaneous respiration, and the requirement for vasopressors, all of which indicate the likelihood of death within one hour after extubation."

For DCD to occur requires the willing participation of the attending physician or their designee, often a critical care physician. This physician has to be present at withdrawal of support and pronounce death. The location where this occurs is different across the country and different OPO service areas. In the Northwest, it is usually done in the ICU and the patient is then rapidly transported to the operating room, but in many locations the withdrawal of support is done in the operating room. Each individual hospital usually sets its own policy regarding how these cases will be conducted. It is important to select potential donors that will expire in a prescribed period of time. This selection process is imperfect and the family must be informed and prepared that the death may not occur in a timely fashion and, if it does not, the loved one will be transported to a comfort care setting for observation. Also, it varies across the country whether the family can be present at the time of death or not, with the ICU setting being friendlier for the family to be present. Once death is pronounced, it is important that the organs be recovered in a very timely fashion to minimize warm ischemic time. If the family is to be present, it is important to prepare them: for donation to

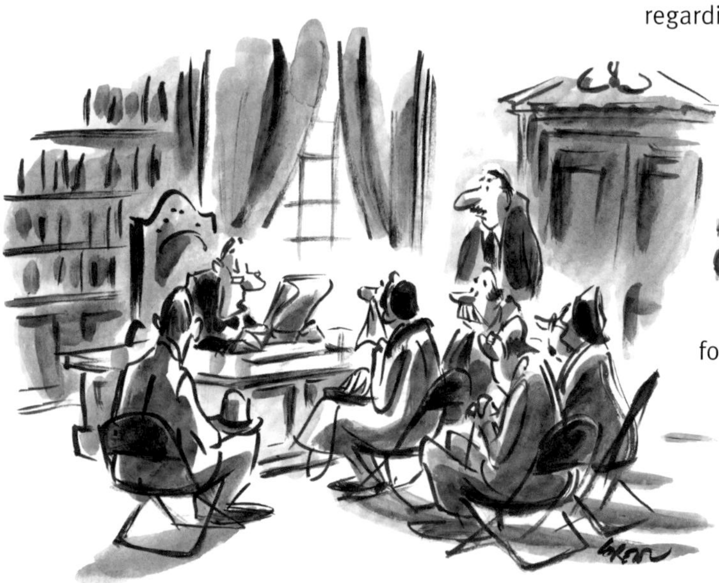

"Not much in the way of hard assets, I'm afraid, but he did leave some highly desirable organs."

be successful they must depart or the patient must be moved upon death declaration.

Organs recovered from DCD donors potentially could make up 10% of organs donated. At the time of writing this chapter, this is only occurring in 3 to 4 service areas. Organs that are being transplanted from this class of donors are kidneys, livers, lungs and in some cases hearts. Kidneys transplanted from DCD patients do almost as well as kidneys from standard donors, and better than kidneys from high risk donors. Livers do not do quite as well with about a 10% decrease in graft and patient survival compared to standard donors.(8) Lungs are being transplanted at several centers with some reports that outcomes are similar to standard donors.(23) At some meetings, it has been suggested that the effects of brain death on the activation of a generalized inflammatory response may not be seen in the DCD donor.

The attending physician plays a key role in communication with families of the potential DCD organ donor patient. It involves coordination and a group effort, bringing together a supportive family, an informed and willing attending physician, the OPO clinical staff, and the recovery team all working together to make the gift of life.

Tissue Donation

Tissue donation improves the quality of the life for many recipients. Most of the time, tissue transplantation is life enhancing. Take for instance the life of one of my most popular internal medicine professors. In his later years, he could not see well enough to recognize who might be speaking to him. As he walked through the halls of the college of medicine, it was apparent that this distressed him because he could not recognize people's faces. I even quit speaking to him to avoid distressing him. One day I slipped and said, "Good afternoon, Dr. Purple," and he said, "Oh, hi Bill, how are you doing?" I then learned that he had received corneal transplants. What a difference that donation made in the quality of his life.

The daughter of another close friend was a scholarship soccer player and she loved soccer. Unfortunately, she blew out her anterior cruciate ligament (ACL) and could not play. Reconstructive surgery was done using a human ACL, and after physical therapy and rehabilitation she was able to return to the sport that she loved. This was very important to her life, her sense of self esteem, and self worth.

An example of tissue transplantation improving both the quantity and quality of life is provided by this case. A teenage girl had severe aortic valve disease. The Ross procedure was performed on her (the diseased aortic valve was replaced with her own pulmonic valve and then her pulmonary valve was reconstructed with a donated human pulmonary valve conduit). This operation gave a wonderful anatomical and physiological result. It also did not require any use of anticoagulation after surgery. She graduated from high school and attended a nationally prominent university where she swam competitively for the swim team. She then went on to graduate from medical school. This operation is also ideal for women who want to have children because the use of human tissue graft removes the risk of thromboembolism and, therefore, the risk of taking anticoagulation. In addition, recent evaluation demonstrates her hypertrophied left ventricle has returned to normal. There is some risk that her human graft will eventually calcify and require replacement, but since it is now on the right side of her heart, the risk of re-operation is reduced.

Tissues that are now routinely recovered include bone, tendons, ligaments, joints en bloc, skin, saphenous vein, iliac vessels, aorto-iliac arteries, heart valves and corneas. There are an estimated 750,000 to 1 million tissue grafts performed in the USA each year.(24) It is commonly done at community hospitals as well as large tertiary care centers. Any hospital that has an active surgery program for orthopedics will likely be doing tissue grafts. The most common human allograft performed is bone. Bone grafts are used by a number of surgical specialties. Skin is recovered and made into a de-cellurized dermal graft. This product is very useful for managing infected abdominal wounds as an alternative to Marlextm mesh. The de-cellurized dermal graft has good strength and can be used for closure of abdominal wounds. It serves as a matrix for in-growth of vasculature and is resistant to infection.(25) There seem to be fewer small bowel fistulas with this closure than with prosthetic material. Aorto-iliac grafts are also useful in infected operative fields for replacement of infected Dacrontm grafts.(26) Other vascular grafts such as the saphenous vein are used for limb salvage when the patient has no usable conduit for auto grafting.

Infectious Disease Transmission

Infectious disease can be transmitted by both organ and tissue transplant.(27) While the best tool for reducing this risk is still a careful medical social history, it may not identify all risks. For example, West Nile virus has been transmitted by organ transplant. In the first report, all four organ recipients developed infection, three had encephalitis and one died.(28) After investigation, it was concluded that the donor received an infected blood transfusion during the donor's resuscitation. The Red Cross now pools multiple units of blood and does nucleic acid testing (NAT) for West Nile along with HIV, HBV and HCV prior to the blood being released. Another case of organ transplant transmission has been reported with two of the four organ recipients developing encephalitis and coma.(29) The donor history was vague, but the donor had spent a lot of time outdoors and had a febrile illness prior to the head injury. Recently rabies was transmitted from an organ donor to all four organ recipients, having a fatal outcome.(30) When this was investigated, one of the donor's friends recalled that the patient had been bitten by a bat. Unfortunately there is not a good laboratory test for rabies that can be performed in a timely manner to screen organ donors.

In 2001 there was a death of a 23-year-old following reconstructive knee surgery from clostridia infection transmitted by allograph tissue transplant. The CDC investigated this case and found 26 other cases of various types of infection probably transmitted by tissue grafts.(31) Many tissue allografts are not sterilized because it would damage the collagen. Some tissue is radiated but the dose to kill clostridia spores may not be achieved. The FDA now requires tissue processors to increase the level of surveillance and to perform many more cultures of tissue during processing to reduce this risk.

A tissue and organ donor in the Northwest that had negative antibodies for HCV later fulfilled Koch's postulates, and multiple organ tissue recipients became infected with HCV.(32) This infection was in the time window between infection and developing antibody. This is always a possibility when using serological test. The FDA now requires that all tissue donors have NAT testing for HIV, HBV and HCV. This can be accomplished on tissue donors while the tissue is being processed and before release. For organ donors there is not yet the capacity to do NAT testing in real time. There are pilot projects going on in California where real time NAT testing is being done on organ donors. At some point in the future this will likely be required on all organ donors. At the time of this writing, NAT testing is not feasible nationally due to the time limitations required for organ transplantation. Regardless of how many screening tests are performed, there is always going to be a small risk of transmitting an infectious disease by organ or tissue transplantation.

Careful examination of the organ and tissue donation process makes clear that a well trained team providing a coordinated communication effort with the treatment team can significantly increase the organ and tissue donation rate and provide much needed support to the family during this end of life stress. The need for donated organs and tissues continues to increase every year. Despite the benefit, there continues to be a real but very small risk of harm (including the risk of death) as a result of receiving an organ or tissue transplant. The heightened stress level for the family increases the likelihood of poor communication of these complex issues. Only optimum communication can bring a positive outcome to a patient death.

REFERENCES

1. Nathan HM, Conrad SL, Held PJ, et al. Organ donation in the United States. Am J Transplant. 2003; 3 Suppl 4:29-40.
2. US Department of Health and Human Services; Health Resources and Services Administration, Office of Special Programs, Division of Transplantation. The Organ Donation Breakthrough Collaborative: Best Practices Final Report. Washington, DC; Sept 2003.
3. Shafer TJ, Davis KD, Holtzman SM, Van Buren CT, Crafts NJ, Durand R. Location of in-house organ procurement organization staff in level I trauma centers increases conversion of potential donors to actual donors. Transplant. 2003; 75(8):1330-1335.
4. Gortmaker SL, Beasley CL, Sheehy E, Grenvik A et al. Improving the request process to increase family consent for organ donation. J Transpl Coord. 1998; 8(4):210-217.
5. Roth BJ, Sher L, Murray JA, Belzberg H, Mateo R, Heeran A et al. Cadaveric organ donor recruitment at Los Angeles County Hospital: improvement after formation of a structured clinical, educational and administrative service. Clin Transplant 2003; 17 Suppl 9:52-57.
6. Siminoff LA, Gordon N, Hewlett J, Arnold RM. Factors influencing families' consent for donation of solid organs for transplantation. JAMA. 2001; 286(1):71-77.
7. Wood KE, Becker BN, McCartney JG, D'Alessandro AM, Coursin DB. Care of the potential organ donor. N Engl J Med. 2004; 351(26):2730-2739.
8. Bernat JL, D'Alessandro AM, Port FK, et al. Report of a National Conference on Donation after cardiac death. Am J Transplant 2006; 6(2):281-291.
9. Siminoff LA, Mercer MB. Public policy, public opinion, and consent for organ donation. Camb Q Healthc Ethics. 2001; 10(4):377-386.
10. Siminoff LA, Lawrence RH, Zhang A. Decoupling: what is it and does it really help increase consent to organ donation? Prog Transplant. 2002; 12(1):52-60.
11. Kubler-Ross E. On Death and Dying. New York: Touchstone; 1997.
12. Shafer TJ, Ehrle RN, Davis KD, et al. Increasing organ recovery from level I trauma centers: the in-house coordinator intervention. Prog Transplant. 2004; 14(3):250-263.
13. US Department of Health and Human Services, Organ Donation Breakthrough Collaborative; 2006.
14. The US Organ Procurement and Transplantation Network and the Scientific Registry of Transplant Recipients. 2006 OPTN/SRTR Annual Report: Transplant Data 1996-2005. Available at www.ustransplant.org/annual_reports/current. Accessed 9-12-07.
15. Shafer TJ, Schkade LL, Evans RW, O'Connor KJ, Reitsma W. Vital role of medical examiners and coroners in organ transplantation. Am J Transplant. 2004; 4(2):160-168.
16. Institute of Medicine, National Academy of Sciences. Non-heart-beating organ transplantation: medical and ethical issues in procurement. Washington (DC): National Academy Press; 1997.
17. Institute of Medicine, National Academy of Sciences. Non-heart-beating organ transplantation: practice and protocols. Washington (DC): National Academy Press; 2000.
18. Recommendations for non-heart-beating organ donation. A position paper by the Ethics Committee, American College of Critical Care Medicine, Society of Critical Care Medicine. Crit Care Med 2001; 29(9):1826-1831.

19. Health Care at the Crossroads: Strategies for Narrowing the Organ Donation Gap and Protecting Patients. Joint Commission on the Accreditation of Hospital Organizations; 2004.
20. Robertson J. The dead donor rule. Hastings Cent Rep. 1999; 29(6):6-14.
21. Siminoff LA. The dead donor rule: not dead yet. Am J Bioeth. 2003; 3(1):30.
22. Lewis J, Peltier J, Nelson H, Snyder W, Schneider K, Steinberger D et al. Development of the University of Wisconsin donation After Cardiac Death Evaluation Tool. Prog Transplant. 2003; 13(4):265-273.
23. D'Alessandro AM, Fernandez LA, Chin LT, et al. Donation after cardiac death: the University of Wisconsin experience. Ann Transplant 2004; 9(1):68-71.
24. Ochs R, Kerr K. Safety, ethics questioned in tissue transplant industry. San Francisco Chronicle. 2006 Jan 22; A-6.
25. Scott BG, Welsh FJ, Pham HQ, et al. Early aggressive closure of the open abdomen. J Trauma. 2006; 601:17-22.
26. Vogt PR, von Segesser LK, Goffin Y, et al. Eradication of aortic infections with the use of cryopreserved arterial homografts. Ann Thorac Surg. 1996; 62(3):640-645.
27. Zou S, Dodd RY, Stramer SL, Strong DM. Probability of viremia with HBV, HCV, HIV, and HTLV among tissue donors in the United States. N Engl J Med. 2004; 351(8):751-759.
28. Iwamoto M, Jernigan DB, Guasch A, Trepka MJ, Blackmore CG, Hellinger WC et al. Transmission of West Nile virus from an organ donor to four transplant recipients. N Engl J Med. 2003; 348(22):2196-2203.
29. West Nile Virus Infections in Organ Transplant Recipients. MMWR 54 Dispatch[1-3]. 2005. 10-5-2005.
30. Srinivasan A, Burton EC, Kuehnert MJ, et al. Transmission of rabies virus from an organ donor to four transplant recipients. N Engl J Med. 2005; 352(11):1103-1111.
31. Update: Allograft-Associated Bacterial Infections-United States 2002. MMWR . 2002. CDC. 3-15-2002.
32. Hepatitis C Virus Transmission from an Antibody-Negative Organ and Tissue Donor. MMWR 52[13], 273-276. 2003. CDC. 4-4-2003.

Children: Monosyllabic Conversations

Marcene McVay, MD; Samuel Smith, MD

> "I'm not Cheryl," she protested loudly, after the surgeon had begun introductions. With that, five-year-old Cheryl marched into the office, leaving her mother in the waiting room. Seeming to ignore the doctor, she began to play, neighing like a horse.

Speaking to children is not particularly difficult, but communicating therapeutically can be a challenge. Communication with people of all ages requires taking into account verbal, nonverbal, and symbolic avenues of expression. Adults generally believe that they communicate about themselves primarily with words. Children, however, are masters at picking up on nonverbal cues. They have been doing so from infancy, when they intuitively came to understand their caretakers' facial expressions, inflections, posture, timing, and mood long before they were able to comprehend the literal content of their speech. At times of stress, such as a medical encounter, children often rely on this previously mastered capacity to determine how to feel about the interaction.

Interviewing children, therefore, is a constant challenge to a surgeon's ingenuity. Certain general principles serve as important guides for fostering meaningful communication and accomplishing the goals of the interview.

One overriding principle in dealing with children and their parents is to respect the child and his or her feelings, regardless of age. As with any patient communication, surgeons need to take the time to watch, listen and try to understand what may not be immediately apparent.

WHO TO INCLUDE IN THE INTERVIEW

Except in the case of adolescents, it is common for the doctor to meet with the parents to obtain their views on what is transpiring. Whether the child is actually present during the initial parent/doctor interview depends on many factors: the age of the child, the type of problem, the health care setting and the preferences of the doctor and those of the parents.

In general, children who understand and use verbal communication can be interviewed along with their parents. Younger children can be allowed to play in the same room. However, surgeons must be aware that certain subjects of inquiry are delicate and should not be broached in front of children.

During a visit to a pediatrics ward to do a consultation many years ago, one of the authors observed the chief of child psychiatry engaged with a child. Oblivious to any adult presence, he was stooped over introducing himself to a young child in pajamas. Then they both settled crosslegged on the floor to chat.

While not every doctor is willing to sit on the floor to accommodate a young patient, this vignette serves as an illustration of the need to meet children at their own level, both in terms of the physical dynamics and the choice of words.

In child psychiatry, where parent interviews are apt to be lengthy and children typically are uncomfortable being talked about, it is customary to see the parents of preadolescent children alone for the initial interview. In these circumstances, there must be a transition between the parent interaction and the interview with the child, and this transition is an important determinant of the tone of the subsequent doctor/child dialogue. An approach used frequently is for the surgeon to make some comments in front of both the parents and the child often in the waiting room. This allows the nature of the parents' concerns or reasons for bringing the child to be detailed, and basically gives the child permission to cooperate with the doctor during the interview.

When conversing with adolescents, the prevailing wisdom is that speaking with them first is an important ingredient in building trust. Teenagers are otherwise prone to believing that the doctor is their parents' agent and has been primed to reflect their parents' biases. Alternatively, beginning the interview with everyone together allows the parents to state their concerns in front of their child. If the surgeon has already been given information or opinions by the teenager's parents, it is often helpful to share this judiciously with the child, who will then realize the surgeon's forthrightness.

An important corollary is that parents must be forewarned of this need to share with their teenager, so that they will have advance notice that communications about their child will not be secret. Typically, personal details about parents' backgrounds and relationships are not automatically shared with teenagers.

An elective umbilical hernia repair of a 15-year-old female is canceled due to a positive urine pregnancy test obtained the morning of surgery. The surgeon is notified and meets with the patient and her mother to discuss the situation.

"Why has my daughter's surgery been cancelled?" asks the mother.

"Well," the surgeon replies, looking at the teenage girl, "although we will certainly be willing to repair your hernia in the future, we won't be able to repair it today."

"What is it?" queries the mother again, her daughter's face also quizzical.

"Well, your daughter's pregnancy test, which we routinely perform before surgeries in adolescent female patients, is positive." An awkward pause is followed by, "We can't do elective surgery today because you're pregnant."

"WHAT?" the mother shrieks, looking angrily at her daughter. An argument between the two ensues ...

Clearly, several other options for handling this difficult situation are possible. Meeting with the daughter first or with a social worker or nurse (who can stay with the adolescent patient for the important moment of telling the mother why the surgery is canceled today), would decrease the public display of emotion. Hopefully, the nurse or social worker can stay behind to answer other questions and help keep things as calm as possible.

BEGINNING FRAMEWORK

Introductions are a basic starting point and set the tone for the exchange. It is helpful to ask children how they wish to be addressed and to find out from them their perceived purpose for the visit. Not infrequently, children will indicate by means of shrugs or blank looks that the reason for the encounter escapes them. In that event, the surgeon may give a brief synopsis of concerns to facilitate dialogue. Examples of such an opening include: "Your parents are concerned that you have been waking up every night screaming and coming into their room," or "Your teacher and principal are worried that you have not been going to school, and your parents don't know what to do." Language should be direct, descriptive and nonjudgmental. Talking down to children is every bit as problematic as talking above their heads. Ask them if they understand and can talk more about what is happening. The degree to which children will engage in direct verbal interchange as opposed to more tangential stories and play depends on the doctor, the setting, and the child's stage of development.

In pediatric interviews, familiarity breeds comfort, not contempt. Surgeons should give children time to get used to the room. Children may want to hold the stethoscope or touch and examine various instruments before they are used.

Surgeons need to speak directly and make eye contact. With younger children, the surgeon may sometimes choose to stoop to their level. A surgeon does not need to talk to children in a regressed and unnatural style. It is also not usually helpful to speak in a gushing or high-pitched way. The choice of words must be both understandable and acceptable to the child. This lays the groundwork for approaching sensitive or embarrassing aspects of their condition or physical examination, which can generally only take place once a basic alliance has been established. Sometimes the surgeon must recognize the need to stop and start over in order to re-establish the relationship with the child.

Eight-year-old Jessica presents to the surgery clinic with her parents after having been referred for evaluation of chronic diarrhea and incontinence. After a junior surgery resident presented the history outside the room, the surgeon enters the exam room to find Jessica curled in her mother's lap. During introductions, the surgeon smiles and offers his hand to Jessica saying, "Hi there, you must be Jessica, I will need to check your bottom."

She immediately begins to cry and loudly protests, "NO!" while burying her face in her mother's body.

Apparent that no cooperation will be gained from his patient, the surgeon continues with interviewing her parents. Jessica continues to cry during the interview, despite the surgeon's best attempts to ignore her. Her parents become increasingly frustrated as the conversation continues. The surgeon finally asks if Jessica always acts this way.

Jessica's mother explains snappily, "She's had so many different doctors stick their finger up her bottom, but no one can figure out what's wrong with her. Are you going to tell us what the problem is or should we just leave now and stop torturing her?"

"I'm terribly sorry, but I think we have started off on the wrong foot here," the surgeon responds, noting that the situation will not likely improve on its present course. "Why don't we try starting over? I will go out and come back in so we can restart from the beginning." Two minutes later, Jessica and her parents hear a knock on the door. "Good afternoon, I am Dr. Jones. What brings you to see us today?"

In new encounters with patients, it is important to try and find out what the hot buttons or cultural taboos are that can cause a clinic or hospital visit to go off the tracks before you find out the hard way. Sometimes apologizing, calling time out and starting over can rescue a bad start.

Young children are very egocentric, and can often misinterpret facial expressions as being directed toward them. For example, a frown of concentration can be misinterpreted as disapproval or rejection. The surgeon needs to pay attention to the patient's and family's nonverbal communications, as well as to his or her own. It is thus vitally important for clinicians to be aware not only of verbal communications but of the many ambient and nonverbal factors which can contribute significantly to the underlying mood of pediatric interviews.

A surgeon enters 10-year-old Jimmy's room on the pediatrics ward of the hospital after his primary physician has requested an excisional lymph node biopsy for possible lymphoma. Jimmy was admitted to the hospital with high fevers and diffusely enlarged lymph nodes, but all tests have been inconclusive regarding the origin of his illness.

Upon entering the room, the surgeon introduces herself to both the child and his parents. Immediately and in hushed tones, the parents ask if the surgeon will speak to them outside of the patient's room. After closing the door behind her, the mother states, "I know that Jimmy's doctor has asked you to take out one of his lymph nodes. She thinks it could be cancer, is that right?"

"Yes," the surgeon replies. "It could be lymphoma or it could only be an infection."

"Well, whatever it is, we don't want Jimmy to know about it. It will only upset him," the mother states firmly.

The surgeon then inquires if Jimmy knows about the possibility of surgery. The mother makes it clear that she does not want him to be made aware of the nature of his upcoming procedure. She especially does not want him to know that surgery has even been scheduled until the day it will occur.

This is a difficult dilemma for many pediatric specialists, but you should always be firm that the child has to be included in the conversation before a procedure or test can be done. It is important to make clear that even a minor child's concerns and questions are important and must be answered in addition to the guardian giving consent.

SETTING

The setting for interviewing a child bears close attention. Regardless of whether the child is in a clinic, private office, or hospital bed, it is usually possible to maximize effective interaction by restructuring the environment as necessary to suit the purpose of the interview, as well as the child's stage of development.

An office or clinic should be bright, cheerful and child-oriented with materials and decorations for preschoolers, school aged and adolescent patients and their parents. If the interview is at the bedside or in the emergency room or any other less controlled setting, the examiner can still bring in some materials to set the child at ease, such as a small teddy bear or animal which clips on to a stethoscope, or small animal figures kept in the coat pocket. A cloth puppet takes very little space.

Preadolescents and teenagers generally are put off by toys, but can often be reached by more adult behavior, such as starting a conversation about recent sporting events, local news or school activities.

PRIVACY

With school aged and older children, it is especially important to respect their sense of privacy, although certain concerns may be more pertinent at one age than at another. While undressing may be excruciating for a second or third grader, confidentiality is less important for this age group since they often assume that all information will be shared with parents. It is often extremely important, however, to be circumspect with information sharing when dealing with adolescents.

Some topics are highly charged and the clinician must discuss and establish appropriate parameters in the early phases of the interview. In some specific cases, patients and parents must be told in advance that solicited information may, or perhaps must, be shared with agencies and other people. This includes suicidal or homicidal intentions, child abuse, sexual abuse or neglect, certain types of delinquency, and dangerous and self-destructive behaviors.

CHILD'S STAGE OF DEVELOPMENT

Careful descriptive research has demonstrated that child development evolves longitudinally according to generally predictable perspectives in several domains. These areas include biological, cognitive, language, psychosocial, psychosexual and moral development. Children do not necessarily progress at the same pace in each domain, underscoring the need to tailor language and approach to the needs of each individual child.

Nevertheless, it is helpful to envision children as undergoing developmental stages in an orderly and sequential fashion, with each stage characterized by underlying developmental themes and preoccupations. The stress of a medical encounter is then superimposed on the normative emotional, psychosocial and cognitive challenges which make up a patient who appears before the clinician.

One of the major developmental preoccupations of young infants is understanding social reciprocity and the subtle rules of social interactions. Therefore, it is important to approach them gently and in a stepwise fashion. The infant should be examined on the parent's lap and it is often more comforting for the infant to be examined in an upright or a sitting position than supine. The examiner may make use of soft vocalizations and cooing sounds and should avoid abrupt large motor movements or facial looming.

With toddlers, where one of the predominant developmental issues is separation individuation, it is very important to allow maternal access when needed and to reassure them that their mothers will not leave the office area during examinations. On other occasions, it is helpful to begin the interview in the parents' presence. When a sufficient level of comfort has been reached for parent/child separation to occur, the child should be reassured that the parents will remain in the waiting room. A matter-of-fact flexibility is often the key to obtaining cooperation.

The surgeon needs to remember that the negativism of the two and three-year-old often serves the purpose of preserving the newly developed autonomy of the child. Therefore, it needs to be respected and not necessarily confronted. Distraction is an important device for this age group. As with the infant, one needs to take time with the toddler and use slow and tentative, rather than forced, interplays.

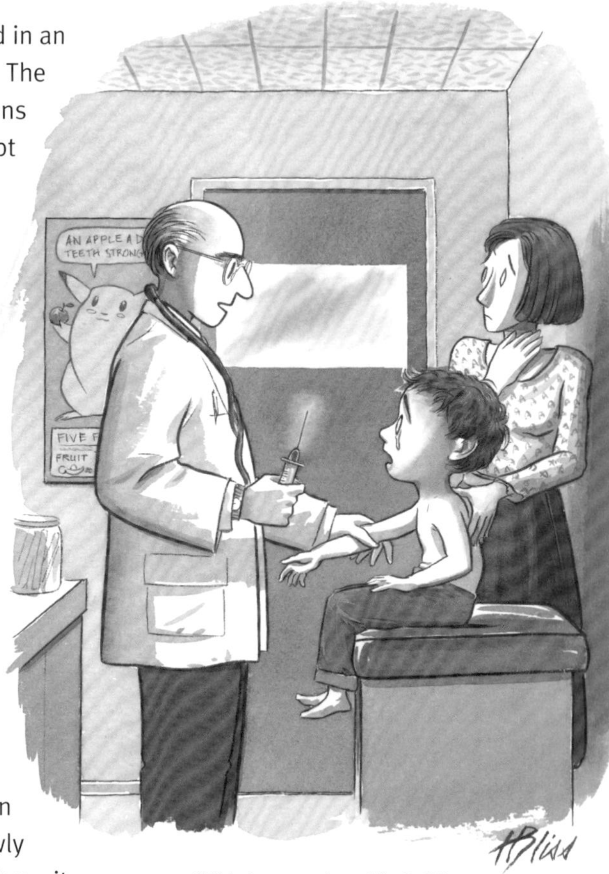

"This is gonna hurt like hell."

For three and four-year-olds, while themes of separation remain important, there are now additional preoccupations with bodily integrity and fears of violation and mutilation. Children of this age need to be reassured that routine procedures will not lead to drastic consequences. Cause and effect thinking for the preschool child is often quite magical and their logic is very idiosyncratic.

While the thinking of school age children begins to approach the kind of cause and effect reasoning of adults, there is nevertheless a preoccupation with fitting in with peers and with the privacy of one's own body. Bodily functions and displays can be quite shameful and must be treated by the clinician with a great deal of respect. School aged children are enormously curious. One of the most important developmental themes of this age is mastery. They clearly want to know explanations of how, why, and what. They are also very concrete and literal. They can be expected to follow rules once they understand them, and to be rather obsessive in their attention to details and categories of objects.

Adolescents, on the other hand, are often much less organized, though better able to deal with abstractions. One of their underlying themes is independence and consolidating a sense of identity about themselves. They can be particularly put off by authoritarian interchanges, while at the same time feeling quite omnipotent and grandiose. They tend to answer questions with monosyllabic words "yeah," "neah," "no" and "yes."

TIMING AND SEQUENCE OF QUESTIONS

Inquiries about psychiatric difficulties, sexual behaviors, and other delicate subjects are better left toward the end of the interview. Showing disapproval, but also sometimes approval, can markedly affect or diminish openness. Kids often keep their worst fears to themselves; imagined outcomes are usually much worse than the real ones. Certain words and euphemisms carry much power with children and it is important to find out from the parents, or from the child directly, their special words for pain (e.g. "Owwie"), genitals, excrement and urine.

Validating behaviors are quite facilitative during an interview, but should usually be considered different from overt approval. Examples of validating behavior include empathic eye contact, nodding and reciprocity in mood and body language. Yet just as validating behaviors may be helpful, children and parents also pay attention to invalidating behaviors such as yawning, fidgeting, or looking at one's watch which creates a negative environment for openness and honesty.

It is important to be aware of and guard against snap judgments and biases. One should develop hypotheses early in the interview and try to clarify them objectively by assembling information clues. It is important not to talk too much, to make use of silences and to observe. In interviewing parents, be aware of repetitions, phrases, striking metaphors, offhanded statements that seem vaguely inappropriate, and discrepancies. When observing young children, be aware of recurrent play themes, and especially what is happening just before or during a break in play and a switch to a different play material. The following case scenario addresses the common difficulty of getting from the chief complaint to the problem of greatest concern to the parents and patient.

Damien, a 12-year-old boy, is brought to clinic by his mother and grandmother for evaluation of breast masses. He is obese and exam reveals symmetrical disk-shaped subareolar masses consistent with benign gynecomastia. It is explained to the patient and his family that this commonly occurs in pubertal males who are obese. The surgeon recommends a weight loss program before surgery is considered. The mother, however, is adamant that the breast tissue be removed, despite repeated objections by Damien. After several minutes of discussion, the surgeon suggests the patient and mother discuss the situation further on their own, taking into consideration the recommendations made to them in clinic that day.

The surgeon hands the mother his business card and starts to leave. His hand is on the doorknob when he pauses and asks the family if there is anything else before he leaves. The patient's mother asks, "So it's not cancer?"

The surgeon turns and reassuringly replies, "No ma'am, very unlikely." He again turns to the door.

"But how can you be sure? I just lost a sister to breast cancer and I am worried that this could be cancer." The mother says with a little gasp.

The surgeon sits back down to explain all the reasons that breast cancer is not a worry in this clinical setting, noting the relief in the eyes of both the patient and his mother.

This is a frequent occurrence with patient encounters and you should never miss the opportunity to address the real reason the family or patient is concerned or worried.

SPECIAL INTERVIEW SITUATIONS

Discussing Pain with Children

When aspects of the examination, tests to be conducted or the course of the illness will be painful, a straightforward approach is best. While it might be tempting to perform the procedure or test first and explain later, such a sequence leads to future fears and mistrust. However disrupting active protests can be, the child will at some level appreciate being told in advance about the pain and rely on the doctor for future warnings.

Similarly, wherever possible, it is helpful to use additional medical support staff for reassurance and calming, rather than trying to "outmuscle" the child. Where restraint is necessary to perform a procedure or examination, it should always be firm but gentle and accompanied by narrative reassurance of what is going to take place. For minor procedures, such as venipunctures and shots, parents are often able to assist. With elaborate procedures, support staff are more appropriate, since parents may become distressed themselves. For many procedures in babies and young children, swaddling is used as a means of restraint. Once again, usually a candid explanation of the sequence is essential and appreciated beyond what the vocal complaints would indicate.

Child Abuse

The complex subject of physical, sexual, and emotional abuse has become almost a clinical subspecialty in its own right. While it is not possible to discuss the subject comprehensively here, some general principles should be kept in mind.

Clearly, the clinician must always be alert to the possibility of abuse. The observation of aberrant parent/child interactions in the waiting room or office should raise the index of suspicion; for instance, a child who displays extreme fearfulness, avoidance, or excessive disinterest toward a parent, or an 8- to 18-month-old who does not demonstrate infant separation protest or stranger anxiety. By the same token, an older child displaying these and the opposite affectations, such as cloying eagerness to please, anxious clinging, over-accommodation and inappropriate guilt, are also worrisome. From the parents' standpoint, marked family dysfunction, vindictiveness, volatility, parental apathy and egocentrism often coexist with abuse and neglect.

In the office, surgeons should be aware of the content of observed symbolic play, such as overly repetitive themes of a doll or animal being naughty, beaten, locked up or sadistically victimized. Compulsive masturbation, eroticized behaviors, precocious preoccupation with sexual matters and frequent runaway behavior in teenagers are suggestive of inappropriate overstimulation and possible sexual misuse. Some typical indicators of physical abuse are bruises and lacerations in various stages of healing, scars, a history of broken bones, vaginal or urinary infections, rectal fissures and repeated unnecessary emergency room visits for infants.

If abuse seems apparent or is alluded to by an older child or adolescent, it is important to take up

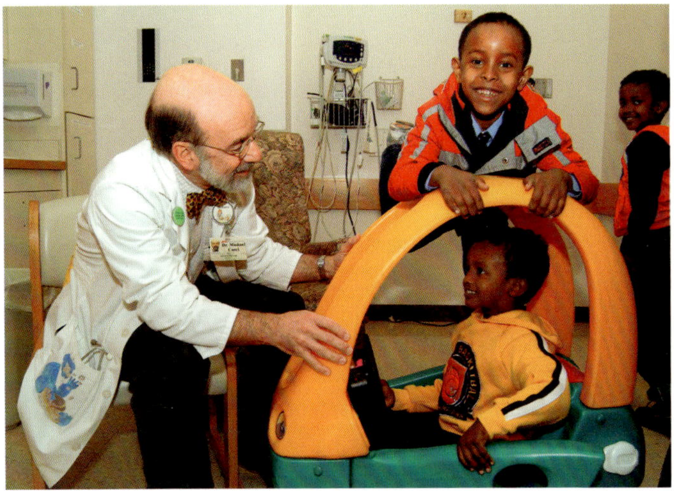

the issue directly in a straightforward fashion, rather than fumbling euphemistically or inquiring at length about peripheral matters. Otherwise, the child will become increasingly anxious or put off by the interviewer's embarrassment and avoidance. On the other hand, if there is a vague suspicion of abuse but it is not central to the interview, the clinician will want to build a rapport before sensitively opening up this area.

In the preschooler and young child, nonverbal and symbolic expressions must often be relied upon more than direct disclosures. Drawings, play themes and behavior aimed at the interviewer over time can often be revealing, but may take several sessions to emerge. Many children who have been abused are frightened by routine pediatric contacts with their bodies. Approach them slowly, asking permission to touch them, and then proceed without sudden movements. Specific inquiry should initially be open-ended, such as "Has anyone ever touched your private parts?" and not directive. Talking about sexual abuse with children often requires considerable rapport because of guilt and shame. Dolls and drawings often allow more comfortable communication.

When strong suspicion of sexual and physical abuse arises, it is important to turn to experienced colleagues to arrange for more definitive investigation.

However, the surgeon should never end the interview without being assured of the capacity of the parents to protect the child in the interim. If the suspected perpetrator is in the family or immediate environment, the safety of the child must be guarded by making emergency contact with the local protective agency or child abuse team.

Using an Interpreter

It's important for a surgeon to use trained interpreters, or at least interpreters who are outside the patient's family but with whom the surgeon is acquainted. Unfortunately, many families bring an older child to do their interpreting for them. When that happens, the surgeon must keep in mind the cognitive and developmental level of the interpreting child. The need for literality of the translation should be stressed. The doctor should watch the person speaking and try to read body language even if unable to understand the actual words. The surgeon should always expect that the family understands some English and therefore, should be careful of what is said to other English speaking people in front of the family.

Giving Feedback to Parents

It is a common saying among parents that they get the blame for whatever is wrong, but are not entitled to the credit for what is right. When dealing with behavior, it seems more helpful to ask if it accomplishes the desired outcome than to label it intrinsically right or wrong. Given that it is most often the parents who bring the child to see the doctor, it is safe to assume something is troubling them. Incorporating the parents' concerns when offering feedback is a powerful means of forging an alliance and getting around the less useful concept of blame.

Parents are motivated to address a surgeon's comments constructively when they genuinely feel the feedback will help them rectify some of their concerns. When faced with nonjudgmental evidence that certain behaviors are not effective, coupled with clear examples of alternatives, parents are typically receptive and appreciative. A practical working alliance can be established with parents by employing this collaborative format. Interestingly, most children are pleased about these negotiations. They view them as a vehicle for modifying problematic situations with which they have been struggling themselves.

CONCLUSION

Interviewing children and their parents can be a challenge, but one that is certainly surmountable. It is essential to understand the dynamics of interviews with children of different ages and make appropriate modifications in the surroundings, involvement of parents and siblings and in the way the child is addressed. Some of the barriers to effective communication are listed in the following table.

It is important to gauge how much the surgeon should talk, neither overwhelming the child nor allowing prolonged silences. Avoid levity or gravity and never be pompous. Listen and inquire to uncover the problem and resist any tendency to premature closure of ideas. Never be condescending, avoid cutting off inquiries or comments from the child or parents and never give pat reassurances. If confronted, do not react defensively. Try to draw out the child and parents to discover the reason for their aggressive stance. Be alert for signs of abuse, but do not let suspicion dominate the interview.

Above all, appreciate the child as an individual. Include the parents to an appropriate degree, thereby making all the parties partners in the evaluation of the problem and the formulation of the treatment plan.

SELECTED REFERENCES

1. Sackett DL, Rennie D. The science of the art of the clinical examination. JAMA. 1992; 267:2650-52.
2. American Academy of Pediatrics Committee on Practice and Ambulatory Medicine. The use of chaperones during the physical examination of the pediatric patient. Pediatrics 1996; 98:1202. http://aappolicy.aappublications.org/cgi/reprint/pediatrics;98/6/1202.pdf. Accessed 10/1/07.
3. Miller, GA. The magical number seven plus or minus two: some limits on our capacity for processing information. Psychol Rev. 1956; 63:81.
4. Price, JL, Cordell, B. Cultural diversity and patient teaching. J Contin Educ Nurs. 1994; 25:163.
5. Miller, WR, Rollnick, S. Motivational Interviewing: Preparing People to Change Addictive Behavior. New York: The Guilford Press; 1991.
6. DiMatteo, MR. The Psychology of Health, Illness and Medical Care: An Individual Perspective. Pacific Grove (CA) Brooks/Cole; 1991.
7. Meichenbaum, D, Turk, DC. Facilitating Treatment Adherence: A Practitioner's Guidebook. New York: Plenum Press; 1987.
8. Waitzkin, H. Information giving in medical care. J Health Soc Behav. 1985; 26:81.
9. Bernier, MJ. Developing and evaluating printed educational materials: A prescriptive model for quality. Orthop Nurs. 1993; 12:39.
10. Bellet, PS, Maloney, NJ. The importance of empathy as an interviewing skill in medicine. JAMA. 1991; 266:1831.
11. Smith, RC, Hoppe, RB. The patient's story: Integrating the patient- and physician-centered approaches to interviewing. Ann Intern Med. 1991; 115:470.
12. Botelho, RJ, Skinner, H. Motivating change in health behavior: Implications for health promotion and disease prevention. Prim Care. 1995; 22:565.

OBSTACLES TO EFFECTIVE COMMUNICATION

1. Talking too much.
2. Being too casual (levity or gravity).
3. Not understanding the problem.
4. Cutting off the parent.
5. Being overly didactic without attention to feelings.
6. Giving pat reassurances.
7. Being defensive when confronted.
8. Not recognizing countertransference.
9. Being polemical and politicizing.

Gerontology: Speaking with the Older Patient

Joan M. Teno, MD, MS

Mrs. C is an 89-year old white female status post right hip replacement with systolic hypertension. Her level of function up to the last year was good, with only assistance in housework and shopping. During her early postoperative recovery period, she developed multiple spinal compression fractures with increasing difficulty walking, to the point of needing a wheelchair. The family was concerned whether she could live by herself. One aunt was pressuring the family to "put her in a nursing home" where she would have proper care.

A hospitalization that involved x-rays, special tests of nerve conduction, and multiple consultants left the family with the diagnosis that she had severe osteoporosis with multiple compression factures. She had to take 27 pills per day. The medicine made her sick and tired. Could she live alone in the community with help? Was the medicine necessary?

Physicians in training often view older patients as difficult and time consuming. The elderly often have multiple problems. Getting an accurate history is difficult, especially if they are cognitively impaired. The usual approach of eliminating irrelevant signs and symptoms in an attempt to reach one unifying diagnosis does not apply in their care. Rather, it is usually multiple interacting pathologies that result in several "chief complaints."

Furthermore, these patients often pose difficult ethical issues for physicians regarding the right of self-determination and the patient's site of residence. However, most geriatricians, hospice physicians and members of outpatient geriatric assessment teams find treating older, cognitively-impaired patients challenging and they provide the professional a sense of accomplishment.

Physicians spend significant time talking to patients, with some form of cognitive impairment, and their caregiver(s) about difficult topics such as the diagnosis of dementia or decisions about the locus of care. Such a discussion should occur with both the patient and at least one caregiver present. Experienced physicians have learned that the time spent with the patient and caregiver(s) in these initial discussions saves time and emotional distress later.

TWO-ON-ONE CONVERSATIONS

These "two-on-one" communication encounters require special attention to the fact that more than one person is involved in the conversation. The physician must balance between the needs of a patient, who may be hearing impaired and the caregiver(s), who may monopolize the conversation. This situation is difficult for the physician but can be equally frustrating for the caregiver(s).

Often, geriatricians may utilize a multidisciplinary team for cognitively impaired patients to:

- Coordinate medical care;
- Decide upon placement during their remaining years; and
- Assess their medications.

In the opening example, the patient's family prepared the patient for the multidisciplinary geriatric assessment. They wanted to know which questions she wanted addressed during the geriatric assessment. Through conversation they discovered that she wanted to know whether she could stop the pills to build-up her bones given that it was causing her to feel sick to her stomach. In addition, much to the family's anguish, she confided to her granddaughter that she did not know if she could go on. She wanted to die. Both were upset as they went to meet the physician and other members of the health care team.

Physician	"Good afternoon, Mrs. Coombs and Mrs. Simmons, I'm Dr. Tripps, one of the new geriatric fellows. Now, what is the problem that you've been having?"
Patient	"I have a bad back and can't walk."
Physician	"How long has this been going on?"
Patient	"Well, since last August when I went to the hospital."
Physician	"What did your doctors do at that hospital?"

Fifteen minutes later, Mrs. Coombs had recounted the results of her x-rays and other tests. As she talked, the physician made a list of her medicines. She did not voice her concern about the number of medicines, their side effects, or her wishes to die. Finally, the granddaughter thought it was time to bring these issues to the physician's attention.

Granddaughter	"Excuse me, I think it's important that you ask..."
Physician	"Wait, I want to finish getting the history from your grandmother and then I will talk to you separately."

From this example, it is obvious how difficult it is to be the caregiver in these "two-on-one" small group conversations. It is frustrating to listen to aspects of medical history while the primary concerns of the patient and caregiver are not being addressed. As a result of the physician's poor interviewing skills, two issues were omitted:

- The patient's concerns regarding the number of pills and side effects of medications: and
- The caregiver's concerns regarding the patient's thoughts of dying.

It is important for physicians to initially address concerns with both the patient and the caregiver. In addition, this discussion should include the goals of the assessment process. In the example of Mrs. Coombs, from the perspective of the caregiver, it was important for the health care providers to address the issue of depression with her grandmother. If these concerns and goals are not assessed, the patient and/or the caregiver(s) will leave the clinical encounter frustrated and dissatisfied.

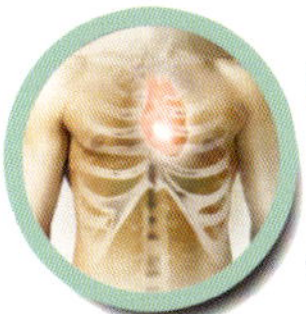

CONVERSATIONS WITH PATIENTS AND CAREGIVERS

An important part of outpatient geriatric assessment is talking with patients and their caregiver(s). The issues to be discussed are emotionally charged, such as the diagnosis of dementia, the decision that a patient can no longer drive, or the decision for treatment goals to focus on the patient's comfort. Sometimes caregivers do not want to discuss concerns regarding the patient's memory with the patient present. As a practitioner, it is important at the outset of the encounter to explain to both parties that, with the patient's permission, physicians will talk to each of them separately and then together.

At the onset of the conversation, physicians should encourage both the patient and caregiver to ask questions regarding terms or statements that they do not understand. When talking to both patient and caregiver, the physician needs to balance both their needs and be positioned so both can be addressed without turning the chair. Occasionally, this is not possible. A patient may have a hearing deficit that necessitates that the physician sit directly in front of the patient. In these situations, the physician should acknowledge that the patient's concerns will be focused on first. Then the caregiver(s) will be given an equal opportunity to voice their concerns. When speaking with the caregiver in these situations, the physician should repeat what was said to the patient so that they do not feel left out of the conversation.

When speaking to both the patient and caregiver, it is important to watch facial expressions. In doing assessments of cognitively impaired patients, the caregiver expressions may clue you in to responses that are inaccurate or about which the caregiver has different opinions. Conversations regarding implications of the diagnosis of dementia may be difficult for impaired patients. Likewise, it is important to watch patients' facial expressions to recognize if they are becoming overwhelmed. In these situations, the health care provider should acknowledge the patient's feelings and offer to stop the conversation.

With the cognitively impaired patient, it is important to adjust the vocabulary, content and rate of speech. Patients may have an expressive or receptive aphasia as part of their dementia, which would interfere with their ability to express their thoughts or understand what is being communicated to them. This can be extremely frustrating for the patient. In these situations, it is important to simplify the content to smaller "chunks" of information and to check the patient's level of understanding. Patients will often answer "yes" to the question, "Do you understand?" Thus, a better check of patient understanding is to ask them to relate their understanding of what has been discussed.

As with any patient encounter, it is important to summarize the salient points and provide patients with simple written instructions or written materials that reinforce what has been said.

DECISIONAL INCAPACITY

Dementia is a permanent and progressive impairment of intellectual function.(1) If patients do not die of other coexisting diseases, they will become unable to make joint decisions with their physician regarding whether to employ or forego life-sustaining therapy. As part of the geriatric assessment process, it is important to undertake advance care planning with patients and caregiver(s), including completing a written advanced directive. Advance care planning is the process of communication and negotiation that formulates patient preferences for medical care and the development of contingency plans that ensure that those preferences will be honored.(1,2) Advanced directives are one outcome of advance care planning. Advanced directives may be formal (e.g., a living will or durable power of attorney for health care decisions) or informal (discussion with a physician recorded in the outpatient medical record). Conversations regarding a patient's wishes and values in the event of future inability to make decisions should occur once a good rapport with the patient and his or her caregiver has been established. Often, the availability of educational materials on formal advanced directives will help facilitate the initiation of the conversation (e.g. http://www.agingwithdignity.org/5wishes.html).

Advance care planning occurs over the course of the patient illness, often starting when the patient is first diagnosed. One may begin the conversations by asking the patient whether they have an advanced directive or living will. For the patient who does not have an advanced directive, ask if they are interested in reading further material about the importance of advanced directives, noting that many patients are interested in learning about them. Often, the first step in advanced care planning is to ask the patient: "If you were too sick to make medical decisions, who would you like your doctor to speak with on your behalf?" From there, the degree of specificity is dependent on where the patient is in his or her disease trajectory, the patient's social circumstances, and whether the patient wants to make plans. Some persons do not want to make future plans; rather, they want a loved one to serve as their proxy decision maker. Often, the health care provider should offer to schedule time with the proxy decision maker to discuss advanced directives.

It is important that health care providers are aware of state laws regarding withholding and withdrawing life-sustaining treatment. Some states such as Missouri or New York require "clear and convincing evidence" prior to withdrawal of artificial hydration and nutrition. In these circumstances, it is important to counsel patients that they should strongly consider completing an advanced directive if they prefer life-sustaining treatment to be withdrawn under certain circumstances.

One approach is to share with the patient and caregiver that many patients are interested in obtaining living wills or advanced directives. The U.S. Supreme Court decision regarding Nancy Cruzan allowed a "clear and convincing evidence" standard for incompetent patients. However, patients should also be made aware of state laws regarding decision making with incompetent patients.(2) If the patient and/or caregiver are not familiar with formal advanced directives, the physician or other health care provider should make available educational material about advanced directives. Then, the health care provider should offer to schedule time with them to discuss advanced directives, keeping in mind that the physician is not the only one who can counsel patients on formal advanced directives. It may be helpful to bring the social worker or other allied health care professional into the discussion.

"They may forget what you said, but they will never forget how you made them feel."

Attributed to Frederick Buechner
novelist and nonfiction writer

Too often, patients and their caregivers can become overwhelmed with decisions that they feel are too technical. One approach is to ask the patient open-ended questions such as:

"What are your concerns about dying?"

Questions like this focus on the type of medical outcomes that are clearly unacceptable to the patient where death is preferred to the life that faces them. The alternate approach, as noted previously, is to ask the patient who should make decisions with their health care provider in the event the patient is unable to. If the patient has formulated preferences and values regarding end-of-life decisions, he or she should be encouraged to discuss these decisions openly with the persons they designated to participate in decision making with their physician.

Similar conversations should occur between the patient and proxy decision-maker about patient preferences and values for life-sustaining therapy. Strategies for this "two-on-one" encounter apply as discussed previously. While it is important to give the proxy/caregiver an opportunity to voice concerns, the clinician needs to make sure the patient understands the implications of treatment preferences. An iterative process needs to be used to make sure that patient's refusals or requests are informed so that the patient understands both the risks and benefits of the decisions. Often, the process is ongoing and accomplished over several office visits. Because preferences may change over time, it is important that physicians review patient preferences on a periodic basis.

COMMON PITFALLS

Mrs. Hill and her caregiver, her adult daughter, Joan, are meeting with a physician to discuss filling out a living will. The patient has mild memory deficits, but has concerns regarding the care that her husband received 10 years prior before he died in an ICU.

Physician	"We are here today to discuss your living will, Mrs. Hill. I'm glad that you could come, Joan."
Joan	"Mother and I feel strongly that we don't want all those tubes and machines that Daddy had. It was terrible; he was in such pain. Mom does not want that."
Physician	"Mrs. Hill, how do you feel about this?"
Daughter	"Go ahead, Mom. Tell the doctor how terrible it was for Daddy..."
Patient	"I would not want to have all those tubes."
Physician	"So you would not want any attempts made to restart your heart if it stopped? Or, to help you breathe?"
Daughter	"That's right. We want none of that."

One interpretation of this conversation is that the patient should be made a D.N.R. (Do Not Resuscitate). A closer look reveals several errors that could lead to decisions being made that do not reflect the true wishes of the patient. First, the daughter monopolized the conversation. The patient may be just agreeing with her daughter. Second, it's unclear what the patient preferences really are and under what context they would apply. How does the patient's situation differ from her husband's? If the patient needed a ventilator for a short time period before returning to her previous functional state, would she still want to refuse this therapy and die? These decisions to employ or forego treatments are situational. It is important that patients comprehend the consequences of these future preferences. Third, terminology such as "machines" or "restart your heart" are vague. Without clarifying their meaning, the advanced directive may be more of a hindrance than a help to future decisions.

Rather than focusing on treatment, a much better approach would be to focus on where the person is in their experience with living with multiple medical conditions, and her goals of care.

Some appropriate strategies in this situation may be to let the daughter ventilate her concerns about how her father died. Then the physician would focus attention on the patient. If the daughter interrupts, the doctor emphasizes that it is important to discuss this with her mother, as well as with her. In some circumstances the conversation may need to be brought up again when the daughter is not present in the room.

CONCLUSION

In caring for frail, older persons with cognitive impairment, health care providers are faced with managing patients within caregiving systems, usually family units. Physicians will often have encounters where sensitive issues will need to be discussed with both the patient and the caregiver. To do this effectively, the health care provider needs to adjust communication skills to these "two-on- one" situations. Particular attention needs to be paid so that the needs of both the patient and the caregiver are satisfied. Often this requires focusing on different parties at different times in the conversation. In talking with the older, cognitively impaired patient, the physician should adjust the vocabulary, content, and rate of speech so that the patient is able to understand what has been said. It is often a good idea to ask patients to summarize what has been said as a test of their understanding. Furthermore, the provision of written material that reinforces main points is helpful. With these efforts to adjust one's style to the patient encounter, compassionate and effective care may be rendered to patient and caregiver(s).

ACTION POINTS

1. In addition to the chief complaint, ask the patient and family, “What is important for you to accomplish with this visit today?”
2. “Two-on-one situations” require physicians to balance the needs of the patient and his or her family.
3. If the patient has either hearing and/or cognitive impairments, acknowledge that you will focus on the patient, but speak separately with the family if the patient agrees.
4. Advance care planning is an ongoing discussion of the patient values and goals regarding medical care. Usually, the majority of patients can name a proxy, someone that they would want to make health care decisions with a physician if they are unable. With progression of chronic illness, some patients will want to make specific statements about their future medical care regarding their values, outcome states they want to avoid, and specific requests regarding the use of life-sustaining treatment.

REFERENCES

1. Teno JM and Lynn J. Putting advance care planning into action. J of Clin Ethics. 1996; 7(3):205-213.
2. Teno JM, Nelson HL, Lynn J. Squam Lake consensus conference: Advance care planning: priorities for ethical and empirical research. Hastings Center Reports. 1994 Special Supplement: S32-S36.

Chemical Interference: Under the Influence

Jeffrey L. Clothier, MD

The core biopsy showed ductal carcinoma in-situ of the patient's left breast. She sits beside her husband in front of my desk. I can't tell which one is exhaling booze breath. She's well dressed and attractive. In-situ cancer. Never an easy discussion stone sober.

She fidgets with her purse. He stares me down and I know he's the one who's drunk. I turn away and face her. "Your biopsy shows what we call pre-cancer. Malignant cells, but they haven't gone anywhere. The tumor's not invasive. That's good news."

Her husband sits up, misses the armrest with his elbow. "When the hell did cancer become good news?"

She studies her fingernails. "Just listen, Mark."

"You hearing what I'm hearing? He motions at her with a fist. "You got cancer. Cancer! Ain't good news no matter what he says."

I let silence creep into my office. Then I say, "Your treatment choices include a lumpectomy and radiation therapy or a mastectomy."

He jumps to his feet this time. "Mastectomy my ass! Doc, you ever say that word again and I'll...nope, no friggin' mutilation, no way."

She jumps up and runs out of my office.

He's leaning over my desk now. The breath and some oil product on his clothes make me push my chair back. He reaches over and grabs a fistful of my white coat. "Now look what you done."

Clinicians frequently encounter patients who are under the influence of legal and illegal substances. The most common cause of chemical impairment is alcohol. This is particularly true for emergency room physicians and surgeons. The magnitude of this problem was revealed by Rivara, et al.(1) They found that almost half (47%) of patients attending a regional level I trauma center had a positive blood alcohol level (BAL). Over a third of these patients (35.8%) were actually intoxicated. Smothers, et al. found that alcohol related problems were present in 40-42% of patients admitted to a nonfederal, short stay general hospital.(2) To underscore the problem, they reported that only 21% of these patients had any substance-related intervention, and only 24% were referred for subsequent substance abuse treatment. Others have reported similar results.(3)

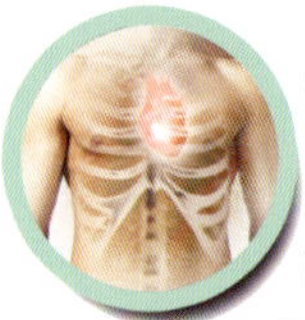

COMMUNICATION BIAS AND ERRORS

Good communication requires a coherent two-way system. Clinical interviewing involves a patient and provider. It is, at the most basic, a reciprocal receiver/transmitter relationship that forms a dialog. The dyadic communication illustration below illustrates the basic communication pathways assuming full fidelity of message. In reality, the data that is transferred as a message suffers from a finite introduction of error. This error introduction results in a degraded message and miscommunication. (4)

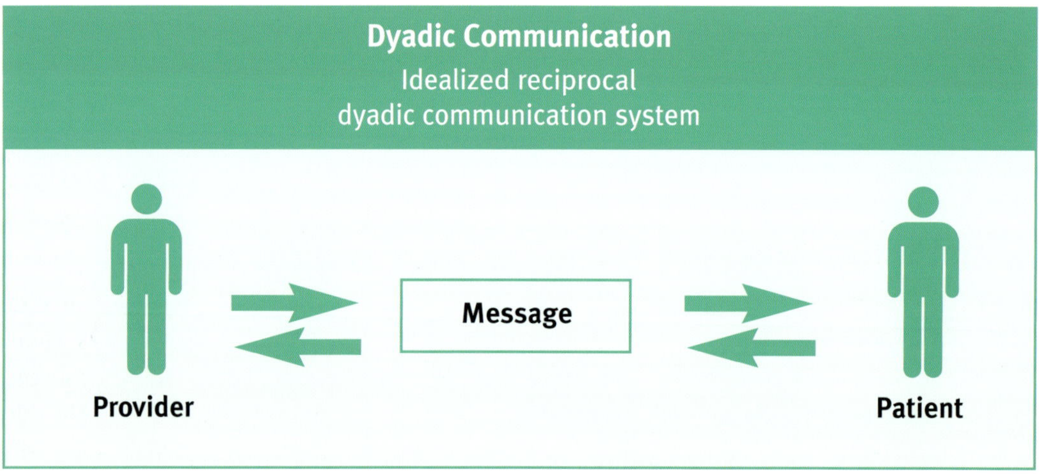

Each member has a filter that codes and decodes the message. In the best of conditions there is also error introduced by passing through these filters. The fidelity of the communication is degraded. The communication filters illustration below expands the diagram to illustrate more fully the multiple transfers of data during the communication process. Chemical interference impairs cognition and communication skills and further introduces error as the message passes through the filters.

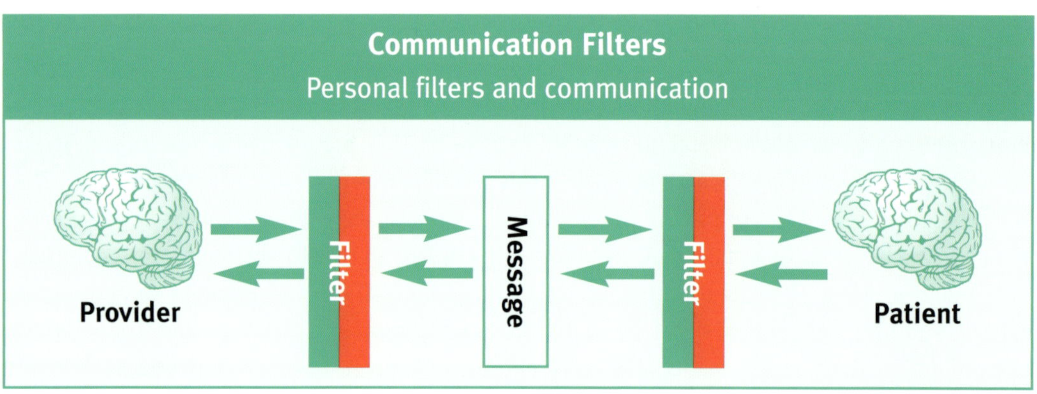

The filters have two major components. The first is related to the sensory and attentional systems. This filter allows you to focus on a specific set of stimuli and to filter out the extraneous stimuli. The second filter functions at an unconscious level of awareness for the most part. This filter results from the biased interpretation of the sensory information. This is because the learned response patterns arising from the normal developmental processes become second nature.

The filters depend on intact function of the sensory and perceptual systems.(5,6) The learned responses interact with the nervous system by introducing perceptual bias. Developmental processes contribute by establishing a pattern of bias in attitudes and understanding. These biases influence our normal interactions. Judgments are made about the relevance and reliability of information at an unconscious or preconscious level. If the provider has attitudes toward a patient that are not consciously addressed by the provider, the message may be misinterpreted or discounted altogether.

The nervous system coordinates the interpretation of the message, as well as elaboration of a message to transmit as a response. Attention is important in this process. There are two components of this attentional system. The first is a top-down modulation of attention from the prefrontal, parietal and limbic cortices and the second component arises from the ascending reticular activating system (ARAS).(6) The parietal and frontal lobes anticipate the message to a degree. This allows "gap filling." This function is most effective in a state of quiet arousal. Therefore, things that interfere with our state of arousal interfere with the functioning of the parietal and frontal lobe.

The flow of thought occurs in relation to cognitive associations that relate one thought to the next. Normally these associations are understandable to the outside observer. This allows some anticipation of the message. The flow of thought relies on an ability to concentrate and maintain the direction of flow. When the nervous system is stressed physically, chemically or emotionally, this ability is reduced. In this setting, we speak of loosening of the association. To the observer, the flow of the communication becomes disjointed and sometimes difficult to understand. The patient with loosened associations may actually forget what they were saying and begin down a different set of associations.(7)

Our brains work to fill in the incomplete data we are presented with. This is revealed by the fact that we are unaware of the ocular blind spot created by the position of the optic disk on our retina. In this regards, perception is not just what we see or hear, but also what we think we see or hear. A basic example of this is seen in our lexical and textual processing. The following is an illustration that was popularized a few years ago.(8)

Word scramble that was popularized on the internet a few years ago illustrating the interpretive power of the perceptual systems.

RDIAENG

Aoccdrnig to a rscheearch at an Cmabrigde Uinervtisy, it deosn't mttaer in waht oerdr the ltteers in a wrod are, the olny iprmoetnt tihng is taht the frist and lsat ltteer be in the rghit pclae. The rset can be a taotl mses and you can sitll raed it wouthit porbelm. Tihs is bcuseae the huamn mnid deos not raed ervey lteter by istlef, but the wrod as a wlohe.

The ability to fill in the blanks works *for us*, as well as against us. Our perceptions are colored by our attitudes and prior experience. These attitudes and experiences influence our expectations. If you have attitudes about certain types of patients, such as alcohol or substance abuse patients, your perceptions may be incorrect or incomplete. This filter bias may unduly influence your ability to communicate with the chemically impaired patient. The result may be miscommunication between provider and patient.(9)

CHEMICAL EFFECTS ON COMMUNICATION

The most straightforward explanation for the chemical effects on communication relate to the specific pharmacologic effects of the chemical on the sensory, memory, arousal, and attentional systems. Pharmacologically there are some differences in the effect of various psychoactive compounds. The table below shows the major classes that may be encountered in an emergency room setting. Additionally, an important rule of thumb is that anything that interferes with cerebral functioning will also cause a behavioral regression.(10) The dysfunction results in a reduced inhibition so that things that would usually be 'edited' by the internal editor, sneak out and are actually expressed.

... anything that interferes with cerebral functioning will also cause a behavioral regression.

Chemical Class and Behavioral Effects

Class	Cognitive/psychological effects
Depressants (includes benzodiazepines and alcohol)	Anxiolytic, reduced inhibitions, increased aggression, reduced concentration and attention, decreased memory, lethargy, incoordination, somnolence, coma and death
Stimulants	Euphoria, restlessness, hyperactivity, exaggerated movements and speech, aggression, racing thoughts, loose associations, paranoia, psychosis and delirium
Hallucinogens	Perceptual distortions, hallucinations, disorientation, paranoia, panic and delirium
Anticholinergic/antihistaminergic agents	Drowsiness, sedation, confusion, reduced memory, hallucinations and delirium
Opiates	Exaggerated sense of well being, lethargy, somnolence and ambivelence

There are three basic effects. The first is a general depressant effect. The impact here is primarily on systems of arousal, attention, memory and motor control. These pharmacologic effects translate into the impairment of the first set of filters and cortex. Alcohol, barbiturates, and benzodiazepines share these effects. In general, the effect progresses as the dose increases. The general progression extends from relief of anxiety and increased talkativeness to reduced inhibitions and aggression, poor motor control and coordination followed by blackouts and ultimately somnolence, coma and potentially death. Agents in this class are synergistic with one another so that, at a low BAL a patient given a small dose of lorazepam will have a greater effect than either alone.

The second general type of effect is a stimulant effect. Agents in this group include cocaine, crack, amphetamine, methamphetamine, MDMA (Methylenedioxymethamphetamine–"Ecstasy") and methylphenidate, among others.(3) Agents in this group have effects that range from increased arousal and alertness all the way to psychosis. As the dose increases, the associations that guide thought become loosened and the person becomes unable to connect the stimuli with the meaning of the stimuli. Things may take on an idiosyncratic interpretation. This is a form of psychotic thinking. At high doses, perception is distorted and the meanings of various stimuli are mistaken. Paranoia can develop. In fact, there is little difference between the cognitions of persons with amphetamine toxicity and schizophrenia at a behavioral level.(7) The exaggerated motor activity makes this group particularly prone to the potential for violence.

The third general effect is related to the hallucinogens. Agents in this group include LSD, mescaline, ketamine, phencyclidine, and high doses of dextromethorphan. The effects of this group of agents are primarily an interference with the perceptual system. These agents typically produce vivid visual hallucinations. In higher doses, however, they may also produce panic, paranoia, agitation and even delirium. There may also be cross modality sensations such as "seeing sounds," "feeling colors," etc.

A GENERAL MODEL OF CHEMICAL INTERFERENCE IN COMMUNICATION

The expressed message is also influenced by the sender's personal bias and unconscious processes. Most of us have certain topics that we would rather not discuss. These topics create an unconscious discomfort described as signal anxiety. This anxiety acts as a signal for the unconscious editor to avoid the topic. Anxiety may interfere with the delivery of the specific information requested. This internal editing may prevent the patient from disclosing some information until trust is formed with the provider. This internal editing is known as resistance.(9)

The reduction of an internal state of anxiety is one of the common features of many abused agents. For instance, we describe alcohol as a social lubricant. The lowered anxiety results in an increased sociability and feeling of ease that results in greater loquaciousness by the drinker. The chemically impaired patient may be more willing to address topics that create signal anxiety. Subjects given other sedative agents such as lorazepam or amobarbital report a greater willingness to discuss difficult topics during the intoxication phase. This has been exploited since the 1930's by psychotherapists and psychiatrists. This facilitated interviewing is also known as narcoanalysis or the "amytal interview." The administration of an anxiety relieving dose of amobarbital IV reduces inhibitions and produces a greater willingness to discuss anxiety-provoking material. This is popularly shown in movies as truth serum. The principle is that removing anxiety helps people talk more freely to some degree.

This effect can be exploited during the interview of a patient under the influence. It is also probably one of the reasons that many confessions of newly arrested individuals occur under the influence of substances. Sigurdsson and Gudjonsson (1994) found that a significant number of offenders confessed during a police interview while intoxicated.(11) The most common report by these offenders was a feeling of confusion. A particularly interesting finding is that it is rare for the confessed criminal to claim a false confession under the influence. Despite this, there is generally a prohibition against interrogating prisoners while they are under the influence since they may not fully appreciate their rights.

Reducing anxiety also has a behavioral dark side. There are some things about which we should be anxious, including displaying aggression or being violent. When the anxiety is lowered, some people may react quickly to perceived threats or personal slights. Because of the intoxicated state, the patient may rely more on contextual and emotional cues to determine the message. For this reason, a neutral tone and pleasant emotional state reduces the likelihood of such reactions.

Impairment of the cerebral substrate by chemicals often interferes with the ability to formulate the message. This results in a temporary thought disorder, which in turn results in tangential and incomplete transmissions. These messages are often loaded with errors. At times, the chemicals may interfere with the internal processing so that the person may appear psychotic and unable to attend to their perceptions. Hallucinogens and various anticholinergic agents are common chemicals that produce this effect. In this setting, the patient may be unable to interpret his or her environment due to perceptual and cognitive impairments. Generally, disturbed orientation will be present.

Chemical Impacts on the Communication Process

1. Reduced anxiety—increases talkativeness, lowers behavioral inhibitions
2. Interference with formation of thoughts—this may range from circumstantial conversations all the way to frank delirium and psychotic thought processes
3. Reduced inhibition—may be more reactive, may be more emotional
4. Impaired memory while intoxicated—may not recall accurately the events that occur while in your care. May not recall discharge instructions.

ERROR CHECKING AND COMMUNICATION

The multiple opportunities for error to intrude on the normal patient-provider communication become evident. If you consider the situation between two computers on the Internet, you have a similar situation. High fidelity communication must include a way of insuring that the message received was the message sent. In computer networking, this is done by embedding a code in the transmission packet that is used to determine if information was lost in transmission. Without this error checking mechanism, communication across multiple computers would be impossible.(4) Normal communication between people includes a message that is explicit and a message that is implied by the behavior of the sender. This set of behaviors is known as prosodic communication. It is basically how you say things. It includes the nonverbal gestures such as facial expression as well as the tone and rhythm of the speech. In human communication, error checking is accomplished by the fact that human communication includes not only the language of the message, but also the prosodic message and a context in which the message is provided. In other words it is not just what you say but how you say it and the context of where it is said that provides the entire message. Normally, all three of these messages are coherent and consistent. This principle is an important principle in dealing with the impaired patient. You must insure that the verbal and nonverbal messages are consistent. Often the chemically impaired individual seems more sensitive to the nonverbal behaviors.

The intoxicated patient is often overly emotional and somewhat reactive. The impairment of inhibition is the result of a reduction in the frontal lobe modulation of expressed behavior. Most intoxicants inhibit the frontal lobe functioning so that there are fewer constraints on behavior. One of the biggest challenges in dealing with an impaired patient who has a lack of inhibition occurs when he or she projects his or her anger onto the provider and staff. This represents an attack on the professionalism and compassion of the staff. At these times it is important to avoid taking such attacks personally. Documentation of the patient's behavior is important and is more powerful if it is not fueled by an attempt to confront the patient with his or her perceived failings. If a confrontational atmosphere is present, the patient often reacts strongly to the situation and may become more difficult.

The impact of substances on cognition can be to such a degree that a formal thought disorder is present. Such a disorder may range from rambling storytelling that moves from subject to subject (loosening of associations) to hallucination-driven psychosis. Some chemicals are more prone to cause such perceptual distortions in patients. In these settings, proper pharmacology may be necessary to restore the ability of the patient to interact appropriately with his or her environment. This is usually accomplished by the use of neuroleptic agents such as haloperidol. On the other hand, the use of low doses of benzodiazepines may worsen the situation by further intoxicating the patient.(9)

DEALING WITH THE BARRIERS

As shown above, the barriers to effective communication with the chemically impaired patient are substantial. The interview style must be adjusted to reflect the impact of the substances on communication. There are some specific interview techniques that can be useful.

1. **Avoid unnecessary conflict**. A simple technique to help with this is to stay pleasant and positive. Describe the desired behavior rather than emphasizing undesirable behavior.

For instance, instead of saying "Don't move" you can say "You need to stay still." A congenial, nonjudgmental approach to the patient may reassure the patient he or she is in a safe and secure setting. This allows the patient to lower defenses and cooperate more fully.

Interviewing the Chemically Impaired Patient

1. Stay positive—avoid blaming the patient. Emphasize behavior you want and not behavior you don't want.
2. Stay calm—slow the pace of questioning. Provide written information.
3. Foster the therapeutic alliance—Externalize the trouble to the world outside the hospital.
4. Use distraction effectively. Often the short attention span can be used to move the patient along in the interview.
5. Provide written and verbal directions—especially treatment referrals and discharge instructions. Always address driving.
6. Be specific in your questions and answers.
7. Reduce environmental stimuli—helps the patient focus on the treatment team.

Expressing a neutral and nonthreatening, nonverbal style is sometimes difficult with intoxicated patients. Recognizing the patient is impaired is an important first step. Avoid accusations. Real behavior change takes time. Maintaining a therapeutic stance reassures not only the patient but also the staff that may be disturbed by the patient's lack of control. The staff will generally follow the lead of the provider. If the provider is calm and nonjudgmental, the staff will usually model this behavior.

2. **Slow the pace.** Slowing the onslaught of questions is a technique that can actually provide you with more information in a shorter period of time. The delayed processing that typically occurs in the impaired patient will often require the rapid questioner to have to repeat the question several times. However, if you slow it down a bit, the patient is able to better interpret the question.

3. **Foster the alliance**. This is done with a combination of verbal techniques as well as nonverbal behaviors. Standing beside the patient and avoiding eye contact is a nonverbal behavior that is less confrontational than standing opposite. It also provides a cue that you understand the patient is having trouble with the "world out there." Showing the patient that you empathize with his or her difficulties beyond the hospital fosters an alliance with the patient. You can do this verbally as well, by acknowledging the problem the patient is having 'out there.'

4. **Use distraction effectively**. Recognize that the impact of chemical impairment on the frontal lobes may impair a person's ability to shift his or her thoughts from one topic to another. The perseveration that occurs limits your ability to effectively gather

information. Usually this presents as the patient focusing on one symptom or another. By learning how to distract the patient from pain or discomfort, you can often gather important pieces of history. This technique requires the interviewer to manage the flow of information. It relies on some of the other techniques described above.

5. **Provide written and verbal instructions.** The impact of the intoxication on memory and processing has therapeutic and medicolegal importance. The patient will require more reinforcement of the expectations during treatment and when he or she leaves the treatment setting. This requires attention to the communication of expectations and plans. Written plans are better than verbal. Written plans given to a caregiver are even better. Whenever dealing with an impaired patient, documentation of the expectations and plans is critical. Drug screens and alcohol levels are some of the most important items to obtain. This provides evidence of impairment in the event the patient claims negligence. However, citing the levels is only minimally helpful. A description of the behavior of the patient, instructions given to not drive or operate machinery, and referrals for substance abuse treatment are critical to complete the therapeutic engagement.

The inherent liability for subsequent claims of negligent care when patients left the treatment setting was highlighted by Simel and Feussner.(12) These authors surveyed attorneys using three different scenarios. The first scenario involved a patient treated and released from an ER with a positive blood alcohol determination who subsequently was involved in an automobile accident. In this scenario, no documentation of advice regarding referral and driving was shown. In the second scenario, the patient was treated and released, without a BAL determination, and no treatment or driving recommendations were made. The final scenario was a patient treated and released, who had a positive BAL and was documented to have received advice against driving and was referred for treatment. The attorneys were asked whether they would advise the patient that he or she had potentially received negligent care. In the first scenario, 43.1% of the attorneys advised that there was perceived liability. In the second scenario, 17.3% advised there was perceived liability. In the final scenario, only 3.5% of the attorneys advised that there was potentially negligent care and perceived liability on the part of the physician. This emphasizes the importance of assessing and properly documenting advice and referral when treating an impaired patient for any ailment.

6. **You should be specific and deliberate in your questions and answers**. The impaired patient may find it easier to give vague and general answers. The use of deliberate and specific questions is a bit different from the general admonishment to ask open-ended questions. However, the impaired patient may not have the concentration or capacity to respond to open-ended questions. Specific questions are better handled when the nervous system is impaired. Likewise, brief, specific answers to the patient's questions are also easier for the patient to process. Brevity and clarity are characteristics that are valuable in this setting.

7. **Reduce environmental stimuli**. Even at its best, a busy emergency room is a cacophony of sounds and visual stimuli. The easily distracted patient may have trouble focusing on treatment. Reducing environmental stimuli can be useful to help the patient focus on the communication process. A quiet room with low level lighting should be used wherever possible. Limiting the accessibility of loose equipment is also important. Patients may become uncontrollable quickly and loose equipment can become dangerous objects.

WHAT TO DO WITH THE CHEMICALLY IMPAIRED PATIENT WHO NEEDS MEDICAL OR SURGICAL INTERVENTION

Chemical impairment will impact almost any co-occurring medical disorder. As a complicating factor, it needs to be addressed. One of the most important pieces of history to obtain from an intoxicated patient is the history of substance abuse. The important points are to identify the duration and intensity of the use, duration and intensity of any withdrawal symptoms in the past and when the last use occurred. Taking this history requires very little time and progresses from questions about typical use to that which may include heavier use. For instance, asking how much a patient usually drinks may not reveal the severity because they may minimize their patterns of use. Following that question with asking how much they can use in a single day is helpful and is then followed by asking how often that occurs. This helps define the intensity of use. Asking how long the use has been occurring gives an idea of the duration of use.

Because withdrawal may be associated with impaired mentation and delirium, it is important to try and obtain the chemical use history before the withdrawal begins. Part of this history is to ask about previous withdrawal phenomena. Obtaining the history prior to withdrawal will allow the provider to initiate proper detoxification protocols before delirium or agitation begins. Withdrawal is usually easier to prevent than to treat. This will reduce the length of stay and provides a better experience for both the patient and the nursing staff.(3)

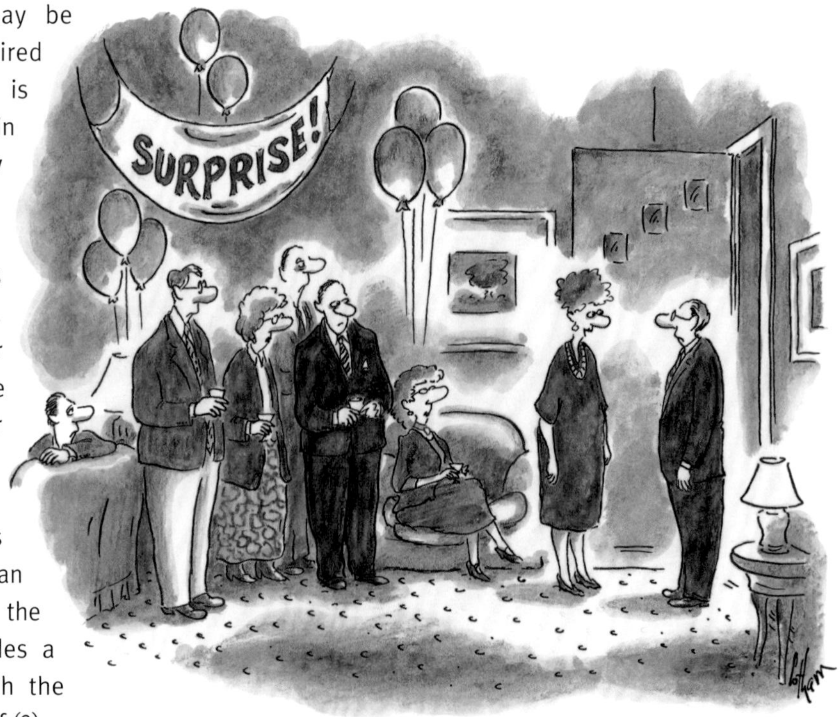

"I invited a few friends over who think you should see a psychiatrist."

This is also the time to obtain a drug screen to identify any unknown agents that might complicate treatment. This is particularly true for patients who will undergo surgery. This helps in the event of a post operative delirium by reducing the potential list of causes.

Assuming that the medical or surgical care is uneventful and the patient recovers, a frank discussion with the patient should emphasize the need for change. This intervention need not be dramatic and time consuming. Intervention is obviously more effective in patients who are ready to change. Wasting time on trying to convince a patient to change a behavior that he or she wants to keep is unproductive. Instead, a simple assessment of the patient's readiness to change may identify those patients where a more detailed referral is appropriate. For some patients who have not reached the point where there is sufficient motivation to change, simple written advice at the time of discharge should be given. This has been shown to be effective in increasing the patient's readiness to change. This means that they will be more likely to accept treatment in the future.(13,14) So, even if the patient is unwilling to be referred from the ER or at discharge, simple written advice may subsequently be helpful.(15)

In the end, the communication process with the chemically impaired patient is fraught with potential difficulties. The barriers are a result of both chemical interference and personal filters that bias expectations and understandings of both the provider and the patient. Recognizing these filters and the specific ways that chemicals impair communication helps reduce errors and misunderstandings. Interventions for the substance abuse patient extend beyond the treatment setting. Providing simple written directions for post discharge follow-up of substance-related conditions is essential in discharging the provider's duty to the patient.

Too often the physician's secret chemical of choice destroys a career before anyone is brave enough to lead a frank and honest discusssion.

PA Rowland

REFERENCES

1. Rivara FP., et al. The Magnitude of Acute and Chronic Alcohol Abuse in Trauma Patients. Arch Surgery. 1993; 128: 907-912.
2. Smothers BA., et al. Detection of Alcohol Use Disorders in General Hospital Admissions in the United States. Arch Intern Med. 2004; 164: 749-756.
3. Holcomb TE, Clothier JL. Alcohol and Substance abuse. In: T.E. Andreoli, C.C.J. Carpenter, R.C. Griggs, J Loscalzo, editors. Cecil Essentials of Medicine, 5th ed. Philadelphia: W.B. Saunders. 2001; 1011-1022.
4. MacKay DJC. Information Theory, Inference & Learning Algorithms. Cambridge: Cambridge University Press. 2003.
5. Joseph R. Neuropsychiatry, Neuropsychology, and Clinical Neuroscience, 2nd ed. Baltimore: Williams and Wilkins. 1996; 118-138.
6. Mesulam, M.M. Attentional Networks, Confusional States, and Neglect Syndromes. In: Principles of Behavioral and Cognitive Neurology, 2nd ed. London: Oxford Publishing. 2000; 174-256.
7. Reed K. Lectures in Psychiatry: The Functional Psychoses : The Schizophrenias and Major Affective Disorders. St. Louis: Warren H. Green Publishers; 1985.
8. http://www.pacificsites.com/~brooke/Learning.shtml Accessed on 9/19/06.
9. MacKinnon RA, Michels R, Buckley PJ. The Psychiatric Interview in Clinical Practice, 2nd ed. Washington DC: American Psychiatric Publishing, Inc; 2006.
10. Lishman WA. Organic Psychiatry 3rd edition. Oxford: Blackwell Publishing; 1997.
11. Sigurdsson JF, Gudjonsson GH. Alcohol and drug intoxication during police interrogation and the reasons why suspects confess to the police. Addiction. 1994; 89: 985-997.
12. Simel DL, Feussner JR. Does Determining Serum Alcohol Concentrations in Emergency Department Patients Influence Physician's Civil Suit Liability? Arch Intern Med. 1989; 149:1016-1018
13. Connors G J, Donovan DM, DiClemente CC. Substance Abuse and the Stages of Change. New York: Guilford Press; 2001.
14. Westreich LM. Turning Alcohol and Drug Emergencies into Catalysts for Change. Current Psych. 2002; 1(12):51-57.
15. Nordqvist C., et al. Can Screening and Simple Written Advice Reduce Excessive Alcohol Consumption Among Emergency Care Patients? Alcohol and Alcoholism. 2005; 40:401-408.

Physicians as Patients: Scared Silly

Parvis J. Sadighi, MD, FACS
Nicholas P.W. Coe, MD, FACS

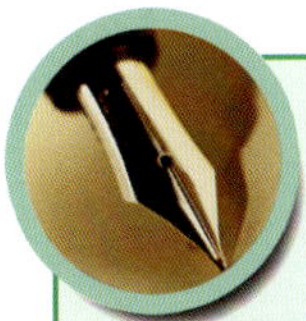

"I have never been operated on. But I have lain on the operating table facing the tearshaped operating lights trying to imagine 'the ultimate horror.' I hope when my time comes, I'm not a whiner. I want to keep my dignity. I'd rather suffer pain."(1) *Richard Selzer, surgeon and author*

Many surgeons have always felt a sense of pride and satisfaction in being chosen to give care to a colleague or his family. With that, however, comes a significant challenge: physicians as patients are at times critical, demanding, expecting more, and expecting to be treated differently—as a VIP. They may say, "Do not treat me like a patient, treat me like a doctor,"(2) demanding respect and consideration. At other times, the expectation of VIP treatment more often than not comes from the spouse. This is much more difficult to deal with and one wonders if this is the sentiment of both the physician and spouse or only the spouse. On the other hand, the treating physician may have the fear and anxiety of not meeting the unexpressed standards set by the patient and by himself.

From many anecdotes, reading and experience, we also have in the back of our minds the idea that physicians are considered to be the worst patients.

In our subconscious, we are always fearful of becoming a patient and we actually have considerable difficulty in being a patient. This should not come as a surprise as we, especially as surgeons, are accustomed to giving orders and dictating the course of treatment.

"Physicians are considered to be the worst patients."

The knowledge about many diseases and their possible complications, including some dreadful ones, creates a greater anxiety and fear than those found in non-medical patients.(3) Anxiety and fear may manifest in two different ways: complete submission and platitude—"I'll do anything you say," or a defensive or difficult attitude toward treating physicians, nurses, lab or x-ray technicians, and subsequently erecting a psychological defensive shield or barrier that is impenetrable.

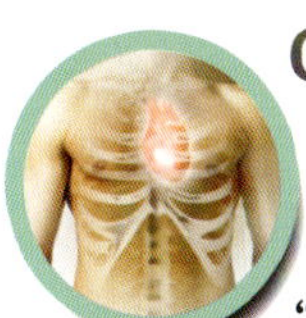

CURBSIDE CONSULT

Minimizing the symptoms and denial are also seen more frequently in physician patients than in non-physician patients. Many physician patients do not wish to "bother" other colleagues with their symptoms. This invariably leads to "self-treatment" or what is known as curbside consult. Both have the potential for serious and poor outcome. "Self treatment" removes the objectivity and distance necessary in the physician patient relationship.(4) The curbside consult deprives the consulting physician of the critical information obtained by a complete history and physical examination, placing him in a very awkward position of having to give advice with incomplete information and facts.

The following examples are helpful in illustrating the point.

Case #1.

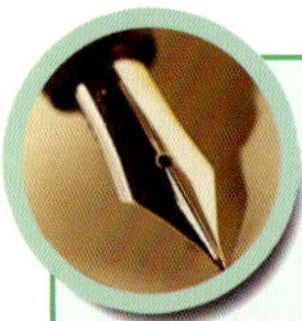

Dr. August is a 76-year-old retired surgeon who called a surgeon he knew at 1 PM. He stated that for two days he had had epigastric pain which is not resolving. He asked if he could come and see the surgeon in his office. About 45 minutes later, the surgeon was able to get a history from Dr. August and examine him. It turns out that the pain came on gradually; there was no nauseous feeling or vomiting, no fever, no chills and no past history of any serious illnesses. The pertinent finding on examination was tenderness in the low epigastric area. Dr August was told that his condition was suspicious for acute appendicitis and he should be admitted. After admission, the white count showed only slight elevation which increased the next morning. Early morning examination revealed increased tenderness in the low epigastric area with rebound, and significantly diminished bowel sounds.

The surgeon told Dr. August that, in his opinion, he needed surgery. His response was, "I'm not sure I have acute appendicitis because the pain has not localized to the right lower quadrant. Don't forget that during my time I have operated on hundreds and hundreds of patients with acute appendicitis, and this is not the picture of acute appendicitis."

The surgeon replied, " If it would make you feel better, I could order a CT scan of the abdomen or an ultrasound of the abdomen, but I still believe the diagnosis of acute appendicitis is the correct clinical diagnosis."

Dr. August's wish was to continue with the observation, and not to go ahead with surgery and not to have a CT scan or ultrasound.

Early afternoon examination once again revealed rebound tenderness in the low epigastric area and the pain was getting worse. At this time Dr. August agreed to have surgery, but he recommended an exploratory laparotomy through a midline incision, which the surgeon did not believe was necessary. The surgeon explained that he would do the standard appendectomy incision, and if it became necessary he could always extend it to explore the rest of the abdomen.

The surgery went uneventfully, and Dr. August had acute appendicitis and did very well postoperatively.

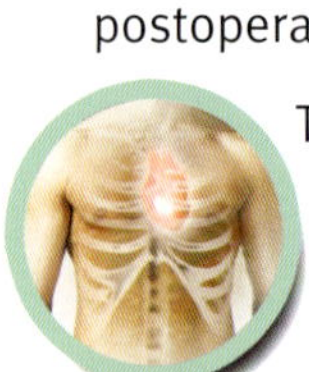

This case illustrates the following issues:

- This retired surgeon had considerable difficulty admitting the fact that he was a patient, and more importantly not acting as a surgeon.
- The surgeon was grateful for the fact that Dr. August gave him an opportunity to do a full history and examination in his office. Quite often, a physician patient satisfies himself by obtaining a curbside consultation from another colleague.
- Downplaying or denial of symptoms are common.(4,5,6)

- The physician patient may present symptoms organized in a way that fits or confirms his own preconceived diagnosis. It seems that prior to obtaining any consultation, Dr. August had already prepackaged all the symptoms and formulated the plan of treatment.

Case #2.

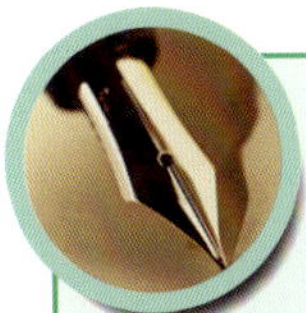

Dr. Borden is a 68-year-old practicing internist who stopped a surgeon in the hospital corridor asking if he could talk for a couple of minutes. He told the surgeon that during his office hours the previous day when he was writing a prescription for a patient, he realized that his handwriting was clumsy and he had lost half of the vision in his left eye.

He said, "I panicked, but fortunately after two or three minutes, the symptoms completely resolved. I started myself on coumadin." He continued, "I am sure I had a TIA. Do you think I should be taking something else in addition to coumadin?"

The surgeon said, "Dr Borden, let's go to my office so I can check you."

Dr. Borden answered, "I can't. I have an office full of patients this afternoon, and there is no way I can cancel them."

At the surgeon's insistence, Dr. Borden agreed to come to his office at 4:00. The surgeon knew that Dr. Borden had been in excellent health. An avid runner who had competed in marathons in the past, he had no previous history of cardiovascular disease or any surgery and was a non-smoker. His examination, however, revealed his blood pressure was 160/80 with a harsh bruit over the left carotid artery, his eye exam was negative, and he had no weakness of his right hand. The surgeon arranged for him to have an urgent duplex examination of his carotid which revealed 90% stenosis of his left internal carotid artery, and the technician called to let the surgeon know that in his opinion, there was a fresh thrombus at the origin of the internal carotid artery on the left side. The surgeon explained the situation in detail to Dr. Borden, telling him about his plans which required him to be admitted, to be on IV heparin, and to have a carotid endarterectomy under local anesthesia first thing in the morning. The possible risks of not doing anything and the risks of the operation were explained to him in detail.

His first response was, "What am I going to do with all the patients who are coming to see me tomorrow?"

Fortunately, his secretary of 25 years was able to take care of that problem promptly. Dr. Borden had an uneventful carotid endarterectomy under local anesthesia, and he indeed had a small piece of fresh thrombus just distal to the area of stenosis. He was discharged home the next day. On the same afternoon post discharge, he resumed seeing his patients. When the surgeon told him he should have taken a few days off, his response was, "I am doing a good job of advertising for you. People are asking, 'What is the incision on your neck?' and I tell them what happened."

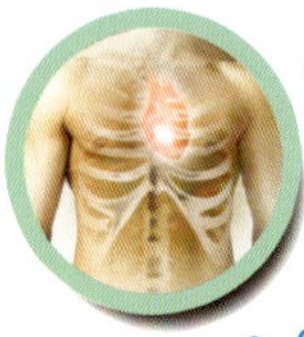

Case #2 illustrates the following issues:

- This is a physician who was treating himself in spite of being aware of the seriousness of his own condition.
- One of every three physicians in the United States does not have a personal physician. This is double the rate of the general population. In a cohort study of physicians graduated from the Johns Hopkins School of Medicine, Gross, et al., (6) found that surgeons and pathologists were significantly more likely to not have a personal physician.

Considering the psychological profile of surgeons, the above finding is understandable although it is difficult to explain why pathologists would be hesitant to have a personal physician.

- The study of illness behavior among Norwegian physicians (7) showed that 75% of physicians provided self treatment in the past three years, and the female physicians were more likely than males to have consulted other physicians (87% vs. 60% $p<0.001$).
- According to Schneck,(3) "Confidentiality issues are a major reason for delay by physicians in seeking personal medical attention; illness may adversely affect malpractice and other insurance coverage as well as hospital credentialing."
- In parallel, Lazare(8) believes physicians, many of whom enter the profession to conquer, master, or control disease, and who are expected to know more about disease and illness than lay people, may be particularly shamed by their own illness. This may explain, in part, why physicians delay seeking help for their own symptoms.

These issues lead to:

- Self-prescribing and self-treating which is also quite common among physicians. A study of young Norwegian doctors revealed that about 90% had self-prescribed in the previous year and the older doctors had a high prevalence of self-treatment.(3,9)
- "Curbside consultation" with its inherent dangers often is associated with the minimizing of symptoms: "I did not want to bother you with this..."
- Financial considerations: "I really cannot afford to have my office closed even for a few days." Younger surgeons may be concerned about the interruption or loss of referral.

"A physician who treats himself has a fool for a patient."

Sir William Osler

First professor of medicine at Johns Hopkins University

MAJOR SURGERY ON SURGEONS

Case #3

Dr. Crowley is a 78-year-old retired surgeon who was referred to his surgeon by his primary care physician for evaluation and treatment of a recently discovered 7.6cm juxtarenal aortic aneurysm.

Dr. Crowley was quite prompt for his appointed time. He had stopped his practice of surgery 10 years prior, after undergoing an abdominal perineal resection for carcinoma of the rectum, which left him with a permanent colostomy. He had no past history of any other illnesses or problems, and he has remained relatively active. He has smoked a pack of cigarettes a day for over 50 years. The pertinent finding on physical examination was the yellowish discoloration of his front teeth, his mustache, and his fingertips indicating many years of smoking cigarettes to their very end. His abdominal aortic aneurysm was readily palpable and pulsatile in the mid epigastric area, and a well functioning colostomy was found in the left lower abdomen. The peripheral pulse was actually quite normal. A review of his CT scan revealed he did indeed have a 7.6cm juxtarenal aortic aneurysm.

The surgeon had a long discussion with Dr. Crowley regarding the findings. Endovascular repair versus an open repair was discussed.

His response: "I am an old fashioned surgeon and I would rather have the old fashioned surgery, but I need to ask you a number of questions. Am I going to make it? Do you guarantee that I am going to make it? "

Dr. Crowley and the surgeon did discuss the risk of doing surgery versus not doing surgery, possible complications, and mortality rate. The surgeon also added, "And let me respond to your question by asking you a question. During all of your years of doing surgery, did you ever give guarantees to any of your patients?"

"No," replied Dr. Crowley, with a softened voice.

"I am asking you to stop smoking completely," the surgeon replied emphatically.

Dr. Crowley looked away, "Save your breath."

Dr. Crowley underwent a retroperitoneal repair of his juxtarenal abdominal aortic aneurysm. Thankfully there were no postoperative complications or problems. He continued to do well and he has continued to smoke.

In his postoperative period, he admitted to the surgeon, "I was scared to death. I did not want you to find out, lest you think that I am a wimp."

Another time, Dr. Crowley told the surgeon that he would wake up at two or three o'clock in the morning thinking about all the possible complications. These concerns were frequently being rewound and revisited in his mind.

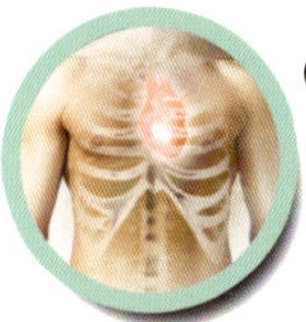

Case #3 illustrates the following issues:

- Dr. Crowley shows the typical exaggerated fear of a surgeon undergoing major surgery.
- In the initial encounter, he came across as a rough and defensive person, both of which were a psychological response of his inner defense to the exaggerated fears.
- He was also the typical example of "Don't treat me like a patient, treat me like a doctor."(2)
- Dr. Crowley downplayed or masked his anxieties for the fear of being embarrassed and signaling weakness, both quite difficult for a surgeon to deal with.
- During his initial phase of his hospitalization his roughness and defensiveness was quite obvious to the nurses and technicians. Once he realized his major surgery was behind him and he was doing quite well, he was a pleasant person. After his discharge, one of his nurses told the surgeon, "Dr. Crowley came in like a lion and left like a lamb."

Case #4

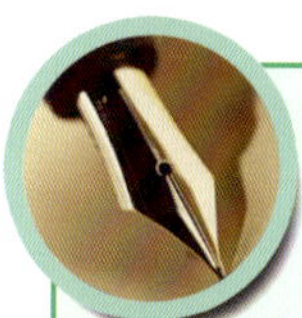

Dr. Dunn was a 63-year-old orthopaedic surgeon with non small-cell cancer of the left upper lobe of the lung, who except for having a pack-a-day history of cigarette smoking had no major illnesses or surgeries. He underwent a left thoracotomy. A tumor of the left upper lobe was crossing the fissure; therefore, a left upper lobectomy and a resection of the apex of the left lower lobe was performed. The surgeon had done a pleural washing for cytology before and after resection. The one prior to resection was positive for non small-cell cancer of the lung. The patient received chemotherapy postoperatively, and he was active and doing quite well for about four years when he developed pain in the posterior part of his incision. His work-up indicated that he had chest wall metastases and multiple other metastases. He initially responded well to another course of chemotherapy and radiation; however, the unremitting pain in his chest wall became quite debilitating, requiring multiple nerve blocks and a considerable amount of medication to give him only relative comfort. For the last few weeks of his life, he ended up needing nursing home and hospice care. The surgeon visited him often and had a number of conversations with him. In spite of being heavily medicated for pain, his mind remained sharp.

"I think this is it, I wanted to see my fifth year mark after surgery, which I did," he told the surgeon.

The surgeon had quite a bit of difficulty coming up with a response; after a long pause, he said, "There is a time for every one of us to go; it is an inescapable fact of nature."

Other conversations were mostly related to control of pain and family visits, or if there was anything the surgeon could do for him. Toward the end, he was so exhausted that he would have difficulty finishing his sentence before his eyes would close.

The surgeon would leave quietly whispering, "Rest well, my friend."

DYING PHYSICIANS

In caring for a dying physician, the following are a few of the myriad issues we need to consider:

- The dying physician abruptly faces a table that has turned which heightens the death anxiety considerably.
- Medical knowledge: we cannot assume that the physician/patients are aware of all the details and intricacies of their disease, especially when it is not in their own field of expertise. This will require considerable patience and explanation.

On the other hand, the knowledge and the awareness of the disease, especially if the patient remains mentally alert, also create considerable anxiety about death. (10, 11)

- Physician patients tend to remain stoic and express more concern for the spouse and family than for themselves.

Of all the stressors of 35 years of practice, including a trial for alleged malpractice, I found caring for a dying colleague to be the most stressful.
Parvis Sadighi, MD, FACS

- What about cardiopulmonary resuscitation? In the study "Physicians as Patients: Choices Regarding Their Own Resuscitation," Hillier, et al., (12) found that for acute myocardial infarction with ventricular disrhythmia, 100% would want CPR at the age of 40 years and 28% would still want CPR at the age of 80 years. The CPR was least desired with advanced Alzheimer dementia with only 11% desiring it at age 40 years, and none at the age of 80 years.

Rivera, et al., (11) in polling the physicians and nurses found that 73 % would accept CPR if complete recovery was anticipated.

- Dr. Dunn, in the last few weeks of his life, found serenity in resigning himself to the fact of dying. To date, that serenity eludes his wife and his surgeon.

Fear of Mistakes

The error rates are frightening when you're the patient, spouse, or parent of a patient. In 2002, a survey by the Harvard School of Public Health reported errors in their own or a family member's care at a rate of 1 in 3.

Dr. Nuland, a Yale surgeon, accepted that his daughter needed a new shunt in her brain. However, due to multiple complications, it took four operations to fix. "I had to be very restrained," he says of his dealings with the other doctors involved. "I knew how badly it was affecting them emotionally," he told reporters for *Time* magazine.(14)

Dr. Robert Johnson, a Southern California orthopedic surgeon, broke the scaphoid bone in his right wrist after he had finished scrubbing for a case. He called a friend to do the repair.

"There is no such thing as minor surgery when you're the patient."
Anonymous

"I felt bad to be a bother," he told his friend on the way to the operating room. During the surgery the rongeur chewed up the scaphoid bone in Dr. Johnson's right hand. He lost his career as a surgeon, but the friendship survived despite a successful suit by Dr. Johnson against the hospital and the surgeon.(14)

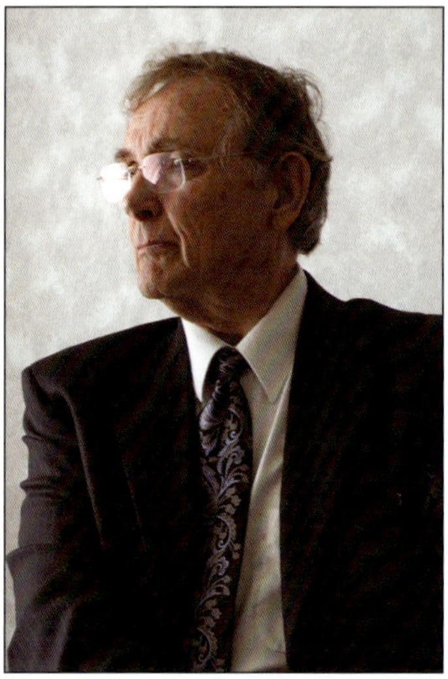

Dr. Robert Johnson

ACTION POINTS

I. IF YOU ARE TREATING A PHYSICIAN

- Examine the physician as a patient, not as a "VIP."
- Do not allow the physician's prepackaged diagnosis to prevent you from performing a complete evaluation and physical examination.
- Do not ignore the 'shame, humiliation and stigma' the physician may be experiencing.
- If confidentiality is an issue in his/her community, suggest that care be given elsewhere, but reassure the physician that you will coordinate the efforts.
- Never assume that physicians' medical knowledge includes a complete understanding of the condition for which you are seeing them.
- Always provide the same quantity and quality of information you would provide to non-surgeons.

II. IF YOU ARE THE PATIENT YOURSELF

- Find a treating physician whom you trust.
- Do not choose an M.D. member of your family as a treating physician.
- Choose an institution with a reputation of quality and proven expertise in the 'area' of your condition.
- Obtain as much information as possible (internet, literature, databases, etc).
- Make sure you have your spouse, a trusted member of the family, or a trusted friend with you when seeking consultation.
- Give consideration to your health care proxy and DNR preferences.

REFERENCES

1. Morin SP, Rowland-Morin PA. Mortal lessons. The Connecticut Magazine. 1984 Nov; 73.
2. Rosenbaum EE. A taste of my own medicine: When the doctor is the patient. New York: Random House Inc; 1988:14.
3. Schneck SA. 'Doctoring' doctors and their families. JAMA. 1998; 280:2039-42.
4. Rosvold ED. Doctor don't treat thyself. http://www.webmm.ahrg.gov/case.aspx?caseID=71. Accessed 6/5/06.
5. Spiro HM. When doctors get sick. Perspect Biol Med.1987; 31:117-33.
6. Gross CP, et al. Physician heal thyself. Arch Int Med. 2000; 160:3209-14.
7. Ness DE, Ende J. Denial in medical review. JAMA. 1994; 272(22):1777-81.
8. Lazare A. Shame, humiliation, and stigma in the medical interview. Arch Intern Med. 1987; 147:1653-1658.
9. Rosvold EO, et al. Illness behavior among Norwegian physicians. Scan J Public Health. 2002; 30:125-32.
10. Fromme E, Billings JA. Care of the dying doctor. JAMA. 2003; 290(15):2048-55.
11. Kane AC, Hogan JD. Death anxiety in physicians: defensive style, medicine specialty and exposure to death. Omega. 1985-86; 16:11-21.
12. Hillier TA, et al. Physicians as patients: choices regarding their own resuscitation. Arch Intern Med.1995; 155:1289-93.
13. Rivera JR, et al. Cardiopulmonary resuscitation: personal choices of physicians and nurses. Bol Assoc Med PR. 1992; 84:139-43.
14. Gibb N, Bower A. What doctors hate about hospitals. Time. 2006 May 01; Sect. Medicine:42-52.

Telemedicine: Without Touch

Stephen R. Smith, MD, MPH
Mary R. Wimberly, RN

Mrs. O'Connell was nervous about taking pills. She had become nauseated, vomited and had chills after taking Aldactazide three years ago. Now the doctor had prescribed Esidrex for her high blood pressure. She took the pill at 11:30 on the morning of May 15th. An hour later she didn't feel well and called the doctor's office. She was told the doctor was busy and that she should call back at 1:00 pm.

By 1:00 pm, she was weak, sweating, and nauseated. She had her 15-year-old niece, Andrea, call the doctor's office because she was too weak to do it herself. When Andrea called she was told the doctor was still busy. Andrea told the office person that her aunt was ill from the prescription she had just taken. She was told to call back later.

Andrea called back at 1:20 pm and spoke to a nurse. She was told that the doctor was still busy, but Andrea insisted on talking to him. Andrea told him that her aunt had taken the pill and was not feeling well. She was having a hard time breathing, was having palpitations, was nauseated and was having hot and cold flashes, she said. Andrea also added that her aunt appeared to be discolored to her. The doctor told Andrea to give her aunt orange juice every half hour and to call back "if anything came up."

After futile attempts to get her aunt to take the juice and seeing her rapidly deteriorate, Andrea called the doctor's office back. She spoke first to a nurse, then to the doctor, informing him that her aunt couldn't even take a sip of juice and that she was having a very difficult time breathing and was turning blue. The doctor told her to "take her to the hospital."

Not knowing exactly how to get her aunt to the hospital, Andrea called her grandfather. When he arrived, Mrs. O'Connell was unable to move and he and Andrea couldn't move her into the grandfather's car. Mrs. O'Connell's son was then called who, when he arrived, called the Emergency Medical Service. This was at 2:44 pm. Mrs. O'Connell was dead on arrival at the emergency room.

Mrs. O'Connell's tragic story is an extreme case of what can go wrong when a telephone is involved in the practice of medicine. In her case, the family sued the doctor and won a major settlement. The goal of this chapter is to provide surgeons with an approach to the telephone practice of medicine that will help ensure that patients receive the care they need, and that will allow surgeons to view the telephone more as an ally than an adversary.

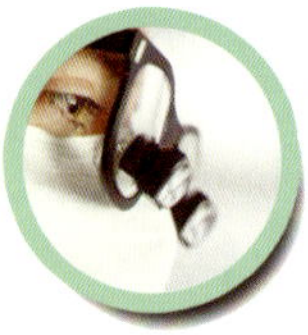

THE IMPORTANCE OF THE TELEPHONE IN THE PRACTICE OF MEDICINE

It is hard to imagine life in the United States without the telephone. Approximately 90 percent of households in the United States have a telephone. And telephones are no longer restricted to home or office. In today's rapidly developing technologies, the telephone is a ubiquitous instrument, appearing in cars, briefcases, trains, airplanes and pocketed in sports jackets.

The telephone has been part of medical practice since its inception, when Alexander Graham Bell placed the first emergency call to his assistant as he spilled sulfuric acid on himself and his invention. Today, 25% of new diseases are reported through the use of the telephone, 24% of all medical care contacts take place on the telephone, and 12.5% of a physician's time is spent on the telephone. (1-3)

About half of the telephone calls received in a surgeon's office during regular working hours are for administrative reasons, while the rest are related to specific medical problems. After regular office hours, however, over 90% of the calls are symptom-related. Curtis reports that the rate at which after hours calls can be expected is 450 contacts yearly for every 1,000 patients in a primary care practice. (4) Greenlick and colleagues (2) determined that 990 telephone calls were placed annually for every 1,000 patients in an HMO, both during and after hours.

The manner in which after hours telephone calls are handled varies in different countries. In the United States it appears that after hours telephone calls are rather frequent, but result in the patient being seen by the physician in about 20% of the cases. (5) In the United Kingdom, New Zealand, and Australia, after hours telephone calls are less frequent, but approximately 80 percent of the calls result in visits. (6-8)

While the volume of telephone calls may appear daunting, the variety of complaints offered by the caller is quite manageable. In one study of four private family practices, the researchers found that five complaints accounted for over half of all the symptom-related calls received during regular office hours, and that 25 complaints accounted for 81.5 percent of all logged complaints. (5)

THE CHALLENGES

Whether during regular office hours or after hours, surgeons often view telephone calls as disruptive. During office hours, telephone calls interrupt the usual patient care flow. After hours, they disrupt the surgeons' private lives. With the exception of some pediatricians who charge nominal fees for telephone calls, most doctors do not receive any direct compensation for telephone calls.

Surgeons have less control over the environment in dealing with patients over the telephone. Much of the data that surgeons use in their clinical decision making is not available. The lack of the physical presence of the patient denies the surgeon the visual clues so important in making a diagnosis. Patients express so much in their body language and facial expression. Gone too is the opportunity to physically examine patients, or to visually judge their reactions to questions, suggestions, or surgical maneuvers.

In a more subtle way, the telephone also restricts the surgeons' use of paralinguistics to understand the patients' meanings. Paralinguistics refers to the way in which we speak, beyond the actual words spoken. The meaning of words can be altered by the intonation, volume, pitch, speed, or other variations in the way the sounds are produced. The telephone may mask some of this paralinguistic communication. Taken together, visual cues and paralinguistic cues account for up to 70% of the social meaning of communication.

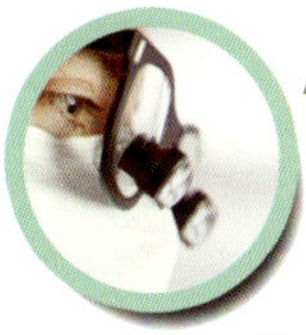

AN APPROACH TO PATIENT CARE

Despite the limitations that the telephone presents, surgeons can provide excellent patient care over the telephone, leaving patients well satisfied.

Surgeons should be sure that all of the office staff shares the same approach to dealing with telephone calls. Standard procedures should be established, preferably in writing, that will guide the office staff in their handling of calls. For example, any office staff person who receives a telephone call from a patient complaining of a symptom should record the patient's name, telephone number, and the reason for the call. That way, the patient can be called back if the surgeon later decides to do so.

Protocols need to be individually tailored to each practice. Those who initially screen the telephone calls need to know what the surgeons expect them to do. In a study of four private family practices, the staff who handled the telephone calls as they came into the office had received no specific training in how to handle the calls. It was noted that when receptionists received a telephone call in which the caller complained of symptoms consistent with an upper respiratory tract infection, an office visit was scheduled for 87% of such patients, while when physicians managed the same complaint, 70% were managed without an office visit.(5)

Much of the enigma in the way telephone calls are treated is due to the lack of clarity in thinking about telephone calls as real health care encounters. The case of Mrs. O'Connell above and the cash settlement that attended it should put to rest any doubt about the reality of telephone calls as bona fide health care encounters. Surgeons are responsible for the way telephone calls are handled in the office by themselves and their staff.

The same care and consideration should be given to patients over the telephone as is given in person. That does not mean that every telephone call should last 20 minutes. Good telephone management should result in fewer calls, with none lasting more than four or five minutes. During that brief time, surgeons should be using the same skills in history-taking and communication that they would use in face-to-face encounters.

Since the surgeon is so dependent on the verbal communication from the patient, it behooves the surgeon to take the greatest pains to elicit the most information possible from the patient. The worst way to do this is for the surgeon to ask a lot of direct questions. Yet this is quite typical of the way that physicians take a history over the telephone. When audiotapes of telephone conversations were analyzed, the physicians did most of the talking.(9) Open-ended and broad questions are more likely to provide the surgeon with the clearest picture of the patient's problem.

Patients should be encouraged to elaborate on the details by asking questions such as, "Tell me more about it." The caller should be given ample opportunity to present a full exposition of the problem. Not only will this shed light on the disease process, it may also serve a cathartic purpose, relieving the caller of much anxiety and apprehension. (10)

Periodically, the surgeon should succinctly summarize what the caller has said. This not only corrects any misinterpretations, but conveys to the caller that the surgeon is respectfully listening. Care should also be taken to have the caller define any ambiguous terms. For example, "high fever" should prompt the surgeon to ask if the temperature was actually taken and how high it was.

If the conversation seems to be drifting, the surgeon can redirect it by asking the caller to fill in more details about the symptom or sign that is of most interest. Only after the caller has had ample opportunity to describe the problem should the surgeon begin to ask more direct, closed-ended questions.

Whenever the opportunity presents itself, the surgeon should offer supportive comments to the caller. Often the caller, be it patient or caregiver, feels overwhelmed, threatened, and vulnerable. They are calling the surgeon because they no longer feel competent to handle the problem themselves. A simple, sincere statement such as, "You seem to have done all the right things so far," can greatly assuage these anxieties. Empty reassurances as, "Don't worry, everything's going to be fine," may not be very helpful.

These general communication skills are not specific to telephone management. They are equally appropriate in face-to-face encounters. In addition to these general communication skills, there is a certain approach that the surgeon should take when dealing with patient complaints over the telephone that are different than that taken in the office setting.

A Specific Approach to Telephone Management

The surgeon should focus more on management decisions rather than diagnostic decisions when handling telephone calls from patients. In the office setting, the surgeon will ask questions that are likely to be helpful in the diagnosis. While on the telephone, the surgeon (or whomever is taking the call) should ask questions that will be helpful in deciding whether or not the patient needs to be seen. Conrath and colleagues (11) describe the way physicians function on the telephone as that of a "decision theorist," while they seem to employ a "gestalt" approach in the office setting.

This approach was used to design a training program at Brown Medical School for third- and fourth-year medical students in which they received telephone calls from standardized patients. The students were told it was a simulated problem and their conversations with the standardized patients were tape recorded. After the first telephone call the students participated in a workshop on telephone management skills. The specific approach to telephone management presented in this chapter was reviewed with the students in the workshop. A week or two after the workshop, the students received a second telephone call from a standardized patient with a different complaint. Again, the conversations were tape recorded and scored. Student proficiency significantly improved between the first and second call. (12)

In most telephone calls, the caller will present a complaint immediately after the usual greeting. At this point, the surgeon should decide if the nature of the complaint is such that the patient needs to be seen. Further questioning about the complaint would only waste time. The opening case of Mrs. O'Connell is an example of this. When the caller states that the patient took a medication and is now having trouble breathing, the surgeon (or whoever takes the call) should follow the "quick sidetrack" of the algorithm leading to a decision that the patient needs to be seen.

While every surgeon will have a different list of what complaints trigger the "quick sidetrack" pathway, certain complaints are likely to be on every surgeon's list. This includes the anaphylactic reaction scenario described in the Mrs. O'Connell case, as well as such complaints as severe chest pain, sudden change in level of consciousness, convulsions, persisting hemorrhage, or very high fever (>106° F or 41° C).

Deciding that the patient needs to be seen does not end the conversation or the questioning. The surgeon needs to communicate clearly to the caller what the next steps are. In general, the instructions should include where the patient is to be seen (office, emergency room, or home), when the patient is to be seen (immediately, within the next few hours, or at a specific appointment time), and how the patient is to be transported (ambulance, helicopter, or automobile).

In the case of Mrs. O'Connell, the surgeon told the niece to bring her aunt to the hospital, but neither told her how to get there, nor ascertained the niece's ability to get her there. Since the niece was only 15 years old, she wasn't able to drive her there herself, nor would this have been appropriate. The surgeon should have told the niece to call Emergency Medical Services, or better still, should have called himself.

It is important for the surgeon to remain calm in such situations. Often, the caller will be in a high state of anxiety. It's easy for the surgeon to become distracted as well.

> I remember vividly one of the first telephone calls I received as a second-year resident while I was taking call on a Sunday. A woman called and said that she found her husband dead on the front porch. I told her that I'd be there right away and got the address on Lake Avenue. As I drove away from my house, I realized that I had no idea where Lake Avenue was. I remembered that we had a large street map of Rochester in the office, so I went there. Fortunately, one of the faculty was in the office that morning and I blurted out the story to him. He calmed me down and reminded me that deaths at home had to be handled by the Medical Examiner's office. Rushing off to the patient's home wasn't going to do much good. More calm and collected, I called the Medical Examiner's office, then called the patient's wife back to tell her of the arrangements.

If the presenting complaint isn't one that triggers the "quick sidetrack," then the surgeon should proceed to collect more information from the patient using the interviewing skills discussed above. Surgeons should ask questions related to the caller's concerns, ask the caller to elaborate on the problem and then, based on the information at hand, focus on specific questions that would tend to suggest the possibility of a life-threatening diagnosis. Surgeons should consider the question, "What diagnoses are consistent with the history given so far that would be a potential threat to life?"

For example, in a child with fever, the surgeon should consider possibilities such as meningitis, epiglottis, severe dehydration, and seizures. Surgeons should then consider what questions they might ask that would point to such diagnoses. Questions that come to mind include those related to stiff neck, changes in the level of consciousness, difficulty breathing, thirst and urination patterns, vomiting and diarrhea, and past history of seizures.

Having received enough information to feel comfortable that no emergency existed, surgeons should then ask specific questions that would suggest that the problem was a benign, self-limited condition for which an office visit was unnecessary. Most common viral illnesses would fall into this category in the child with fever. Questions that might reveal this include inquiries related to runny nose, cough, rash and mild diarrhea.

At this point, surgeons should have a good idea of what the problem is. They should summarize what the caller has related, check to see that the caller agrees with the accuracy of that summarization, then offer the assessment of the situation. For example, in the case of a fever in a 4-year-old child, the surgeon may say:

> "Let me see if I've got it all straight. Your daughter woke up today and seemed to be out of sorts. She was listless, didn't eat breakfast, and has a temperature of 101° F. She's had two episodes of diarrhea since getting up, and complains of some abdominal pain. She hasn't vomited, doesn't have a stiff neck, and has no other symptoms or problems. Is that right?"

(Caller confirms summary.)

"It sounds like she may have a virus that's causing her diarrhea. You did the right thing keeping her home from nursery school. Keep giving her liquids. If the diarrhea lasts more than another two days, or if she stops taking the liquids or starts vomiting, then bring her in to be seen."

Most of the time the caller will not object to the surgeon's formulation of the problem. However, at times the caller may either disagree outright, or more likely suggest some doubt about the diagnosis. This may be expressed by remarks such as,

"Are you sure?" or "I don't know..."

If disagreement or doubt is expressed, the surgeon should collect more information, then either reformulate the diagnosis or reiterate the original diagnosis with an explanation of what led to that conclusion. If disagreement or doubt persists, the surgeon should arrange to have the patient seen.

Having offered a formulation of the problem, the surgeon should next offer a treatment plan. Many times this can be in the form of reassurance and advice on self-care. The instructions for self-care should be simple and straightforward. The caregiver or the patient should be told to call back if problems arise rather than being given a potentially confusing set of contingencies. Patients should always be given some instruction on what to look for and under what circumstances they should call back. For example, in the case of a child with diarrhea, the caregiver should be told to call back if the diarrhea persists longer than two days or if the child stops taking liquids, starts vomiting, or shows signs of dehydration. The specifics of the instructions will vary from surgeon to surgeon. Some may ask the caregiver to call back if the diarrhea lasts more than three days instead of two; others may ask that they call back in one day just to give a progress report. The important thing is that the surgeon convey to the caller that he or she shouldn't hesitate to call back if things aren't going right.

Prescriptions may be given in addition to self-care instructions. In one study, physicians gave prescriptions to patients calling with a complaint 26% of the time without seeing the patient.(5) Surgeon practices vary considerably in this area. The recommendations to the students in the earlier study is that antibiotics should rarely, if ever, be prescribed over the telephone for suspected infections. Usually the patient needs to be seen in order to confirm the diagnosis and to do appropriate laboratory tests. Actual practice differs from this recommendation. Antibiotics are frequently prescribed for what the physician believes is otitis media. Yet, a study by Nickerson, et al.,(6) showed that 21% of children initially diagnosed over the telephone as having otitis media subsequently were found to have either no disease or another illness.

Controlled substances generally should not be prescribed as a result of a telephone call. Non-narcotic cough syrups can be recommended if that is the caller's complaint, as can non-narcotic analgesics if pain is the complaint. If the caller states that non-narcotic analgesics are not sufficient, then that level of pain justifies seeing the patient before narcotics are utilized. Sedatives and narcotics should not be prescribed over the telephone as a general rule.

If the questioning did not result in a determination that the problem was a benign, self-limited process, then the disposition decision should be to see the patient. Further questioning is not likely to change matters. A more definitive diagnosis will have to await physical examination and laboratory testing. For example, in the case of the child with fever, if the history for diarrhea had been negative, and there were no other positive findings, then the child probably needs to be seen. As noted earlier, a diagnosis of otitis media cannot be reliably made over the telephone.

If a decision is made to have the patient seen, then the where, when, and how elements described above need to be determined and communicated to the caller.

Just as the offering of the problem formulation may result in the expression of doubt or disagreement from the caller, so too may the offering of a treatment plan. This most often occurs when the surgeon believes that a visit is not necessary, yet the caller is not convinced. Many patients will be reluctant to press the surgeon directly, so careful attention must be paid to clues that the caller is not satisfied with the proffered treatment plan. A statement such as,

> "Are you sure she doesn't need to be seen?"

clearly indicates the caller's discomfort with the disposition. Left unaddressed, this may result in a visit to the emergency room or a more frantic call at an even less convenient time.

The most direct way to assess the caller's comfort with the treatment plan is to ask. After presenting the plan, the surgeon may ask:

> "Are you comfortable with that?"

A tentative:

> "I guess so..."

should be understood as "No." At this point the surgeon may wish to pursue the nature of the discomfort or reluctance further, or to offer an alternative plan. If the presenting problem is one in which the judgment of whether a visit was needed was a close call, it makes sense just to offer to see the patient. If, on the other hand, the problem seems minor and easily managed without a visit, then the surgeon should pursue the matter further. The surgeon should acknowledge that the caller seems uncomfortable and sensitively inquire to find out what's causing this discomfort. This allows the caller to express concerns previously unstated which, in turn, may permit the surgeon to provide more specific reassurance or information.

The surgeon should try to ascertain the motivation for the call, especially if the problem has been going on for some time. Was it that the patient reached a limit of tolerance of the symptoms, or that the patient or the caregiver reached a limit of tolerance of anxiety? In the latter case, all that might be necessary is assurance that the problem is following a normal and expected course of events. The caller can be told what to watch for that would indicate a deviation from normal and be told that what is being done is the appropriate treatment.

A typical example of this is the complaint of low back pain. The caller will state that the patient woke up with low back pain so severe that he or she could barely get out of bed. History usually reveals that an unusual amount of exertion had occurred on the previous day, but the patient did not experience anywhere near the pain present upon arising that morning. The patient has taken to bed, is using a heating pad, and is taking analgesics. Bowel and bladder function is normal and the patient is reasonably comfortable while in bed. The best course of treatment in this case is reassurance and information on the natural history of low back pain. Unless the surgeon is willing to make a house call, having the patient come in for a visit would be a far less desirable course of action than letting the patient stay in bed for a couple of days.

If agreement can't be reached between surgeon and caller, the surgeon should be willing to see the patient.

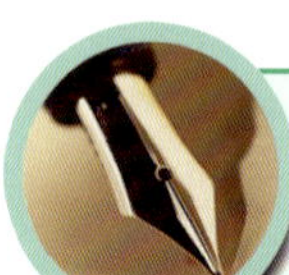

On one cold, blustery, snowy night, a physician who practiced in the upper peninsula of Michigan received a telephone call from a mother about a child with a moderately high fever. Though not seriously ill, the physician thought it best to see the child and asked the mother to bring the child in. "What? On a night like this?" she asked incredulously. Taken aback, the physician asked her why then, had she called? "So someone else could worry besides me," was her response.

Managed Care

The telephone was made for managed care. Surgeons tended to under-utilize the telephone in the old fee-for-service system because they generally could not bill for their time over the telephone, though some pediatricians have begun to do so in recent decades.

Managed care has changed all that. Surgeons could increase their productivity, and thus their income, by the judicious use of the telephone. Both initial visits and follow-up visits for acute, self-limited problems could be avoided in many cases by using the telephone.

Surgeons who use the telephone in this manner should view the telephone encounter just as if it were an office visit. A note should be entered into the patient's record including the date and time of the call. All pertinent positive and negative historical information should be included. The surgeon's assessment of the problem and plans must also be included. The plans should include the advice given to the patient, especially instructions on follow-up. Using the telephone in this manner should not be an afterthought. As a powerful tool of productivity, the surgeon should include time for telephone calls in the office schedule in place of an office visit. Notes should be written or dictated contemporaneously.

TELEMEDICINE

Until recently, telemedicine technology was solely within the realm of the military. Now there are tiny internally placed transmitters designed to relay physiological data through portable notebook computers to satellite phones, which are relayed to a satellite and back to a videoconferencing earth station. From there the message is sent to specific sites for evaluation by surgeons. Experiments using pill-size PED body core temperature monitors, which are swallowed by the patient, transmit body temperature readings. The potential for normal use of this technology in medical centers is tremendous and its use for protecting humans in extreme environments is already being tested. No longer will patients who travel be someone else's responsibility. According to Michael Hawley of MIT:

Physicians will be monitoring and contacting their own patients for compliance issues and providing them with feedback regarding their physiological status. This will be a major challenge to the traditional physician-patient dyad. The basic guidelines for cellular telephones regarding security of information will still apply. However, the guidelines for surgeons contacting their own patients for feedback will need to be developed and studied over time as the virtual house call becomes reality.

Another option for the surgeon to manage the care of his post-op patient is with the use of a portable telemedicine device. Most telemedicine devices will in some way connect to the patient's land line phone. They range from very simple to operate to the more intricate. There are many makes and models and one's choice is based on what is being monitored, ease of use and of course cost. The most basic model requires the patient or caregiver to be able to read, follow instructions, and push a button. The complexity of the instrument may be increased by having attachments of peripheral devices such as a blood pressure machine, weight scales and/or a glucometer. Some even monitor heart activity or may have a camera attachment to allow pictures to be transmitted so that wound healing can be monitored. Transmission over regular phone lines does not yet have the resolution necessary to do an accurate wound assessment, such as looking at depth and measurements, but improvements in the technology are continually being made.

So far, medicine has focused on fixing you when something breaks. This is about finding out how the body works all day. It will become as simple as strapping on a wristwatch and creating a day-to-day medical chart.

The information that is transmitted via these devices will vary based on the complexity of the device. Some may require patients to answer questions related to their diagnosis. The questions are based on symptoms, behavior, and knowledge that the patient has regarding diagnosis. The information is then "risk stratified" which means the patient's answers are flagged as being high risk, medium risk, or low risk. With the information received from structured interactions, the surgeon can better manage the care of the patient and will not have to rely solely on what the patient or caregiver says over the telephone.

Many facilities utilize these telemedicine devices by designating someone to train the patient or caregiver how to use them. That person also is responsible for disseminating the information to the caregiver and also acting upon it as needed based on a predetermined protocol.

While it may appear that the use of such devices places the physician farther from the patient, the opposite is true. This technology places the patient closer to physician access based on their real needs. It empowers the patient to control a part of his or her care. In addition, patients feel more secure because someone is "keeping an eye" on them. When there is a care coordinator, the patient also benefits from having someone readily available that they can call and then if need be, the physician is contacted. It is a reassurance for the physician that someone is watching out for the patient and able to see trends in data in time to keep the patient from a crisis situation.

A 64-year-old COPD patient was very ill for several years. His wife helped care for him. He had repeated ER visits and hospitalizations. In one year, he was in the hospital 13 times and in the ER more than that. He was given a telemedicine device that his wife could operate. After using this device for a year, he only required hospitalization nine times and visited the ER only three times. During this year, he had no unscheduled clinic visits which were quite frequent the prior year. Neither he nor his wife felt the panic that many times would prompt them to either make a phone call to their provider or visit the ER. By having this constant reassurance that there was someone they could call, even if it was only on weekdays, their fears were allayed and that meant less stress for both of them and for their physician. While this appears to be a small reduction, consider the cost savings of one hospital stay for a COPD patient. This patient's costs were high because he was usually admitted directly to the ICU for a few days before being moved to an acute care bed.

Appropriate communication is still critical to good patient management and the telemedicine devices provide the physician with more tools with which to do that. The surgeon who is competent in his ability to communicate needs to develop a variety of methods for using technology effectively. No longer able to treat patients solely in the office or consult with colleagues directly, these new tools are a necessary addition to the surgeon's patient care armamentarium. The caution is clear with their use—these new technologies require new rules to make sure the surgeon understands the whole message from the patient. Otherwise, the patient's care, the patient-surgeon relationship and the surgeon's career may be placed at risk.

CELLULAR TELEPHONES

Some surgeons might be tempted to use cellular telephones in their automobiles as another way of increasing productivity in the managed care environment. Surgeons should resist this temptation. It is dangerous in two ways. First, using a cellular telephone while driving has clearly been shown to increase the risk for motor vehicle accidents. Second, surgeons increase their risk for medical malpractice by using their car as an office. Unlike the real office situation, the surgeon-driver does not have the patient's record to review and the surgeon is not likely to write the kind of detailed note necessary for a good malpractice defense in case of a lawsuit.

A 'safe' rule of thumb is to always use a hard line telephone when you have to discuss sensitive data.

Unless the surgeon is willing to stop the car and park while making the telephone call and be willing and able to write a detailed note, the use of a car telephone should be discouraged. Instead, the surgeon could make better use of the time in the car by listening to medical audio tapes or, better yet, soothing and relaxing music!

When using a portable cell phone outside of the privacy of your car, be careful that others are not able to hear the details of the discussion. This includes trains, buses, subways or the underground, and public and private waiting areas at the airport or train stations. You never know who may be listening.

CONSULTANTS

Often a colleague may not be able to contact other physicians via the telephone for a consult when they are with patients or at the hospital. When this occurs, some prefer to send an e-mail message with the important data and ask the physician to return the call later in the day to discuss the case. Although seemingly professional, there are serious considerations to make before discussing the data contained in the e-mail. First, the information in the e-mail message may not be secure and so the patient's name and address should not be contained within the message. Therefore, in the beginning of the discussion, physicians should establish where this patient is being treated. If the patient is not being treated in a state in which both physicians are licensed to practice medicine, serious issues regarding professional liability need to be reviewed. It is not advisable for physicians to discuss the care of patients in a state in which they are not licensed to practice medicine.

LAPTOPS

The Veterans Healthcare System has mandated a paperless medical record system since the year 2000 but completion of this process has been slow. Most medical delivery systems throughout the United States are continually struggling with patient information that is not well organized. In addition, it is difficult to read due to poor copying techniques, the age of the paper source and the illegible handwriting of numerous authors. These systems are becoming much more complex due to the demands of insurers, managed care administrators, evidence-based mandates, research protocols and costly screening wrapped around high technology tests.

Use of a laptop should not mean more work such as having to double chart. Information should be entered as soon as possible after interaction, if not during that time. The advantage of utilizing the laptop at point of care is the time savings and increased accuracy. Rather than jot down a few things then later try to remember everything to transfer into the chart, the physician can "jot" on the laptop so that what is being entered stays as part of the documentation. It wouldn't be electronically signed until after the interaction when the physician can expand on what has already been documented and make any necessary changes.

Although the evidence varies for incorporating the laptop into the traditional dyadic surgeon-patient interaction, the following guidelines are based on a study of major academic institutions pre/post investments of laptops in clinic settings.

ACTION POINTS

While in the clinic room, the physician should **DO** the following:

1. Explain to the patient the process of using the computer and what will take place during their interaction. If possible, turn the screen toward patients so they can see what is being viewed. Try to look at patients as often as possible, and particularly when you are trying to explain or describe their problem. When you are not able to look at the patient, let him or her know what is being looked at or what information is being documented at that moment.

2. Look up lab results or completed tests in front of the patient. Sometimes these will be color coded to indicate low, normal, and high ranges. If so, and they are easy to read or see, let the patient also look.

3. The physician can also use the laptop to educate and inform. For example, pictures could be stored on the computer and shown to the patient to illustrate what a wound might look like at postoperative day (POD) #1, POD #5, etc.

4. The patient's face should be observed, though, to see his or her reaction to the pictures. Is she curious, reassured or frightened?

While in the clinic room, the physician should **NOT**:

1. Scan the entire note in front of the patient, leaving the patient in silence. If possible, while reading a note, read aloud or talk about some of the information. That will not only relieve the silence, it allows a chance for the physician to explain, confirm, or express her opinions if indicated.

2. Ask questions while looking at the computer screen. Most eye contact should be on the patient when a question is being asked. If not, the important nonverbal clues will be missed, as well as signal to the patient that the computer outranks him or her in importance.

"Enter a hospital when it is in the process of introducing more computers, they say, and you can hear the sound of nurses growling. Doctors using laptops sometimes have to wrestle with incompatible systems, manually retyping lab results from one computer into another."

"What Scares Doctors?"(14)

Some specialties find that simply noting values while in the patient room and then entering these numbers immediately into the template at a work station outside the room works efficiently.

Templates can be developed that work for both patient and physician. The more the surgeon can have available in templates, the more time will be saved. Also, they serve as a "prompt" or "trigger" for the writer to inquire about and/or document specific information that meets outside an accrediting agency's guidelines. In addition, templates should be flexible enough to allow physicians room to document what they believe to be important.

> WARNING:
>
> Surgeons are task oriented. Completing patient electronic records in a timely fashion may please administrator types, but if you sacrifice the loss of personal human interaction, it may destroy your career or damage your patient-physician relationship.
>
> PA Rowland

What does not work as well are computer work stations that are permanently mounted to walls in clinic rooms where the physician faces the screen and away from the patient.

Often, patient satisfaction scores will decrease when an experienced physician begins to convert to the paperless record. However, once the surgeon develops a new interaction style with the computer and patient, the scores will improve and the interaction will be less stressful.

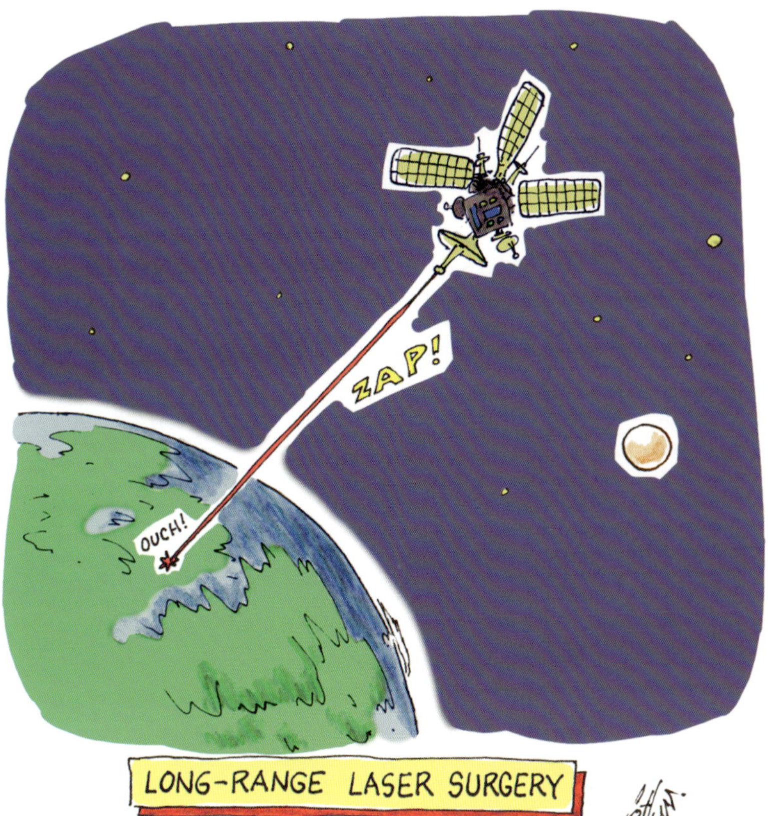

REFERENCES

1. Pope CR, Yoshioka SS, Greenlick MR. Determinants of medical care utilization: the use of the telephone for reporting symptoms. J Health Soc Behav. 1971; 12:155-162.
2. Greenlick MR, Freeborn DK, Gambill GL, et al. Determinants of medical care utilization: the role of the telephone in total medical care. Med Care. 1973; 11:121-134.
3. Bergman AB, Dassell SW, Wedgewood RJ. Time-motion study of practicing pediatricians. Pediatrics. 1966; 38:254-263.
4. Curtis P, Talbot A. The telephone in primary care. J Community Health. 1981; 6:194-203.
5. Fischer PM, Smith SR. The nature and management of telephone utilization in a family practice setting. J Fam Pract. 1979; 8:321-327.
6. Richards JG, Campbell D. Out of hours calls. NZ Med J. 1976; 83:101.
7. Webster GL, Ritchie AF, Morrell JA, et al. Night calls in general practice. Br Med J. 1965; 1:1369.
8. Perry JR, Caine N. General practitioners' knowledge about patients and use of medical records in out of hours calls. Br J Gen Pract. 1990; 40:190-193.
9. Harrigan JA, Gramata JF, Lucic KS, Margolis C. It's how you say it: physicians' vocal behavior. Soc Sci Med. 1989; 28:87-92.
10. Davidhizar RE, Wehlage DF. Telephone 'emergencies': how to respond appropriately and effectively. Postgrad Med. 1987; 81:61-68.
11. Conrath VW, Buchingham P, Dunn EV, et al. An experimental evaluation of alternative communication systems as used for medical diagnosis. Behav Sci. 1975; 20:296.
12. Smith SR, Fischer PM. Patient management by telephone: a training exercise for medical students. J Fam Pract. 1980; 10:463-466.
13. Friend T. Taking Telemedicine to the extreme. USA TODAY. 1998 Apr 21; 6D.
14. Gibb N, Bower A. What doctors hate about hospitals, TIME. 2006 May 01; Sect. Medicine:42-52
15. Balas EA, Jaffrey F, Kuperman GJ, et al. Electronic communication with patients. Evaluation of distance medicine technology. JAMA. 1997; 278:152.

Chief Complaint Profile for Receptionist-Managed Calls in Four Family Practice Offices (N=1,533)

Complaint/Symptom	Percent
URI	24.2
Fever	15.9
Ear pain	4.4
Rash	3.7
Flu	3.5
Abdominal pain	3.5
Nausea, vomiting	2.8
Back pain	2.5
Swollen glands	2.4
Skin infection	2.1
Headache	1.9
Diarrhea	1.9
Joint pain	1.6
Eye infection	1.5
Lumps, masses	1.3
Chest pain	1.3
Dysuria	1.1
High blood pressure	1.0
Sprain, strain	1.0
Question of fracture	0.9
Dizziness	0.9
Dyspnea	0.9
Fatigue	0.9
Laceration	0.9
Urinary frequency	0.8

Algorithm for Managing Medical Problems on the Telephone

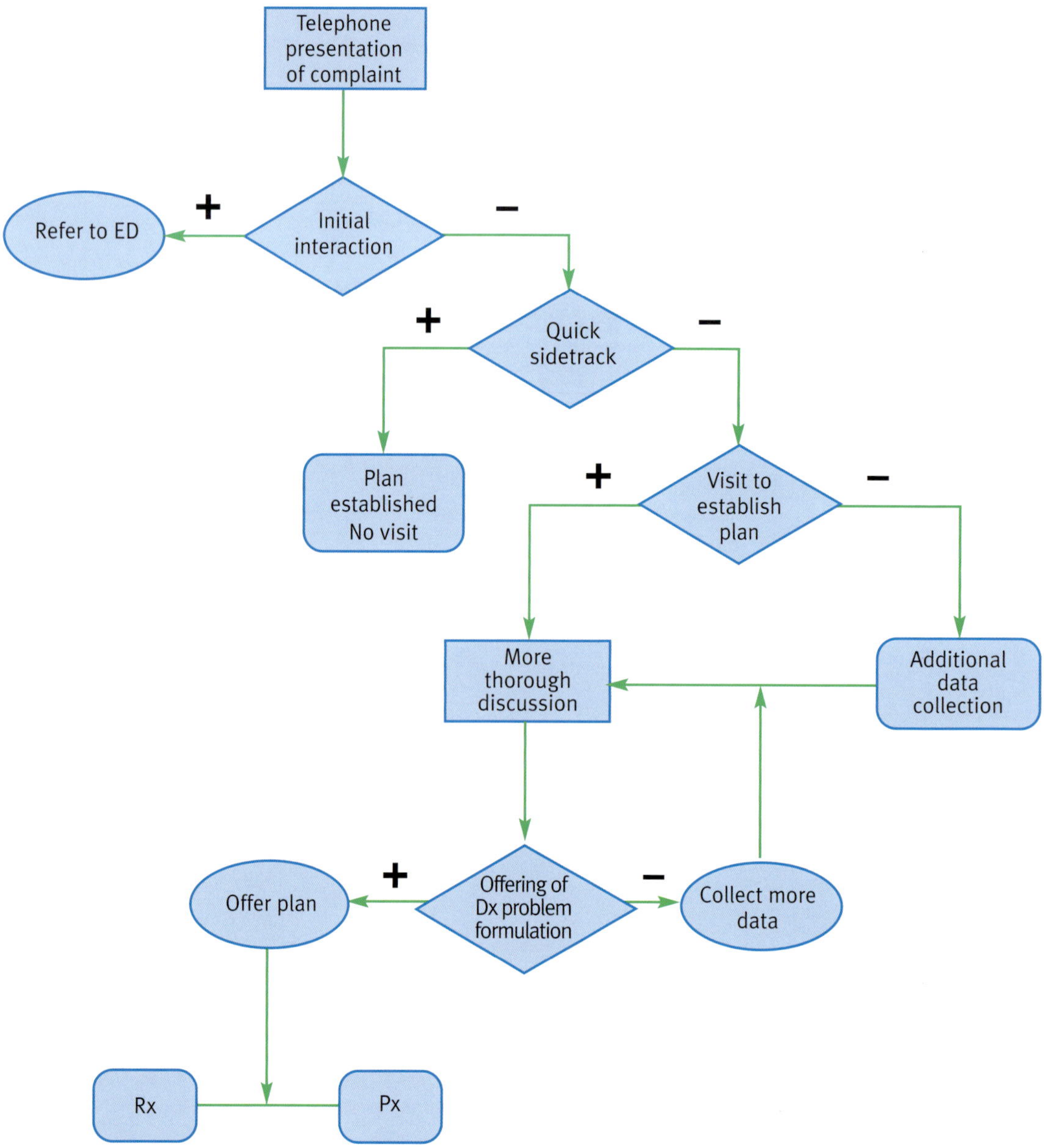

Bad News: Speaking Clearly

David W. Page, MD, FACS
Joseph Melino, MDiv
Nicholas P. Lang, MD, FACS

The family waited in the surgical floor lounge with its bright colors, hopeful decorum and mindlessly blaring TV. The family stood as the surgeon entered, then sat together in a circle. The matriarch, to whom the surgeon's remarks were directed fidgeted with her rosary.

Moments before, the surgeon had felt the cancer rocks embedded in her husband's liver. Disorganized chunks which studded the liver surface converted its tan smoothness to a moonscape of unresectable disease. Deep in his abdomen the seminal rectal cancer had grown to fill his pelvic bowl like thick gruel. The surgeon was forced to perform a colostomy and knew the man's ureters would soon be encased with cancer and obstruct as well.

"He's in the recovery room," the surgeon began. "He tolerated the surgery quite well. However, the tumor was extensive. I couldn't remove it all. I just did a biopsy to prove what it was."

"Is he all right?" the matriarch asked.

"Yes, he's stable. I had to perform a colostomy."

She wept softly. Her family closed in around her on the couch, crowded her and touched her in comfort, as if to cut off the surgeon's presence.

"Tumor you said, doctor?"

"Yes. Quite extensive. In his pelvis and liver. I'm sorry."

"Yes, well, tumor," the old woman sighed. "Thank God it wasn't cancer."

Several mistakes occurred in this postoperative discussion. Attempting to soften the impact of the man's diagnosis, the surgeon unwittingly began optimistically, walked too gingerly over the diagnosis, and misled the family by assuming too much. Important high impact words (such as cancer) were avoided.

This chapter presents the basic elements of delivering bad news. It covers methods, mistakes and directions for improvement. These guidelines will serve as a compass to help clinicians negotiate the perilous waters of clinical decision-making and its related obligation – an honest discussion with the patient and family of treatments and expected outcomes. Their reaction to bad news will vary with their individual life experiences, education, social status, and expectations making it difficult to generalize a single management style. For example, the result of a pregnancy test may be greeted with emotions ranging from shock or disbelief to extreme happiness. A surgeon's communication behavior with one patient may result in rejection of a recommendation, or acceptance and satisfaction with another. Members of different cultures respond differently to bad news. Adhering to the basic principles suggested in this chapter will provide insight into successful communication strategies.

First, there has been a dramatic change in information-sharing between doctors and patients in the Western world (US and Western Europe) from 1961 to 1979.(1-2) For example, a reversal in surgeon attitudes toward telling cancer patients about their diagnosis has occurred. Revealing a diagnosis of malignancy has gone from 90% against disclosure in the 1960s to over 95% in favor of telling patients their diagnosis today. This change occurred because of the emergence of a now widely held belief in patient autonomy and a conviction that patients have the right to make their own decisions about health care issues.

Despite these changes, many patients from other cultures still do not want to be told bad news by a surgeon. In Japan, informing a patient of a serious or fatal condition such as cancer is deferred because of a concern this bad news may damage the spirit, and thereby prevent any hope of recovery.(3-4) Another ethnic group, the Ethiopians, have a strong family structure designed to help cushion and protect the patient. To tell an Ethiopian patient of a bad diagnosis is considered harmful and undesirable. These culturally-based differences confirm the difficulty inherent in making generalizations about giving difficult news. This problem is further aggravated when the bad news occurs after only a brief contact with a patient, such as in the emergency department.

When surgeons, medical students, and patients are surveyed, there is agreement that surgeons need additional training in giving bad news. (5-6) While there are very few formal training programs, the courses that are available seem to be well received by trainees. Early surveys suggest these courses impart increased confidence in the surgeons regarding their ability to deal with bad news. (7-8)

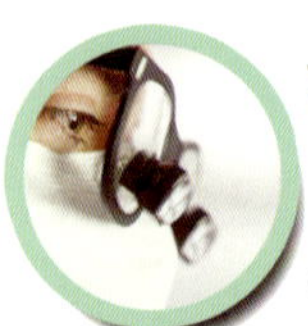

WHAT IS BAD NEWS?

Bad news is information about patients or their loved ones which predicts pain, suffering and/or death in the future. This information opens up a gap between the patient's expectations of a safe and long future and the reality of a life-altering new truth. The judicious delivery of bad news is a necessary part of the practice of surgery. Communicating distasteful information requires compassion, insight and clarity. It also requires information, preparation, and timing.

"I am aware of the Greek program. If you go with an expectation of a miraculous cure – you'll be disappointed. However, if you go to Greece and celebrate your life together and, by-the-way, stop in to visit the clinic – and then make your own assessment, then I think you'll have a great trip."

NP Lang

Eight Steps for Delivering Bad News

Step 1. Turn off your cell phone and beeper, look in the mirror and confirm a professional appearance.

Step 2. Reflect on your goals for the meeting, as well as your patient's goals; review the chart and obtain the latest information before starting the meeting.

Step 3. Select a quiet room, ask who the patient would like to be present, and ask all to sit down.

Step 4. Ask the patient (and other family members what they understand of the situation (how much does the patient know about her condition?); how much does the patient want to know?

Step 5. Provide information about your diagnosis, planned treatment and your expectations regarding outcome; use simple language and wait for a response; do nor use jargon! Assess your patient's level of understanding.

Step 6. Acknowledge your patient's feelings about the bad news; give time for reactions and questions; ask if you have clarified your message.

Step 7. Determine your patient's wishes and the direction he/she wants his or her care to go: align yourself with your patient's wishes.

Step 8. Jointly plan for future meetings and follow-up sessions.

Surgeons must prepare for the frustration, anger, and despair a bad news discussion will provoke. Basic to speaking clearly is the goal of transferring distressing information with no change in the message. Even so, the surgeon should expect questions such as:

"What do you mean you couldn't get it all out?"

"Why did he need a bag?"

"Will you take it off later?"

"Can X-ray treatments cure it then?"

"Should we get another opinion?"

"How long will he be in the hospital?"

"What do you mean he may not make it?"

Misunderstanding magnifies the impact of bad news. Always assess the patient's educational background and the family's ability to understand what is being said. All too frequently, surgeons lapse into jargon instead of interpreting medical terms in ways that listeners can understand. Jargon too often leaves the patient and family nodding politely as the discussion bogs down into a meaningless one-way exchange.

Bad news discussions usually require the use of high impact words. The patient may flinch at language fragments exploding like shrapnel that leave gaping wounds in the listener. Careful word choice is necessary and the clinician should think through the discussion beforehand. Words become symbols of bad disease. The surgeon may envision the patient's breast cancer as occult and curable, but the postoperative discussion may leave the patient imagining a vicious mass of tumor tentacles ravaging her body. High impact words like cancer must always be qualified, the message repeated, clarified, and often diagrammed.

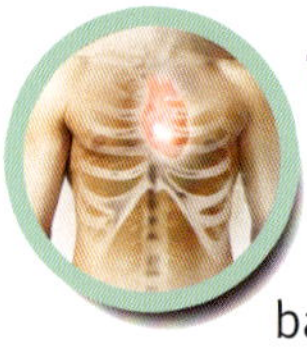

The anatomy of a bad news discussion

Conditions requiring a discussion of bad news include: unexpected death, near or imminent death, pain, prolonged physical and mental suffering; debilitation, and, loss of personal autonomy. Some diseases present catastrophically, others insinuate themselves into a patient's life. In either situation, the illness may become fatal quickly. Alternatively, the patient's clinical course may be prolonged, anguished, and uncertain. Thus, the temporal profile of clinical events shapes the bad news discussion and the need for repetition. Regardless of the setting, certain canned phrases must be avoided.

Bad news discussions often anticipate radical treatment options not initially considered by the doctor or the patient. The discussion often reveals the patient's lack of understanding about the fallibility of modern medicine. Optimistic about cure, patients often aren't prepared for possibilities such as:

- re-operation is needed for bleeding, leaking anastamosis, etc., and a further surgery may be necessary;
- the disease (cancer, coronary heart disease, arthritis, sepsis, etc.) has reoccurred;
- the patient has failed to respond to treatment (infection, multi-organ system failure, metastatic cancer, etc.)
- there is organ failure not related to the primary disease (acute renal failure, acute respiratory failure, etc.).

Perhaps the most important aspect of patient-doctor conflict is patient expectation. Much anger and subsequent litigation evolves from a mismatch between what a patient anticipates (heard) the outcome would be and what the surgeon actually offered (said) as treatment. In this regard, it must be noted that the manner in which surgeons handle the delivery of bad news may determine their medico-legal

When Does News Become Bad News?

Death	
Completed	patient dies suddenly
Imminent	patient's course deteriorates suddenly; little possibility of successful intervention
Probable	clinical events make survival unlikely; marginal status means the time course to death is hours or days
Possible	clinical events have deteriorated or have not responded to interventions
Negative diagnosis	
At consultation	after initial clinical assessment the likelihood of a serious disease arises
After work-up	an intervention or exploratory surgery may be required to confirm the diagnosis
After emergency	severe abdominal, chest or extremity surgery/pain may signal serious disease
Negative outcome	
After surgery	all of the above possible time course events for death may apply to the patient operated upon for what proves to be an incurable disease; complications or a negative outcome may occur days or weeks following surgery
After an intervention	high tech procedures carry risk of complications, as well as the possibility of discovering cancer, etc.
After medical therapy	short or long term medical treatment (e.g. chemotherapy) may prove fruitless; alternative options may or may not hold promise.

liability. Therefore, bad news should be repeated in more than one format. This may include preop informed consent discussions as well as postop briefings about what was actually found and what it means for the patient.

For example,

"Surgery won't help his brain injury, the damage is too severe."

Later, "We don't expect the coma to clear."

Later, "You should at least consider the possibility that we may eventually discover your husband meets brain death criteria."

Later, "Have you considered organ donation?"

A discussion of treatment options must include information about the potential for bad results. Document the discussion. Full disclosure of all possible results of surgery is the foundation of informed consent. The difference between the surgeon's and the patient's perception of a given treatment option is the surgeon's insight into all potential clinical profiles. The surgeon must explain up front (preoperatively) the potential for a bad outcome.

In the critical care unit, patients often become progressively more and more ill and may plunge into a rapid downward spiral of multi-organ failure. The task of informing the patient's family becomes a progressive discussion or snowballing of bad news. Consider the case of a patient who undergoes an elective total colectomy and who subsequently develops sudden onset of chest pain. Imagine the work-up reveals a postoperative pulmonary embolism. The patient is transferred to the intensive care unit, suffers a cardiac arrest, and is intubated. The family must be taken quickly from the context of safe, elective colon surgery to the reality of potential death.

The skillful clinician anticipates this pattern of bad news and "layers" in evidence of the patient's clinical decline in repeated conversations. In this fashion (often referred to by house staff as "hanging black crepe") bad news is offered in small digestible doses. For example, in the surgical intensive care unit a surgical patient may exhibit early signs of multi-organ failure following surgery for a perforated viscus. Experienced surgeons will explain the possibility of uncontrolled sepsis, despite their efforts to surgically repair the bowel and clean the abdominal cavity.

Thus, patients and their families receive distasteful information in numerous niches of the hospital. These include the emergency room, postsurgical waiting rooms, intensive care waiting rooms, hallways, and the surgeons' offices. All of these settings are unfamiliar, threatening, and may reinforce the negative impact of the message. And, of course, patients and their families often harbor preconceived ideas, misunderstanding, fear, anger, and possibly resentment when asked to join a bad news discussion. The surgeon must be sensitive to the complex milieu in which all concerned parties find themselves.

HIGH IMPACT WORDS

There are many reasons to prepare carefully for a bad news discussion. Surgeons who choose words indiscriminately will be perceived as insensitive. If bad news is delivered in a rushed manner, the patient and family will always recall the surgeon's crass demeanor and haphazard remarks. In addition, the lay impact of common medical terms a surgeon may toss off casually is often explosive and loaded with hidden meaning for the patient or family. Frequently, jargon is misunderstood. Several high impact words deserve further discussion.

Dead

Several years ago a medivac crashed while transporting a patient from a rural hospital to a medical center. On board was the pilot, an emergency surgeon, a nurse, and the patient. The pilot was killed instantly in the crash. The patient and the nurse escaped with only minor injuries, but the surgeon, David W., received serious internal injuries to his chest and abdomen which required emergency surgery. He arrived at the hospital with a trauma score of 8. Within minutes he was sent to the operating room and the chaplain was left to 'take care of the family.' Within the hour, the surgeon's parents and his wife, Joan, who was also a surgeon, arrived and began an anxious waiting period.

Two hours passed before the chaplain's beeper called him to the surgical intensive care unit. There, a look from Dr. Morris, one of the trauma surgeons who had taken David to the operating room, made it plain that David had died. The surgeon nervously asked who was in the waiting room as he turned and walked toward it. The chaplain tried to give him all the pertinent information about the patient and his family, blurting out the fact that the patient's wife was herself a surgeon. The news seemed to ease the surgeon's anxiety. As they entered the room, he mumbled, "This isn't going to be too bad."

The situation became tense. Dr. Morris stood before the family and identified himself to Joan. He asked her about her training, but ignored David's parents. He began listing David's injuries, identifying all the possible procedures available to correct them, explaining why each had failed. Then, as he explained the failure of the last procedure he concluded, "And with that we had to stop."

Joan, looking from behind the table, said softly, "Are you telling me he's dead?"

Dr. Morris answered, "Yes, he died from complications of multiple trauma."

Joan looked at Dr. Morris with horror and disbelief and, with one sweep of her arm, an array of coffee cups went flying from the table spraying everyone and everything in the small room.

Shocked at the reaction, Dr. Morris stammered, "Get a hold of yourself. After all, you've lost patients before."

Death cannot be cushioned. Sudden death is an even more painful reality. It will invoke feelings of abandonment, anger, loss of control and guilt. No matter how death is announced, regardless of what euphemism is chosen to soften the blow, the word "death" is crippling. But the word must be articulated. No substitutes are acceptable.

"We've lost him," sounds as if there's still hope that "he" might be found.

The surgeon in the example above inappropriately assumed he had an ally in the wife/surgeon and that this professional alliance would protect him from her emotions. What he failed to understand was that, despite their shared profession and his objective clinical presentation, her reaction was that of a wife, a lover, and a mother. He missed her humanity. He delayed telling her the truth about her husband's demise by burying it in clinically irrelevant detail. He hid behind verbal trash.

There are several overused clichés (meaningless expressions) to avoid in your attempt to cushion bad news. Here are a few:

"He's gone to a better place."

"We had to stop."

"His suffering is over."

"She has expired."

"She's finally resting."

By anticipating the likelihood of death, the surgeon may help soften the ravages of loss for a family. It is useful to provide the family with an ongoing recital of the team's expectations for survival or death as the clinical picture evolves. Here are three examples of how a growing expectation of death can be presented:

- "Your mother's progress is minimal. I now don't believe she can survive her many medical problems. We'll continue to treat her as we have been. But, she may die at any time despite our treatments."
- "He has deteriorated in the last six hours. I now do not believe he will survive. He may die at any time. You may wish to notify other members of your family."
- "The operation was successful, but I am concerned about the amount of infection I saw. With this much infection, there are many patients who die despite the operation. She is critically sick and her course may change for the worse at any moment. I will keep you informed."

When death looms on the horizon, it is wise to encourage the family to take comfort in their personal belief system. This is the time to contact the clergy, for example, who may assist grieving families as the hopeful acute care phase ends and withdrawal of active treatment seems appropriate.

Normal grieving takes many forms. For some, grieving entails outbursts of emotion, pounding on walls, falling to one's knees, or just repeating the name of the deceased over and over again in a piercing voice or a whisper. Some folks are stoic. Some are private. Some need to grieve in public.

However, there are extreme cases where the grieving individual may attempt to inflict injury on himself or attempt to harm others. A bereavement counselor or security personnel is often needed. Intervention may include sedation and physical restraint. Frequently, someone from the family will arise as a leader and help with the out of control person.

Some emotional outbursts are cultural and are an accepted and necessary part of the grieving process. These are not extreme. They may test a surgeon's emotional control. Simply being present during these difficult moments is probably the best medicine.

For families who are experiencing death for the first time, some basic information as to what will happen next is often helpful. Providing information about the medical examiner, organ donation (if the case warrants), handling personal belongings, and a call to an undertaker will help families to cope.

CANCER

Cancer poses a variety of challenges to a surgeon's communication skills. Cancer is not one disease. Nor can the heterogeneity of a particular malignancy, such as breast cancer, be easily described. To most patients, cancer is frightening and unpredictable and treatment is potentially mutilating and ineffective. Clinicians must present in understandable terms the complex ideas of stage, grade, and prognosis. For example, surgeons may state,

> "The cancer is all out. I did not see any spread to your liver or elsewhere. We'll wait for the pathology report to decide if further treatment is needed. It looks good for now."

If a cancer has metastasized as in the opening scenario, a clear presentation of the concept of *incurable* as it applies to the patient must be made.

> "The cancer has spread to your liver. There are many deposits, more than we could safely remove. This was not a curative operation. We can offer you other treatments to give you as much time as possible."

Diagrams often help to demonstrate the scale of aggressiveness of a cancer and are useful in conveying the idea of a poor prognosis. Treatment options should be listed and the concept of adjuvant treatment (often chemotherapy) explained as "additional treatment." Survival percentages may be offered if requested. Often patients or family members will ask surgeons to define the length of survival for a terminal patient. Experienced surgeons hesitate to do this because precise assessments of survival usually prove to be wrong. In fact, doctors almost always offer excessively favorable prognoses. But families deserve the best estimate of remaining life in order to plan end-of-life care.

Avoid the word ***malignancy***. After using the word cancer, clarify what it means for that patient. If the prognosis isn't clear, then say so. Emphasize treatment and leave the projected clinical course open-ended.

PAIN

Pain is a private torment. It can cause patients to writhe in silent, sweaty forbearance, or bitterly complain about discomfort another might consider paltry. Whatever the setting, surgeons must bear in mind the subjective nature of pain. Untreated pain is undoubtedly modern medicine's most magnificent shortcoming.

Surgeons tend to downplay pain unless it's their own. Medical journal editorials by surgeons suffering postoperative agony clearly depict this double standard. For example, the man with persistent back pain after disc surgery must not be discarded by his busy neurosurgeon. Surgeons should help their patients understand the role of the peripheral and central nervous system and the role of emotions in coping with pain. A woman who understands that her breast pain is probably not associated with cancer frequently discovers she can handle the ache. Few patients should be counseled to live with pain.

Surgeons tend to downplay pain, unless it's their own.

Many other high impact words form the latticework of daily dialogue with patients. These include colostomy, radiation, chemotherapy, coma, AIDS, Alzheimer's, stroke, anesthesia, peritonitis, and diabetes. Surgeons should keep in mind that words are symbols of the patient's concerns about death, pain, suffering, disfigurement, disability, and loss of autonomy. The primary focus of bad news discussions should be to discuss the patient's specific concerns about these issues. By far, the most frequent lament of the unhappy patient is,

"The surgeon didn't tell me this could happen..."

POTENTIAL RESPONSES TO BAD NEWS

The patient's personality, prior experiences, and expectations determine how he or she will react to bad news. Family dynamics are also crucial in how other members of the support team will handle the surgeon's news. Unresolved family conflict places additional demands on a surgeon's communication skills. Careful explanation of the work-up (including the role of special tests and procedures) is best done in the presence of the entire family. When patients can't communicate or are deemed temporarily incompetent, the family should designate one spokesperson. Surgeons can expect several common reactions to bad news:

Disbelief	Bad news only happens to someone else.
Surprise	Patients who have not permitted themselves to imagine the possibility of an adverse diagnosis or result.
Reluctant Acceptance	Knowing the presentation to be true, patients (who may have suspected bad news long before seeking help) agree there's a problem.
Willing Acceptance	Most patients, many of whom delay seeking medical advice, cooperate without protest when the surgeon pronounces possible bad news. Patients with strong belief systems similarly rely on God's, not the surgeon's, wisdom.

Regardless of the manner in which patients or families react, the message should always be repeated one more time. Whether delivering potentially bad news or describing an unfortunate, completed complication or poor result, surgeons must assume that a portion of the message was not received. In ideal situations, people only retain 4 to 5% of what they hear. Preoccupation with something said earlier in the discussion often compromises the reception of the full report. Repeating the message helps the patient and the family focus on the meaning.

"We can do something about the brain met that caused the seizures but we can't change the fact that she is going to die soon of breast cancer."

CONCLUSION

In summary, employment of eight principles of delivering bad news will vary with circumstances. These include the length of time the surgeon has known the patient, the surgeon's familiarity with the patient's personal and cultural beliefs and the type of bad news being conveyed. Central to all of these suggestions is an acknowledgement of the seriousness of the bad news and how the patient and family may feel about it.(7-8)

Don't postpone giving bad news. Speak in clear, declarative sentences and use high impact words appropriately. For example, in the opening scene the surgeon should have told the family the disease was cancer (instead of "tumor") which spread (not "metastasized") and was not curable, but treatable.

Plan what to say ahead of time. Redefine the disease. What is the stage? What does this mean regarding treatment? What are the options? What's the possible course in this particular patient?

Expect and deal compassionately with frustration, anxiety, anger and lack of comprehension.

Repeat the message with each new question. Expect a significant period of time after each dose of bad news to allow the recipient to think about what was said. State the essence of the bad news in more than one form.

Avoid cushion words: "tumor," "growth," "essentially," "relatively," "sickness," "demise," "passing," and "piece of cake." Avoid medical jargon.

As the patient's clinical course deteriorates, begin to "layer" in elements of the emerging bad news. Recurrent intraabdominal sepsis, sequential multi-organ failure, progressive metastatic cancer, organic brain syndrome, congestive heart failure all represent clinical courses well recognized for their downward, inexorably fatal course. Surgeons understand this, but need to make certain the burdened family and patient (on request) can also see the long view.

If the patient's status begins to deteriorate quickly, explain to the patient and/or family that the outcome is uncertain and changing rapidly. Encourage the patient and family to seek counsel with their clergy. Offer to have hospital personnel (nursing supervisors, chaplain, grief counselor, psychiatrist, etc.) talk with them. Timing is critical when recommending emotional and spiritual support to a patient and family.

Even when a surgeon believes the patient and family understand the remote possibility of bad news, the message should be repeated one more time. To fulfill the moral obligation of providing an unfettered message, the surgeon must communicate an unambiguous message of bad news to the patient and family in succinct language that everyone can understand.

"There are no atheists in fox holes."

William Thomas Cummings

March 1942

Sermon to the troops at Bataan in Philippines

REFERENCES

1. Cassileath BR, Zupkis RJ, Sutton-Smith K, et al. Information and participation preferences among cancer patients. Ann Internatl Med. 1980; 82:832-836.
2. Novack DH, Plumer R, Smith RL, et al. Changes in surgeons; attitudes toward telling the cancer patient. JAMA. 1979; 241:897-900.
3. Asai A. Should surgeons tell patients the truth? West J Med. 1995; 163: 36-9.
4. Long S, Long B. Curable cancer and fatal ulcers: Attitudes toward cancer in Japan. Soc Sci Med. 1982; 16:2101-2108.
5. Gillard JH, Dent THS, Aarons EJ, et al. Preregistration house officers in eight English regions: survey of quality of training. Br Med J. 1993; 307:1180-1184.
6. Sardell AN, Trierweiler SJ. Disclosing the cancer diagnosis. Procedures that influence patient hopefulness. Cancer. 1993; 72:3355-65.
7. Cushing AM, Jones A. Evaluation of a breaking bad news course for medical students. Med Educ. 1995; 29:430-5.
8. Garg A, Buckman R, Kason Y. Teaching medical students how to break bad news. CMAJ. 1997; 156:1159-64.
9. Buckman, R. How to Break Bad News – A Guide for Health Professionals. Baltimore: The Johns Hopkins University Press; 1992.
10. Surbone, A. Zwitter, M. Eds. Communication With Cancer Patients – Information and Truth. New York: The New York Academy of Sciences; 1997.
11. Iserson KV. Pocket Protocols – Notifying Survivors about Sudden, Unexpected Deaths. Tucson (AZ): Galen Press; 1999.

Religious Phrases to Avoid Saying

"It was God's will..."

"God picks the most beautiful flowers first..."

"This will make your faith stronger..."

"God needs ________ more than you do..."

"Now you have an angel in heaven watching over you..."

"You can talk to ________ anytime you want. She/he will hear you ..."

"God relieved his/her pain..."

"It was actually a blessing because..."

"God has a reason for this..."

"Only the good die young..."

"God never gives us more than we can handle..."

"You shouldn't feel/act that way..."

Adapted from Iserson:

Notifying Survivors about Sudden Unexpected Deaths (11)

Phrases to Avoid

"Death happens. Get over it!"

"Be grateful that you still have your other children..."

"Be grateful that you can have other children..."

"Aren't you lucky that at least..."

"You must be strong for your other children, spouse, etc."

"You must get hold of yourself...."

"The healthy must go on..."

"She/he's gone and you'll just have to make the best of it."

"Don't take it so hard."

"You'll get over this..."

"You're young....you'll find someone else."

"So you think you'll get married again?"

"You must focus on your precious memories..."

"You can always find someone worse off than yourself."

"It's time to buck up and get on with life..."

"Go back to work. It will distract you..."

"I don't want to make you cry..."

"You have to keep busy..."

"You don't need to know that."

"What you don't know can't hurt you."

"I can't tell you that."

"Let's not talk about it."

"It just must have been her/his time to go."

"Things always work out for the best."

"This will make you a better, perhaps stronger person."

"He/she was holding you back."

"The kids are young, so they'll most likely forget him/her..."

Adapted from Iserson:

Notifying Survivors about Sudden Unexpected Deaths

Safer Phrases

"I can't imagine how difficult this is for you..."

"I know this is very painful for you..."

"I'm so sorry for your loss..."

"It's harder than most people think..."

"It must be hard to accept..."

"You must have been very close to him/her..."

"How can I be of help?"

"Let's spend some time together..."

"You are not alone, I'm here to help you..."

"I know this must feel like a dream to you..."

"Tell me how you're feeling..."

"I know you will miss him..."

"She/he was very special to you..."

"I know you are feeling totally overwhelmed right now..."

"I'll call you tomorrow. Until then, if you need me, here is my pager number."

"May I just sit here with you...?"

"Tell me about _____ and your life with him/her..."

Adapted from Iserson:

Notifying Survivors about Sudden Unexpected Deaths

Conflict: The Skilled Response

Francis X. Aumand, III, MSA;
Pamela A. Rowland, PhD

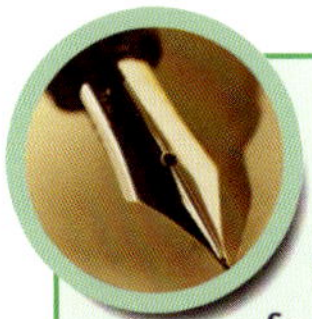

Dr. Jones went to preop holding to see the first patient scheduled in his room for the day. Jack Williams was not there. Dr. Jones asked about the patient and was told by a nervous nursing assistant that he was supposed to come down from the fifth floor, but she did not know why he wasn't here. "We called for him an hour ago."

Forty five minutes later, a frowning Dr. Jones returned to preop holding to see Mr. Williams being rolled into the area by two nurses from fifth floor. "Can't you people ever do anything on time? Your failure has caused a delay in the schedule. We'll have delays in other cases and we'll need to use overtime or to cancel some cases. You just don't care!"

One nurse began to cry and the other stomped off, clearly very angry.

Had Dr. Jones been able to inquire in a less abrasive way, he would have discovered these two nurses and the patient had been trapped for two hours on a malfunctioning elevator and that both nurses had volunteered to stay past their scheduled shift end to help transport Mr. Williams because they wanted to help get the OR schedule started on time.

Surgeons will inevitably witness or be involved in a variety of conflicts throughout their training and careers. It will begin before any words are spoken.

In a professional setting, conflict is a struggle between or among staff, surgeons, residents, students and professionals whose tasks are interdependent, who feel angry and who perceive the other(s) as interfering with their goals.

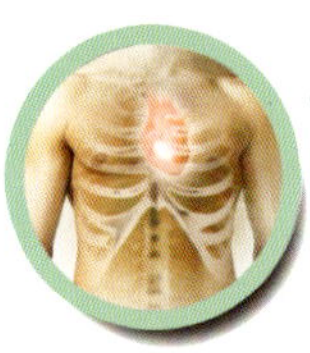

Conflict is rooted in all parts of human nature. Some people actually enjoy conflict while others avoid it. Therefore, it is critical for surgeons to understand that they can't avoid conflict. However, the communicatively competent surgeon will be able to manage conflict. The result—a better decision and outcomes.

1. Recognize that there is conflict.
2. Decide how to respond professionally.

Too often "*conflict*" is commonly used as a label to situations that are not really conflicts. Often conflict is confused with:

Indecision

Disagreement

Stress

These behaviors may be caused by conflict, but are not the causes of conflict alone.

CONDITIONS THAT PRODUCE CONFLICT

Certain conditions produce conflict:

Incompatible Goals

One member of the OR team wants to finish quickly because he has a date. Another member wishes to work late because she will get paid overtime if the case goes beyond the end of her shift. She has recently purchased a new car and is worried about making her payments.

Unrealistic Expectations

Dr. Thomas schedules his Whipple operations for three hours even though the OR records indicate he has never performed this operation in less than six hours. As a result, the staff are angry and later cases are cancelled because he runs over.

Differing Rates of Relationship or Growth

PGY-3 believes he is competent to do breast biopsy simply because he is a PGY-3, but the attending does not.

A highly trained new faculty member challenges the decision of a senior member of the faculty.

> Dr. Muhamad had undergone a surgery residency in his home country and came to the US, where he completed another surgery residency by working at two different programs. His attitude toward everyone was that he was highly trained, very skilled and deserving of a high salary and respect. While his clinical productivity was good, his questions at weekly conference and his academic productivity belied his claims of greatness. He eventually moved to another university because he felt he was not respected by the department chairman.

Inaccurate Perceptions and Attributions

A resident came into the program after he was eliminated from a program in New York. While he did have strong recommendations from the Program Director, he had gone to medical school in a Central American country. Even though he was accepted in this program based on his former program director's recommendations, everyone was concerned about his knowledge base, skill, language and cultural adaptation. Dr. Gomez proved to be one of the best residents (knowledge, skill, technical ability and interpersonal communication) ever trained in this program. He outperformed all others (who had benefited from a medical school training experience in the US) and was easily placed in a very competitive post residency fellowship.

Cultural Differences

Different cultures respond to conflict in either a direct or indirect approach. Many cherish the relationship more than the goal (Japanese, Latin) while others focus more on the goal (Swedish, German). This is critical when conflict involves more than one culture.

Take badly behaving persons off 'the stage.'

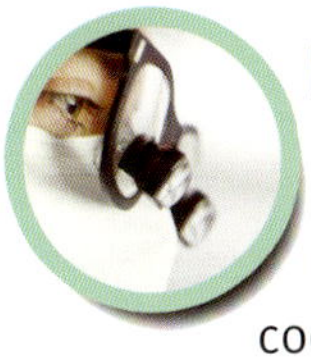

BEHAVIORS THAT INDICATE CONFLICT

Certain behaviors create conflict. The behaviors that may indicate that there is a conflict are recognizable and may define your conflict style. They vary on the amount of cooperativeness and assertiveness you demonstrate.

Passive behaviors—avoiding personal contact

- Writing memos and e-mails rather than direct communication
- Withholding needed information
- Not returning messages, e-mail
- Delay in providing required support

Competing behaviors—getting others to take sides

- Increased volume
- Pre-empting
- Undermining the opponents reputation
- Minimizing the opponents technical skills

Avoiding behaviors—signals of stress

- Sweaty palms
- Nervous gesture
- Closed body posture
- Crying
- Clenched jaw
- Fisted hand

Competing and *passive* behaviors are strategic decisions that we make in our attempts to deal with conflict. They are similar to the old **fight or flight** behavior patterns. These old patterns of **fight or flight** are major inhibitors in our ability to resolve conflict. Within our current professional environments, such as the hospital or office setting, our behavioral patterns have been modified to be less intrusive and aggressive than "**fight or flight**." These patterns have been replaced with the more civilized "**distancing or coercion**" which are now our modern professional behaviors for "fight or flight."

Distancing refers to avoiding contact with our adversaries, just as if we were fleeing.

And **coercion** is a means where we ensure our safety by force or threatening our enemies into submission. Again, in our professional surgery settings distancing and coercion are civilized forms of behaviors of our ancestor's way of dealing with conflict through fighting or fleeing.

In summary, we tend to either **Fight (coercion)** or **Flight (distance)** when trying to resolve conflict.

"Getting' good players is easy. Getting' 'em to play together is the hard part."

Casey Stengel, Baseball Manager

Conflict Types	
TYPE-A	**TYPE-B**
Writing memos & e-mail	Encouraging others to take sides
Withholding needed information	Increased volume
Not returning e-mail messages (within 24 hours)	Not returning voice messages
Pre-empting	Avoiding personal contact
Undermining the adversaries' reputations	Delaying giving required support

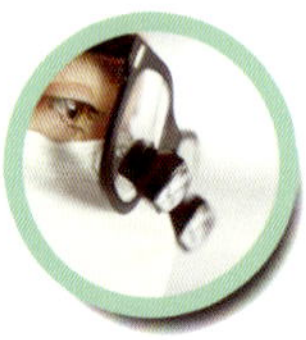

METHODS TO RESOLVE CONFLICT

Once surgeons observe or are told of conflicts within their teams, they must decide whether to take action. The American Medical Association's (AMA) policy states that disruptive behavior as an interaction style with physicians, hospital personnel, patients, family members or others that interferes with patient care, could be grounds for Board discipline. To reduce errors by increasing teamwork, all surgeons must take an active role to identify and manage disruptive behavior.

If the conflict does not look like a struggle between or among staff, surgeons, residents, students and professionals whose tasks are interdependent, then you can simply wait for a while.

If the conflict involves people who do depend upon each other, then the issue needs to be resolved soon.

If the problem involves an emergency situation, then the immediate problem needs resolving and the issue needs to be revisited within a week.

There are three basic methods for resolving conflict

Power Contests

Those involved use their status, volume, promises, verbal aggressiveness or other surgeons, residents and nurses as their allies.

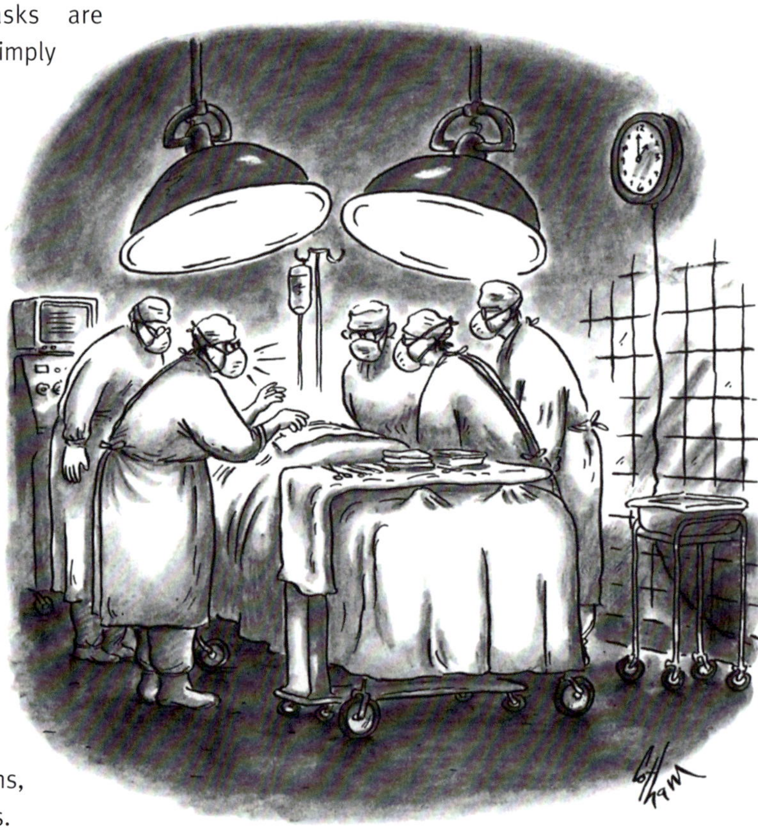

"If I knew where I'd lost the sponge, it wouldn't be lost, now, would it?"

Results: Winners and losers

In the long term, this may prove to be detrimental to morale and effectiveness. No one likes to be a loser, especially surgeons.

Rights contests

Those involved appeal to a higher status person (hospital administrator, nurse supervisor, chief resident, medical affairs officer, risk management) to settle the conflict.

Results: Winners and losers

Although a more structured way of dealing with conflict, it tends to produce a clear outcome where one party will win and one party will lose.

"(OR) nurses learn that the best way to get out from under the spotlight is to prove someone else is the weaker link."

Outpatient Surgery

Some will argue it is necessary in emergency situations, it is not appropriate for long term solutions. Staff will remember the incident and pass stories of your behavior on to the next generation.

Interest reconciliation

Participants are asked to reframe the conflict by verbalizing alternate solutions other than their own. Then they can argue the increased value of one over another.

Results: Win-win

This is the more positive approach. Although meetings that allow others to argue and debate their positions take longer and require more effort, the long term results are better. This method is considered "productive conflict." Small groups that use this method are more likely to buy in to the decision the group develops rather than ignore a mandate.

Since surgeons are often perceived as the leaders of the team, they are often expected to address and solve the conflict. The key to competence for the surgeon is to be able to choose to communicate in specific styles for specific situations.

GETTING TO THE WIN-WIN

There are specific steps to follow when solving conflict issues:

Step 1 Find the time to talk with all involved. Arranging meetings across specialties and sections is always difficult, especially if some are avoiding any form of confrontation.

Step 2 The approach (when/how you or an appointed secretary approaches the other person and asks for the meeting).

Step 3 The request statement (the reason you need to talk).

Step 4 Apply the KISS technique ("Keep it simple, surgeon") to the request statement.

Step 5 Resist the other's requests to "Let me tell you what happened now" via telephone.

Step 6 Resist the other's demand to "Tell me NOW."

Rules: The purpose is not to enforce only one solution. Remember that to be a good leader, you must be willing to be a good soldier. The time and place should be convenient for all parties.

Facilitate the discussion according to the following criteria:

Dialogue that is:

- Directly between all disputants.
- Limited by the professional behavior.
- Only about the immediate issue to resolved. Don't let issues from the past into the discussion.
- Long enough to find a solution.

Professional Behaviors:

- Must stay at the meeting until it has ended—no pagers or telephone interruptions.
- Must consider alternative solutions to the problem.

GUIDELINES FOR THE FACILITATOR:

Step 1 Are the participants staying on the topic? If yes, do nothing, if no then guide them back.

Step 2 Are participants responding to all reasonable alternative solutions to the problem? If not, ask all to respond to the merits of the suggestions.

Step 3 Encourage settlement on a solution before the end of the meeting. Do not allow 'hallway consults.'

Step 4 Encourage 'promises,' not threats.

Step 5 Encourage professional, healthy debate.

Step 6 Discourage defensive behavior or verbal aggressiveness.

THE SOLUTION MUST BE:

- Balanced: each person (nurse, resident, administrator, and surgeon) must see the benefit from the solutions. It must pass the **WI-FM** test "**W**hat's **i**n it **f**or **m**e?"
- Behaviorally specific: defines in clear detail **who** does **what,** by **when** and for **how long**; and
- Written: the solution needs to be recorded and signed by all present at the discussion.

Success is measured when the discussion changes from a **me-against-you** to **us-against-the-problem**. Everyone wins something.

True professionals focus on issues in conflict, not personalities.

VERBAL AGGRESSIVENESS

There are personality traits associated with conflict.

Verbal Aggressiveness

Those who are verbally aggressive focus the attack on the individual rather than an issue. This is often referred to as a 'personal attack.' Clearly, this is a negative trait and considered nonprofessional behavior.

Argumentative

Those who are argumentative enjoy arguing issues and focus on topics that are considered more controversial, provide evidence to support their position on topics and try to refute the other person's position. This trait is not focused on the person, rather the topic.

Communication Apprehension

Those who do everything to avoid conflict often have high communication apprehension scores. Although they may have excellent arguments, they do not want to communicate their ideas in a verbal format. Their level of apprehension in communication conflict situations is very high. Often these folks will walk to the other end of the hospital to talk with someone rather than call or page the person.

Verbal Aggressiveness

Most will react to verbal aggressiveness in one of four ways: a counter attack, pleading, silence or debate. All are counterproductive and take time away from other tasks.

You cannot *not* communicate.

Even silence and turning away is a message to the attacker. These are not safe responses for surgeons. Instead, surgeons need to learn and practice a few techniques so they will be able to respond to verbal attacks with skill and control.

Although surgeons should learn to respond to verbal aggressiveness professionally; they should NEVER be the source of this behavior. Verbal aggressive behavior by the surgeon may be considered harassment and unprofessional.

William Colgate is a 50-year-old male who has come to the emergency department at a university teaching hospital on a Sunday afternoon with his 13 year old daughter, after driving rapidly for 50 minutes from a walk-in clinic near a ski area. He is quite visibly agitated. He was told at the outside clinic that she had broken her wrist during a snow boarding lesson and that they would 'call ahead.' After waiting for over an hour, he is lead into a bay with his daughter. Her vital signs are blood pressure 100/70, pulse 100, respirations 16, and temperature 98.0. The attending physician is asking about her pain level when the father starts challenging the pain medications. Just then a code is called and the physician leaves. Twenty minutes later the resident returns to find an angry father pacing in the room. "Where have you been? My daughter's just lying here in pain and all of you take off! I thought this was a first rate medical center. Don't you give a damn about us? Even a resident should show some caring for a child in severe pain."

Americans learn methods to verbally attack others, rather than respond physically, as part of their communication development. Often children are taught 'not to hit' and to verbalize their feelings at a young age. Over time, adults adopt successful methods of verbal response to conflicts. Police officers are trained to use verbal statements to reduce violence in critical moments. But surgeons also need to develop professional methods to respond to verbal attacks and not respond emotionally. As parallel to technical training, it is critical that surgeons develop methods to diffuse any form of verbal aggressiveness.

In the example, the patient used a common verbal aggressive pattern and said,

"If you really wanted to help me, you wouldn't have gone off and left me!"

The "If you really ..." example is a direct attack. Most surgeons are likely to respond to this personal attack by explaining why they had to leave.

"Mr. Colgate, I was called to help with a serious trauma from another snowboarding accident."

This is not helpful to the surgeon. Mr. Colgate's daughter is in pain, he's scared and he doesn't understand the hospital system. This verbal aggressive pattern has two parts: the personal attack and an attack in the form of an inference.

The inference occurs often in conversations that involve conflict. It is anything that is inferred, including all fallacious statements. These inferences, also called 'verbal traps' will never be eliminated, but we can prepare for how to respond to them professionally.

The appropriate response to the above example is:

"Of course I really want to help you,"

The "even a..." is another form of attack:

"John, even a medical student could pass that exam."

This TRAP is simply a fallacious statement. It infers that the resident (John) is not that smart.

When dealing with verbal aggressive patterns, two rules apply:

Rule One: Ignore the personal attack or fallacious statement

Rule Two: Respond directly to the real issue

"The basic science section of the ABSITE really does test what was taught in medical school."

The most essential part of an effective apology is acknowledging the offense. It correctly identifies the parties responsible for the grievance, as well as the parties to whom an apology is owed. It acknowledges the offending behaviors in adequate detail and it recognizes the impact these behaviors had on the victim. It confirms that the grievance was a violation of the social or moral contract between the parties.

On apology – Aaron Lazare, MD
Professor of Psychiatry

Similar to the Colgate example, the response focused on the examination, not John's intelligence.

The following verbal responses to verbal conflict will allow the surgeon to proceed with the examination instead of continuing the conflict with the patient.

Patient #1:

"Even a resident ought to be able to tell I'm in pain!"

(Inference: You're stupid.)

Resident:

"There are those who don't think residents offer the best care. I'm sorry to hear that you feel that way."

Patient #2:

"Don't you even care if my grandmother is dying?"

(Inference: You don't care about my grandmother.)

believe the nonverbal

Surgeon: Most surgeons/nurses would respond with,

"Of course I care about your grandmother..."

However, just assume your caring is not being examined and don't respond to the "care" part of the sentence.

Instead:

"Now, let's see what the problem is..."

"You must be worried; let's have a look."

Incorrect responses include attempts to explain and justify what the surgeon is doing, or responding with phases that will simply escalate the conflict:

> "Don't assume you're her doctor! Of course your grandmother's not dying..."

Or:

> "I assume you stayed at a Holiday Inn Express last night?"

Or:

> "Did you watch ER reruns on TV last night?"

To determine if you are actually dealing with verbal aggressiveness, look at the patient for nonverbal clues. If the nonverbal message conflicts with aggressiveness, believe the nonverbal message.

A statement of reassurance, followed by medical action:

Surgeon: "I'm very concerned about your grandmother, and I'm here to help her. Now, let's take a look..."

The key is to treat the patient normally while ignoring the personal attack. Never take attacks personally! You will lose. The strategy is for the surgeon to demonstrate that the accusation is false by his or her nonverbal behavior.

Never take attacks personally.

Patient #3:

"Why don't you ever treat your patients like you really care?"

Inference: You don't ever care about your patients.

Professional Surgeon: "Tell me what's bothering you right at this minute."

or "Show me exactly where it hurts..."

In every case, the patient/family member/officer/colleague expects the surgeon to respond to the inference and participate in a verbal or physical confrontation. The professional refuses to take the comment personally and responds professionally.

AGREEING WITH THE ATTACK

Fallacious statements are those which may seem true on the surface or in a few cases, but are false when applied to entire populations or products.

In the William Colgate example, the father is showing the effects of stress. The father is probably scared. Nonverbal cues, such as aggressive posture, direct eye contact, increased volume, and increased rate tell you that he is focusing his attack toward you. He is inferring that:

You are refusing to care for his child.

Mr. Colgate has attacked the resident with his nonverbal behavior and vocabulary. When he adds a follow-up statement, "I should sue this hospital!" the resident should recognize the fallacious comment and consider:

> "There exist some hypothetical fathers who would sue some hypothetical hospital if the surgeons completely ignored some hypothetical child in pain."

Surgeons should not respond to the inference or explain their behavior. Instead, the resident should take advantage of the father's decision and respond to the fallacious part of the statement with:

Father: "Some parents would consider suing a hospital that ignored a child in pain!"

Professional Surgeon: "You're absolutely right. Now, let's take a look at her entire arm."

By saying, "You're absolutely right," the surgeon is agreeing with the inference of a hypothetical situation. The "some parents would sue" is simply a fallacious statement which may be true in one case, but not true for all. However, once the resident has agreed with this statement, it is possible to continue to care for the patient. Whenever verbal aggressiveness can be diffused by agreeing with the fallacious statement, it is an effective technique. For example:

Patient: "This isn't the only emergency department in this state, you know!"

Professional Surgeon: "You're absolutely right..."

This is also a good skill to develop in a physically dangerous situation. It can provide you with some time to negotiate your safety.

Patient: "Everybody understands why you can't get along with anybody in your section, you know!"

Another fallacious statement. There are a few close friends that you've shared your problems with, but you trusted them not to tell others.

Professional Surgeon: "I want you to know that I appreciate their concern. Our section is one of the best teams in the area."

This verbal aggressive pattern focuses on the surgeon's right to privacy. The aggressor is trying to provoke conflict as:

> "What! What do you mean, everybody understands why I can't get along with anybody in my section? I have a lot of friends here!"

This type of response gives the aggressor a chance to bring up a laundry list of complaints answering the "What do you mean..." in the surgeon's response. The surgeon should never escalate the conflict.

Patient: "Even if I do lose my leg because you delayed my surgery, my family would never sue you!"

Professional Surgeon: "When did you start thinking you were going to lose your leg, Mr. Jones?"

This is a common verbal attack pattern, especially from older patients, who are frightened and making great effort not to show it. The surgeon should avoid taking it personally. There are times when patients desperately want to know the seriousness of the injured limb, but aren't able to verbalize their fears. They hear that vascular, orthopedic and general surgeons are involved and don't know who's in charge. The proper response is to ignore the inference *(The surgeons don't know what to do and I will probably lose a leg as a result of it)* and reply as above. This response to this type of verbal aggressive pattern gives patients a safe way to verbalize whatever it was that caused their concern.

What they really want is the answer to the questions:

> "Will they have to amputate my leg?"
>
> "Am I going to die on the operating table?"
>
> "Will I live?
>
> "Will I be able to walk?"
>
> "How will I be able to work?

It would be better if patients simply asked the question, but they may not be able to. They are the patients; surgeons are the professionals, and language is one of their most powerful medical tools. The surgeon must make it possible for patients to say what is really frightening them. A "when" question is the most appropriate and effective way to do that.

> "When did you start thinking your mother was going to die?"
>
> "When did you start worrying about work?"

The question with "when" is entirely neutral; the "why," and "what makes you" questions may challenge the patient's knowledge base and borders on shame or humiliation, resulting in conflict.

Simply increasing your volume or changing the tone of certain words within a statement may also be perceived as aggressive by patients, residents and families:

"If you really wanted to pass your in-training exam, you'd go to Grand Rounds."

"If you really cared about passing your recertification exam, you'd go to Grand Rounds!"

"Even an intern should know about potassium levels."

"A resident who really wanted to move forward wouldn't object to a small issue like our dress code."

"Why don't you ever consider the feelings of the other residents?"

"Some attendings would seriously consider taking action if their colleagues behaved in this manner."

The result: I know you just attacked me. Don't do it again. It won't work.

Once a verbal aggressive pattern is identified, the goal is to diffuse it so there won't be a verbal or physical confrontation that would interfere with the health care process or continued conflict.

There are other verbal aggressive patterns. All can be recognized by their structure, intonation and choice of words accompanied by conflicting body language. Understanding the principles involved allows surgeons to handle any verbal aggressiveness they may encounter. It is important to remember that in verbally aggressive confrontations, the exact words are often not the issue. Nonverbal behaviors will always speak louder than words!

PROFANITY

Much of the time, profanity is part of a verbal aggressive attack. Some family members or patients may use profanity so constantly that they're hardly aware that they are doing it. This is easy to recognize because of redundant use of profanity as an adjective every two or three words.

"All you $#@@ surgeons are $#@@ alike. No one gives a $#@@ whether I live or die."

"Do you think I give a *#** whether you've had any sleep...."

Often profanity is an example of poor communication skills, stress and limited vocabulary, not a vicious attack.

In other cases, the profanity may well be deliberately directed at the surgeon to cause hurt and anger. In these cases, the curses and obscenities are nothing more than another kind of inference, and should be dealt with accordingly. The more attention the attacker gets from the surgeon, the more delighted the attacker will be and the more profanity will be used—because it works. Only when and if the profanity is causing distress to innocent bystanders should a surgeon grant it attention. However, the attention should focus on the behavior, not on the speaker.

"Many people are distressed and alarmed by swearing, you know. Swearing in a medical setting is not a good idea."

Verbal response skills to conflict and verbal abuse are tools that every surgeon needs to develop.

Some believe that all they need to do is simply say: "Please do not talk like that" or "That is not very professional; don't talk to me like that, it offends me."

Occasionally, someone will apologize and it may work, but rarely, and add, "I'm sorry, I forgot there were ladies in the room." But usually, the verbal aggressor just becomes more motivated to do it again.

Other times, people may simply respond in kind.

"You're just a *#*# jerk and never meet any deadlines."

"No, you're the *#*# jerk!"

All this does is escalate the conflict. A surgeon can never argue that since the patient/tech/father/physician/nurse initiated the profanity, it's acceptable to respond in kind.

However, if you address the "noun" and the "profanity" as two topics in your response, you can diffuse the situation. This method also tells the person who is verbally aggressive to stop.

"Dr. Patrick, you have just brought up two topics – which would you like to talk about first – the deadline or %$#@?"

NONVERBAL AGGRESSIVE BEHAVIORS

It is considered quite rude to add certain nonverbal behaviors to your conversation:

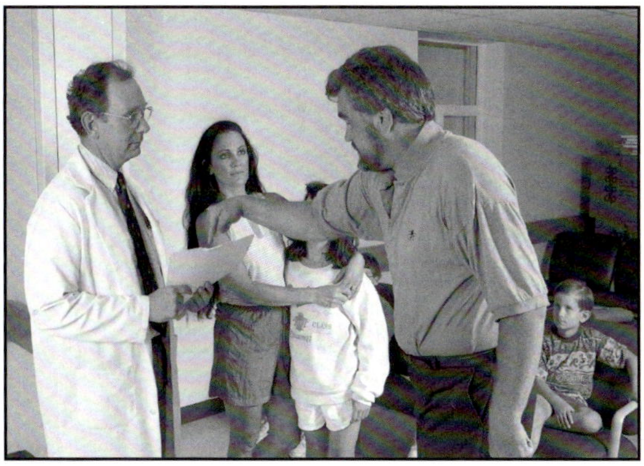

Finger Pointing

Never point a single index finger at another person. This is considered quite rude in many cultures. If you need to demonstrate with your fingers, always use two fingers or the entire hand. Often flight attendants use two fingers to demonstrate aisle path lighting 'in case of an emergency' at the beginning of each airline trip.

Space

Be sure your use of space (proxemics) does not conflict with the topic. For an intimate topic, use intimate space, and use professional space for professional conversations. If the space and topic clash, it will induce conflict. Often, one person creates conflict by simply being too close (intimate space) to the other person in a professional setting.

Touching

Professionals never touch each other except with hands during a handshake, at the shoulder or top of the back. There aren't any acceptable reasons for touching a colleague, student or staff member below the waist. Professional settings yield professional behavior. If you want to give a hug to a resident, colleague, or staff member to demonstrate how happy you are with their success, birth of a child, fellowship offer, etc., the safest statement is,

"Do you mind if I give you a hug?"

before touching.

Health care professionals are allowed to touch patients in specific settings only if there is an accepted provider-patient agreement.

ACTION STEPS

- Avoid aggressive verbal or nonverbal behaviors that lead to conflict.
- Involve all parties throughout the process when resolving conflict.
- Aim for WIN-WIN decisions. Although it takes more energy and time, it will be better supported and longer lasting.
- Don't wait! Too often nurses, surgeons and staff all recognize but don't deal with poor behavior until there are serious consequences.
- FOCUS on the behavior, not the person.
- Watch for patterns that require intervention. Recognize when others need to be involved in the process.
- Remember that profanity is **never** an acceptable behavior for surgeons.

CONFLICT ACTION STEPS

- If the attack is mostly verbal, consider whether the patient or family member may be scared.
- Repond professionally if they say:
  - You didn't care...
  - If you really...
  - Most surgeons...
  - Why aren't you doing anything to help?
- If profanity is used by someone, NEVER respond in kind. Develop a professional response.
- Never take the attack personally.
- Behave professionally.
- Always behave as a gentleman or gentlewoman, no matter how the other person is behaving.

SELECTED READINGS

1. Outpatient Surgery Staff. Make your OR a bully-free zone. Outpatient Surgery Magazine. 2006 May:34-41.
2. Waisel DC. Developing social capital in the operating room: The use of population-based techniques. Anesthes. 2005; 103(6):1305-10.
3. Ridky J, Sheldon GF. Managing in academics: A health center model. St. Louis: Quality Medical Publishing; 1977.
4. American Medical Association [homepage on the Internet]. Chicago: The Association; Physicians and Disruptive Behavior; AMA PolicyFinder. Available from: http://www.ama-assn.org/ama/noindex/category/11760.html.
5. Chervanak FA, McCullough LB. The diagnosis and management of progressive dysfunction of health care organizations. Obstet Gynecol. 2005; 105:882-7.
6. Chervenak FA, McCullough LB, Baril SR. Ethics, a neglected dimension of power relationships of physician leaders. Obstet Gynecol. 2006; 195:651-6.
7. Lang N, Rowland-Morin PA, Coe NP. Identification of communication apprehension in medical students starting a surgery rotation. Am J Surg. 1998; 176(1):41-45.
8. Andriole D, Jeff D, Rowland-Morin PA. Communication apprehension in the third year clerkship. Acad Med. 1999; 74(11):1256-7.
9. Lazare A. On apology. NY: Oxford University Press; 2004

Recognize who or what pushes your buttons and develop a coping plan.

Litigation: When Things Go Wrong

Barry M. Manuel, MD, FACS;
Richard W. Moore, JD, CPCU

> "…..jurors will usually favor doctors if the doctors don't go out of their way to alienate them. All things being equal, jurors tend to believe the doctor, and contrary to popular opinion, jurors don't vote on the basis of sympathy for the victim. The biggest problem physicians have is arrogance. They're irate at the very idea of being sued, and then they act arrogant and are condescending to the jury. They say and telegraph, 'How can this jury understand anything? They're not doctors.' "(1)
>
> Harvey F. Wachsman, MD, FACS, JD
> Neurosurgeon-turned-lawyer

Jurors take their role in the courtroom very seriously. They use every tool available to them to decide the case. Since trials may last two weeks or more, jurors have a lot of time - and they spend a lot of it observing the defendant. Even before hearing the defendant's testimony, jurors watch the defendant's demeanor and make judgments on the person's competence, professionalism, apparent solicitude and concern. According to the feedback from jurors, if the defendant seems to be a caring, concerned professional, the jury will be more likely to assess the facts of the case in a light favorable to the defendant. Jurors believe that surgeons who are invested in their work and their patients make better judgments about the care they deliver. Jurors want to like and believe the defendant. They relate this surgeon to their own surgeons. And in judging the defendant, the jury ask themselves, "If I were in need, is this a person I would trust to help me?"

Being sued for professional liability causes great anguish to surgeons and their families. Surgeons who are sued often experience depression and anxiety, and sometimes, even physical illness. Since it is the process itself, and not just the affront to surgeons' professional competence that is so stressful to them, these effects are noted even in surgeons who ultimately prevail on the merits of their cases.

> "There is an unseen cost to a physician sued for negligence: some studies estimate five years lost of professional, economic, social and psychological productivity. The fear accompanying a claim can change the way a practitioner practices. Worry about the professional and financial impact of a suit can weigh heavily upon the practitioner and his/her family. And self doubt can wreak havoc with sleep patterns, thought processes, initiative and drive…while diversion and denial may work for the physician in the short term, over time these tactics inhibit healing long after the legal and insurance aspects of a claim or suit have been put to rest."(2)

Given the inherent stress of litigation and the inevitable questions of professional incompetence and self-doubt, it may be tempting for surgeons who are sued to avoid even thinking about litigation, let alone becoming actively involved in their own defense. Since approximately 67.6% of all claims brought against surgeons in the United States are closed each year without making an indemnity payment on behalf of the surgeon, and less than 10% of all claims will ever go to trial,(3) it may be easier for surgeons as a group to focus their discussions on issues of quality medicine and methods to avoid litigation rather than on issues which arise for that small minority of individual surgeons who are sued. However, a general overview of the litigation process and suggestions on how to communicate effectively may alleviate some apprehension for those surgeons who find themselves embroiled in litigation. The ability to understand the litigation process and therefore, to intelligently and effectively contribute to the defense process can have a positive impact upon a surgeon's emotional well being and, consequently, on their practice. In addition to the impact on the individual surgeon, malpractice litigation affects the entire medical profession and especially the particular specialty of the surgeon sued, since insurance premiums for medical malpractice coverage are based upon the past losses in their specialty.(4) Just as the medical community cannot tolerate incompetent medical care, it cannot continue to pay judgments and settlements for individual surgeons who are reluctant to take the needed time to prepare their own case, work cooperatively with the defense team, and develop the kind of unique communication skills that will be necessary during the course of litigation.

The ideal time to develop an understanding of the legal system as it applies to the practice of medicine is during medical school and residency. In fact, many medical schools now offer formal classes on medico-legal issues. While it may be more difficult for surgeons to find the time once they are engaged in practice, there are now many useful courses on risk management, claim management, and legal preparedness sponsored by medical subspecialty societies, state medical societies, medical school CME departments, surgeon insurance companies and hospitals. It is essential for surgeons to avail themselves of the opportunity to keep current on the changing medico-legal environments.

Most surgeons and medical students no doubt would agree that it is important to develop basic communication skills to assist them in their practice. Some may argue that a good bedside manner is particularly important for general practitioners and internists who tend to have more personal interaction with their patients than more specialized fields. However, regardless of a surgeon's specialty, if they are sued for medical malpractice, the impact on them, their family, and their livelihood will feel the same to all. And, rather than describing a procedure to patients who know and trust surgeons, surgeons will be faced with justifying their professional conduct to a medical review board, their malpractice insurer, lawyers, and ultimately to 12 strangers who most likely will have no medical training or expertise.

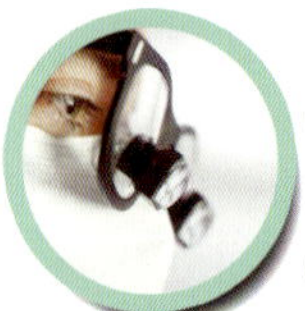

When a claim is brought against a surgeon, ideally the surgeon experts evaluating the case will work with him or her on the medical aspects of the defense. Meanwhile the surgeon's attorneys, who are experts on the legal system and on the specialized communication skills necessary to successfully litigate the case, work with the surgeon to improve his or her ability to communicate those medical aspects of the incident in question to a lay jury. However, the ability of surgeons to effectively communicate their defense is ultimately up to them. It is their responsibility to educate themselves and to remain actively involved in the litigation.

The truth is in the eye of the beholder.

DIFFERENCES IN COMMUNICATION

In those unfortunate situations where a malpractice claim is brought, surgeons who are trained to observe and make scientific judgments frequently find it difficult to effectively communicate in a legal system where simply being "right" is not enough. For example, surgeons may know that their treatment was consistent with accepted practice within their specialty and their defense experts will testify to that effect. However, another surgeon hired by the plaintiff will say something quite different. Who will the jury believe? Although perhaps difficult to accept, the jury may believe the side which is more *convincing*, not necessarily the side which is *medically correct*.

A trial often is truly a battle of the experts. Which side seems the most knowledgeable and the better prepared? Does the expert's explanation of the incident and medical facts seem plausible? Since the jury is not composed of the professional peers of surgeons, the jurors are unable to draw informed judgments about the medical aspects of the case from their own experience. Rather, they may ask themselves which testimony and, specifically, which medical experts make the most sense to them and whether the accused surgeons appeared to "care" for the plaintiff-patient.

Another example of differences between communication in the context of medical treatment and that of subsequent legal proceedings is in the use of the medical record. Surgeons view the medical record's primary purpose as documenting and communicating patient care to all members of the health care team. Plaintiff and defense attorneys and ultimately juries, however, may view it quite differently. Some surgeons think that if something negative is not in the record, its absence will protect the surgeon. As a general rule, this is not true. A complete, legible, and timely recorded event with documented adverse incidents or outcomes will answer many questions and help the defense team. Although there may be many valid medical reasons to supplement a medical record, from a legal perspective it may be costly. Words squeezed into the text after the fact may appear to a jury to have been added to cover an error or omission. If additional thought needs to be entered, it should be written as a late entry bearing the date of entry, not the date of its occurrence. Should a correction to an error be necessary, surgeons must do so in strict accordance with hospital guidelines, surgeon practice, or other applicable rules and regulations. They should never correct an error by erasure, the use of correction fluid, or deletion on an electronic record. Rather, it is recommended that they draw a single line through the incorrect entry, date and initial it, and continue with the correct information.

Surgeons should never amend a medical record once an initial contact from a plaintiff's attorney is made

In particular, surgeons should never amend a medical record once an initial contact from a plaintiff's attorney is made. While they may be tempted in their review of the record to fill in missing information that was inadvertently omitted, they absolutely must not do so, no matter how poor they think the record is in retrospect. Rather than strengthening the case, it will usually weaken the defense and in some cases may cause the jury to want to punish the surgeon for a perceived cover-up. At the very least, the change in the medical record could increase the credibility and the value of the plaintiff's case. Remember that the electronic record contains all entries even though some may not be visible to the clinician.

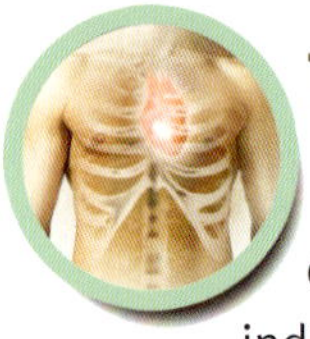

THE SURGEON AS DEFENDANT

Although the facts of a case are critical, juries are often swayed by appearances and other subjective factors during trial. Moreover, it is likely that the jury will have no individual or collective medical expertise. In the interest of impaneling an impartial jury, if the jury pool were to include persons with a medical background, they would probably be excluded from the jury panel because that knowledge may be considered unfair or prejudicial. Likewise, if during the course of the trial a juror were to refer to a medical book from home which had not been admitted into evidence, a mistrial may be declared.(5) Consequently, in order to communicate effectively to a lay jury, it is imperative for surgeons to learn how to be more credible witnesses.

Once surgeons are sued for medical malpractice, expert help should be available to them from their insurance company claims staff and their defense attorney. The defense attorney will determine the individual legal strategy and will tailor the general communication techniques recommended in this chapter to fit the needs of the case. It is important to note that these general guidelines may not be appropriate in all circumstances; therefore, it is only through a close review with their attorney that their particular case may be effectively prepared. Surgeons can ill afford to sit back with the attitude that the defense of their case is the sole responsibility of their lawyer. Since they are the ones who know both the facts of the case and medicine, they are an indispensable part of the defense team, no matter how experienced their lawyer is in handling malpractice cases; ultimately, it will also be them on the witness stand and their responsibility to effectively communicate their own defense to the jury.

You're Contacted:

- **About your care of a patient**
- **Because you're part of a team of providers**
- **Because you provided subsequent treatment to a patient**
- **Because a literature search contained your name**
- **Because you are listed on the WWW as an expert.**

The Beginning

Many medical malpractice claims first begin with the filing of a lawsuit. In that instance, surgeons typically receive a summons and complaint, which generally set out rudimentary facts of the incident. When they receive the summons and complaint they should read it thoroughly and review the facts with their attorney or claims representative. They may find that the complaint states facts that are incorrect, names the wrong person as defendant, or misses the mark entirely on the question of negligence. However, do not become complacent simply because some facts may be incorrect. No matter how poorly written a complaint may be, the plaintiff attorney may correct these defects at a later time.

Before a malpractice claim is formally made against surgeons, they may receive a request for the records of a particular patient. Neither surgeons nor their staff should ever release patient records to the patient or plaintiff's attorney without first obtaining an original signed authorization by the patient. A written authorization from the patient is essential because of the physician patient privilege that generally prohibits a surgeon from disclosing a patient communication without a waiver of or 'exception to the privilege.' In addition, surgeons should preserve the original record and deliver copies only. Although the same generally applies to any films, in certain circumstances it may not be feasible for surgeons to make copies because of the number of films and expense involved for those that aren't digitized. In those instances, they should carefully catalogue and deliver the files directly to the requesting party along with a return receipt identifying each individual file. They should also make an arrangement to have the original files returned to their office. Any procedure of this type should be agreed upon ahead of time and done only with the approval of the claim representative assigned by the surgeon's insurance carrier.

No matter how poorly written a complaint may be, the plaintiff attorney may correct these defects at a later time.

Before speaking with counsel or any third party, surgeons must ascertain whether they have received a signed release from the patient. If in fact, they have not obtained a release, they should say:

> "I cannot comment on any portion of the treatment until I have a signed release from the patient."

Even if they have received a signed release, they are best advised not to speak with anyone except as instructed by their attorney. They should simply say:

> "I am sorry, but I do not think it is in my own best interest to comment. You may contact my attorney who will assist you."

Naturally, when surgeons receive any notice of a potential claim or suspect that one is imminent, their first responsibility is to notify their insurance carrier claims staff and seek their advice. They will also need to get copies of all relevant medical records. The company will advise them not to discuss the facts of the case with anyone other than their insurance company and their attorney. This is to avoid creating additional witnesses who may be subpoenaed to testify about statements made about the case by any surgeons or staff. This does not mean, however, that surgeons should not fulfill their obligation under the regulations and by-laws of the hospital in reporting a particular incident within the context of a formal peer review. Whether or not statements in a peer review are discoverable in outside proceedings depends upon the jurisdiction in which they practice. Moreover, there may be additional statutory reporting requirements which may vary by state. It is the responsibility of each individual surgeon to remain abreast of their reporting obligations.

Worker's Compensation

If the patient has filed a worker's compensation claim, a separate patient authorization is NOT needed.

Your Claim Representative and Defense Attorney

The claims staff of a surgeon's insurance company have two primary and distinct responsibilities.

The first is to investigate the claim. Although medical malpractice carriers are organized in different ways, a standard investigation may involve a representative of the company meeting with surgeons to discuss the allegations, interview other witnesses to the incident, and gather other information in relation to the claim. This process helps the company evaluate the claim, determine whether it should be settled or defended, and organize the information for use by the defense team. The claim will be much more effectively investigated if the surgeon takes the necessary time to assist their team in the investigation. This may include writing a comprehensive summary of the facts of the incident as they recall them, including facts which may not be contained in the medical record or their office notes; sharing applicable written policies and procedures; and demonstrating the use of medical equipment pertinent to their case. Be sure to explain to the investigator, in clear and concise terms, the medical aspects of the case.

The second responsibility of the claims staff is to administer the claims process. The company will appoint defense counsel for the surgeon and continue to work with the attorney to prepare their case. A crucial part of administering the claim process is selecting defense experts to review the case and prepare for trial. Although subjective matters such as appearance on the stand and the ability to communicate the facts of the issue are clearly important considerations to the jury, the initial decision on whether to defend or settle is based mainly on the reports of defense experts. Just as plaintiffs are dependent upon a medical opinion to make their case, a surgeon's defense is largely based on the strong testimony of knowledgeable experts in their specialty.

The second responsibility of the claims staff is to administer the claims process.

Although the company and defense counsel assigned to surgeons will have a number of experts to draw from, defendants' input in suggesting experts who are knowledgeable about the particular procedures involved in the claim is imperative. Good experts will be not only acknowledged in their field and able to work effectively with surgeons, but also will make a strong appearance on their own behalf. Since credibility is the key issue in a battle between experts, surgeons' attorneys and claims staff will evaluate experts' presentations as well as their credentials.

Obviously, the key communicator other than the defendant and expert surgeon is the defense attorney. The defense attorney (or defense team) is primarily responsible for the surgeon's defense, including preparing them to testify at a deposition and trial, cross examining plaintiff-witnesses, determining litigation strategy, and presenting and arguing their case to the jury. Although the insurance company selects attorneys for surgeons, the attorneys' primary obligation is to the surgeons who are sued. As a matter of ethics, their attorney must not take positions that are adverse to or in conflict with defendants' interests, even though they are being paid by the insurance company.(6) Therefore, surgeons should question the attorney about anything that appears in conflict with the attorney's relationship with the insurance company, such as the representation of co-defendants.

During the course of the litigation, surgeons will work closely with their defense counsel. It is critically important that they are able to work well with their counsel on the basis of confidence and professionalism. If they believe that the attorney is not adequately representing them, or that there is a personality conflict, immediately contact the insurance company, explain the problems and discuss the possibility of appointing another attorney if warranted. It is the insurance company's duty to appoint an attorney who is not only qualified, but also is someone with whom an individual surgeon is comfortable.

Circumstances may arise, either because the potential award is above the limits of insurance available to protect them or because there are potential conflicts in representation, where they may choose to hire personal counsel to help monitor the progress of the claim and trial. In most instances, surgeons will not need to retain personal counsel. However, if they do so it is important that their counsel has experience in medical malpractice cases given the specialized nature of such litigation. In addition to choosing counsel with expertise, it is important that they have confidence in them. Moreover, the role of their personal counsel should be clearly defined and limited, for example, to monitor the progress of the claim and offering advice. In most cases it may not be necessary to have a personal attorney directly involved in the actual litigation.

The uncertainty of the situation may begin to take a psychological toll on a surgeon and his or her family.

With the backlog of cases under the current legal system, it may be years before a claim against a surgeon actually goes to trial. "The average time from the date of the incident to the resolution of suit... increased from 49 months in 1985 to 54 months in 1995. For claims that resulted in payment, the time lag was even greater."(4) In 2006, the pain and suffering for surgeons was stretched to 3 to 5 years according to the ACS review of closed claims between 2004 and 2006. Although both the defense attorney and the representatives of the insurance company have an obligation to keep surgeons informed of the progress of their case, it is imperative that surgeons remain actively involved. If, for example, the defense attorney does not communicate to the defendants as often as they think necessary, the surgeon should call their defense attorney or company representative periodically for an update on where their claim stands.

During the long wait between the initial flurry of activity surrounding the investigation and the actual trial of the case, the uncertainty of the situation may begin to take a psychological toll on surgeons and their families. It is not unusual for surgeons' initial confidence in themselves and in the standard of the treatment rendered to begin eroding, despite strong expert support and quality legal representation. During this stage of the litigation, an important source of help may be surgeons' support groups. These may be organized by a medical society, insurance company, or private group to provide a valuable outlet for sharing this type of anxiety. It is important for surgeons to talk with other physicians or surgeons who have been through the process, to realize that their situation is not unique and to get advice in dealing with the uncertainty.

DEPOSITION AND TRIAL

Although each individual medical malpractice case is unique, there are universal tips that may assist a surgeon-defendant who is preparing for deposition and trial. Before testifying at a deposition or trial, thoroughly review the medical records and meet with the defense attorney to discuss the facts of the case, the defense plan, and potential testimony.

A **deposition** is an examination of a witness under oath conducted by an attorney in accordance with certain procedural court rules.

Through a deposition, the attorney can discover the facts of the case and preserve the witness' testimony for use at the trial. The deposition is also the primary opportunity for plaintiff's counsel to assess both surgeons' credibility and their potential defense.

A lawyer has six major purposes at deposition:

- Discover what the witness knows about the case
- Look for evidence favorable to the plaintiff's case
- Commit the witness to statements under oath
- Look for ways to discredit the testimony of the witness or other defense witnesses
- Attempt to learn the defense of the case; and
- Preserve the testimony of a witness who may later be unavailable to testify at trial.(6)

Since most medical malpractice cases are either settled or dropped prior to trial, surgeons' preparation for their deposition is critical to the ultimate outcome of the case.

In many respects, preparation for testimony at a deposition is similar to preparation for trial, but there are some differences. In both instances, surgeons' primary obligation is to tell the truth even if they believe that the truth may hurt their case. You must also be fair and accurate. Unlike a trial, their testimony at a deposition generally will be limited to the facts and will not be an opportunity for them to justify the treatment, since there is no judge or jury present to decide whether malpractice has been committed.

During your pre-deposition meeting, ask your attorney to not only review with you the facts and legal defenses of a case, but also to explain the mechanics and formal and informal rules of a deposition. For example, if the plaintiff's attorney does not ask an important question about the treatment or other areas of the case, you should **not** volunteer or provide more information. The fact that they failed to ask an important question is the plaintiff's responsibility, not that of defendants. Surgeons must keep in mind that the plaintiff's attorney is attempting to elicit information favorable to the plaintiff, not to defendants. However, plaintiffs' attorneys may decide that the additional information is important to their defense, and that it will need to be brought out. For example, if information critical to the defense is not mentioned in the deposition, at trial plaintiffs' attorneys might make it appear that the surgeon's story has changed. If during a deposition surgeons find themselves in the position of wanting to volunteer information, they should tell their attorney during a break. Attorneys will decide whether it is advisable for surgeons to volunteer any additional information at that time.

In addition to demanding surgeons' appearance to testify, the notice of deposition may also require them to produce documents and other evidence at the time of the deposition. Surgeons should make sure that they bring only the records that have been subpoenaed. Do not provide supplementary information such as journal articles or textbooks. Surgeons should ask their lawyer in advance what to bring to the deposition and make sure their lawyer has reviewed them before they are brought into the deposition room. Before testifying about records or other documents, they should read them fully to refresh their recollection. Do not be trapped into the challenge of attempting to answer a question from memory without looking at the document, since opposing attorneys are hoping surgeons will give inaccurate answers that may be challenged later.

There are simple guidelines concerning documents:

- **Never** testify to the contents of a document if you are not familiar with the document, unless it is before you and you have been given a chance to read it;
- Always **read** the document again before testifying and keep it with you while you testify;
- **Do not** assume facts about the document—check it first;
- **Insist** that the lawyer provide you with a complete copy of the document; and
- **Take your time** and read the document at your own pace.

Don't forget your reading glasses when on the stand. Surgeons who need to put their noses on the paper to read suffer a tremendous credibility loss.

PA Rowland

Surgeons should always pause a moment (2-3 seconds or normal reaction time latency) prior to answering a question posed during deposition. This allows you time to carefully consider your response and also gives your attorney an opportunity to object if the question is inappropriate. The absence of an objection, however, does not indicate that the surgeons' attorneys are not doing their job, since the purpose of many of the questions in a deposition is to develop the facts. Also, even when the attorneys object, surgeons may be required to answer the question.

Errata Sheets

All of the deposition testimony will be recorded and transcribed by a court reporter. You will have the opportunity to review the transcript and make corrections on an errata sheet (Latin for "assigning error and the reply therein").(8) Very carefully review this written testimony to make sure that it is an accurate transcription of what was said in the deposition and immediately notify the attorney of any errors in the transcription or in your testimony.

Finally, remember a deposition provides the opposing attorney with the opportunity to assess not only the facts of the case and, specifically, surgeons' potential defense, but also their demeanor and credibility as a witness in the event of trial. Consequently, how surgeons communicate at the deposition may affect the plaintiff attorney's evaluation of the case and a good presentation may dissuade a plaintiff's attorney from pursuing the case through to trial.

All surgeons make mistakes, but all aren't sued. The difference is communication skills.

PA Rowland

TRIAL

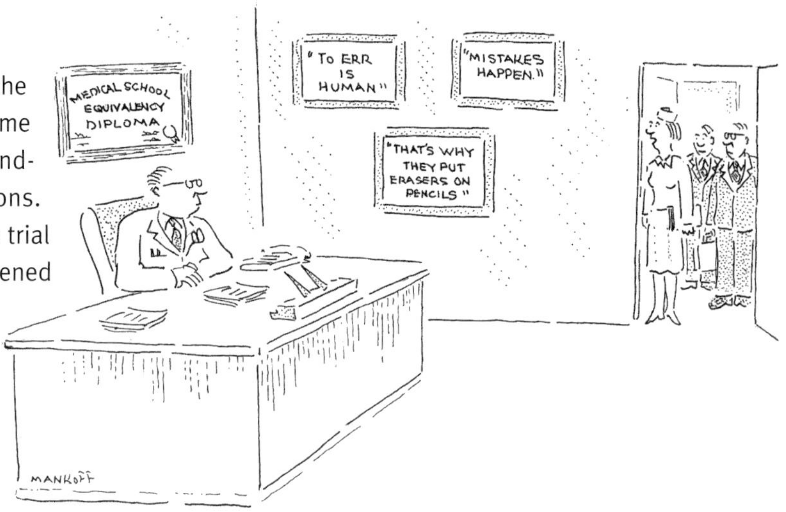
MEDICAL SCHOOL EQUIVALENCY DIPLOMA
"TO ERR IS HUMAN"
"MISTAKES HAPPEN."
"THAT'S WHY THEY PUT ERASERS ON PENCILS"
MANKOFF

"Some guys from the state board of medicine are here to see you."

A trial is a traumatic incident in the life of surgeons, who may become depressed and begin to second-guess their practice decisions. However, once a decision to go to trial is made, surgeons should be heartened to know that good preparation, a credible appearance, and a straightforward explanation of the incident to the jury may very well result in a defendant's verdict.

While it may seem obvious that it is important for them always to tell the truth when testifying under oath, it may sometimes seem difficult when they believe that the truth may hurt their case. However, much like the situation of an altered medical record, reluctance to face up to the facts that are damaging to the case will be readily apparent to the jury. Even if a particular fact is not critical to their case, their lack of candor concerning it will damage their credibility with the jury, who then may dismiss other more important aspects of their testimony.

Additionally, sometimes it may be difficult for surgeons to get the facts across to the jury in an articulate and credible manner. That is, as "scientists," surgeons no doubt strive to be precise in their speech at all times. However, as scientists, they know that it is not always possible to be 100% correct and, therefore, may be accustomed to qualifying their responses. Consequently, when testifying, it may be difficult for them (especially if they are not an experienced witness) to articulate the facts of the case clearly without qualification. Therefore, they may appear to a jury to equivocate during testimony. To jurors, equivocation can create a negative implication and may discredit their testimony. For instance, suppose the medical record indicated that they performed a complete neurological examination on a child who had suffered a fall. If they are asked whether they examined the child's pupils, they may be tempted to say:

"I think I did..."

because they have no actual memory of doing the evaluation in this particular instance. However, if the chart indicates that a full neurological examination was performed and it is their practice to always examine the pupils in conjunction with a neurological exam, then this really adds up to an affirmative answer of:

"Yes, I examined the pupils on this patient."

Frequently, the opposing attorney will simply proceed to the next question. If, however, surgeons are asked about their specific recollection, they must admit that they do not specifically recall performing the particular test but then should proceed to explain why it was in fact performed. Of

Aim for humble, patient and serious.

course, had the record clearly noted all of the elements of the neurological examination and their results, the question may never have been raised.

A similar situation frequently may arise where a question is posed concerning the acceptable standard of care. In determining negligence, surgeons' conduct will be measured against the average qualified surgeon in their specialty, in the context in which the treatment occurred. For example, if most schools of thought, with the exception of one institute, indicate that the treatment rendered conforms to a certain standard, it might nonetheless be true for the surgeon-witnesses to testify that the standard of care is not always that of their treatment in the particular case. However, such testimony might confuse the jury as to the appropriate standard against which to measure the conduct. The jury could interpret this answer as being equivocal on the defendant's part. For a definitive response, surgeons only need to weigh the probabilities and then answer in accordance with the weight of probability and ignore rare exceptions, except in situations where they honestly believe that it is necessary to qualify their answer.

When answering a complicated question, be thoughtful and careful. Quick answers will suggest to the jury that surgeons are either being careless in their response or have memorized the answer to the question. An important rule is never to guess at the answer to a question. It is perfectly okay to say:

> "I do not remember."

Frequently with medical malpractice cases there are questions which an attorney may ask that do not make sense because either the attorneys are trying to lure surgeons into a particular response or they simply do not understand the medicine. Before making any attempt to answer such a question, surgeons should state that they do not understand it rather than trying to be helpful in guessing what is being asked. The plaintiffs' attorneys may ask broad, general questions such as:

> "Generally speaking, Doctor, doesn't good medical practice require...?"

While it is tempting to give an affirmative response without elaboration, this is one instance where it is important to make clear that, while generally true, each individual situation depends upon the circumstances involved. Always be careful about questions that are asked which do not appear medically correct or contain medical ambiguities. Frequently, neither the opposing counsel nor the attorneys for surgeons will recognize the problems in the question. In that instance, surgeons should politely point out the ambiguity to examining attorneys and ask them to clarify the question. Therefore, if surgeons are required to answer the question as posed, they should voice an objection and define the difficulty with answering so that it will be clearly noted in the deposition transcript.

Although it is necessary to explain medicine in a way that can be understood by laymen, surgeons should assume that jurors are intelligent; therefore, it is important that they do not talk down to them. Remember that juries are the ones that ultimately decide the case. It is up to the surgeon to convince them that his or her testimony is correct. To help accomplish this, the surgeon should face the jury when testifying, and speak loudly and clearly. Also, surgeons must control their temper at all times even if they believe that plaintiff's counsel is badgering them. Moreover, do not express exasperation or show boredom with the question. Remember, it is up to lawyers to object to questions, not the surgeon.

Always be vigilant and circumspect during cross-examination. Be particularly careful of opposing counsel who appear to be too friendly. Surgeons should not become too relaxed or casual about questions that they agree with, since they may be caught off guard. For instance, plaintiff's counsel may attempt to get surgeons to agree that a particular treatise is "authoritative," when they may not agree with all the opinions contained in the treatise. Therefore, it is better to indicate that the source is "helpful," but like any other source of information, may not be the final word in any particular area, especially since the facts of each case are somewhat different.

EXPERT WITNESS

Surgeons may find themselves called upon to review a case of alleged medical malpractice, write an expert report, and perhaps testify as a medical expert at trial. The expert should report the medical facts and interpret the result without any concern for the interests of the plaintiff or defendant and without being an aggressive advocate. The report should relate all the facts that have been garnered as a medical summary of the chart and should include the prognosis of the patient, the future life expectancy where appropriate, the question of whether there was a deviation from the accepted and proper standard within the specialty, and a statement based upon "reasonable medical certainty or probability" as to whether the specific injuries resulted from the treatment. In most cases, experts receive the medical information from one of the attorneys. They need to make certain that they have, in fact, received all of the records. It is very important in rendering a written report, which will eventually be used by both sides, that not only the case facts be correct, but also the typing, spelling, and grammar are accurate since it could bear upon your credibility as an expert. If you are eventually called upon to testify, there undoubtedly will be questions about your fees and the time which you spent in reviewing the record, developing your report, and preparing for trial. Surgeons should not get defensive about answering questions about fees from opposing counsel and should answer them in a straightforward and complete way. It is anticipated that preparation is necessary in every step of the legal process and the jury will expect that you spent significant time in reviewing the case prior to trial. The same kind of preparation that is necessary in giving a deposition or testifying at trial is equally important for the expert.

Paid Medical Experts

- Need to have scheduling flexibility
- Be able to handle the stress of being challenged publicly
- Realize that their testimony may be used against them at a later date
- Maintain professional boundaries and not appear to side with those that are paying their bills.

SUBSEQUENT TREATING AND COVERING

In many situations surgeons may think that they are only indirectly involved with the actual treatment—giving rise to a malpractice action. The covering or subsequent treating surgeons are, of course, responsible for meeting the standard of care in the treatment which they render. The plaintiff's attorney may sue everyone involved in the patient's treatment in order to increase the number of policy limits available to pay the claim. Even after an initial review of the medical records, the plaintiff's attorney may be unsure about a number of things, including the medical aspects of the case, whether allegations of medical malpractice against any of the treating physicians or surgeons can be supported, and what the various treating and expert physicians may say about the treatment.

The situation where physicians are not immediately brought into the suit presents a number of interesting communication issues. The plaintiff's attorneys may seek to use surgeons as experts to support a claim of negligence against another treating surgeon or a defense attorney may contact them to strengthen the defense of another surgeon. Since the plaintiff may not have waived rights to confidentiality for their treatment, surgeons should contact their insurance company for advice before speaking to attorneys representing either side. If you still have questions, ask the insurance company to assign an attorney to discuss your course of action. Additionally since a surgeon generally can be added to a suit at almost any time, it is critically important when speaking to an attorney to be very careful in deciding your course of action and what to agree to say.

Because of your special relationship to the incident-giving rise to the suit, it is particularly important that you are careful that your opinion is soundly grounded in the facts as well as the medicine. As the subsequent treating surgeon, you may in fact be the surgeon who discovered a mistake by the previous physician or surgeon, although that mistake may not constitute negligence. There are many times when hindsight reveals that a physician or surgeon did not make the best possible decision. In cases involving even minor errors, the primary physician or surgeon may become defensive about it and seek to divert blame on to another, the subsequent treating physicians and surgeons, thereby making them a target for the medical malpractice action.

SUMMARY

Whenever surgeons communicate, it is important for them to keep in mind their audience. Whether they are providing assistance to defense counsel in the preparation of the case, or testifying before a jury of laymen on a complicated medical issue, the greater their ability to put themselves in the other person's place and provide the information about the incident in a comprehensive manner, the better they will be able to defend their position. Through careful preparation, surgeons can improve their testimony greatly. They should use defense counsel as a resource to answer questions about the litigation process, prepare themselves for their deposition or trial testimony, and critique their own efforts in a positive way. The more they know about the legal system and effective methods of communication, the less intimidated they will be by the process.

The possibility of being sued and perhaps ultimately going to trial can be a terrifying blow to anyone's professional confidence. Nonetheless, it is important to remember that surgeons have a responsibility not only to defend themselves and their actions, but also to represent the medical profession in a competent and professional manner.

Penalty of perjury – any legal testimony in court or deposition

REFERENCES

1. Wielawski I. Avenging Angel or Archenemy. Sunday Journal Magazine. 1998 May; 08(11).
2. Medical Professional Mutual Company. Emotional Support, The Claims Process III, Boston, MA; 3.
3. Physician Insurers Association of America. Medical Malpractice Claim Expenses, Annual Increases Outpacing Indemnity Growth. 1997:4-6.
4. Manuel B and Greenwald L. Using medical malpractice closed claims data to reduce surgical risk and improve patient safety. Bull Am Coll Surg. 2007; 92(3):28.
5. Fitzpatrick v. Allen, 410 Mass. 791; 575 NE 2nd 750 (1991).
6. Opinions of the Massachusetts Bar Association Committee on Professional Ethics: 463-465.
7. Blacks Law Dictionary, 6th ed; 1990.

SELECTED REFERENCES

1. Rowland, PA. Commenting on another colleague's care with patients [Video-DVD]. Hanover (NH): Medical Communications; 2003.

TESTIFYING AT A DEPOSITION

1. Remember the name of the game. ($$)
2. Never volunteer information.
3. Make sure you understand the question.
4. Take time to think before you speak.
5. Never guess at the answer to a question.
6. Remember, sometimes you can't remember.
7. Be patient.
8. NEVER lose your temper.
9. Be polite, but firm.
10. Speak clearly.
11. Always finish your answer.
12. You can always correct an inaccurate or incorrect answer.
13. Always read the fine print of a document upon which you are asked to comment.
14. Listen to the questions.
15. Don't fall for the plaintiff lawyer's style.
16. Your answer sometimes should be as precise as the question.
17. Ask your lawyer in advance what documents to bring. NEVER bring any that were not requested.
18. Never assume falsely.
19. Be consistent.
20. Be comfortable; control your emotions.
21. Don't fear fear.

Common Questions During a Deposition

Demographic

1. What is your full name and office address?
2. Where were your previous practice addresses?
3. In what states are you licensed?
4. When and how did you become licensed?
5. When and from what medical school(s) did you graduate?
6. Where did you do your internship and residency? What were the dates that you attended? Did you successfully complete training?
7. What, if any, specialty do you practice?
8. Are you board-certified or qualified in any specialties?
9. When and how did you become board certified? Did you fail any part of the examination the first time? Why?
10. What ailments or conditions does your specialty deal with?
11. To what medical societies and professional associations do you belong?
12. What must be done to become a member of these organizations?
13. What offices, elected or appointed, have you held? To what committees have you belonged? Have you published or contributed to any medical publications? Were the publications based on research you performed? Describe the research and its results?
14. What research do you have in progress? How much of your time does it take? How much are you compensated for your research?
15. What hospitals and medical schools are you affiliated with?

Patient Care

1. Describe how you met this patient?
2. What do you remember about this case without reference to the records? Do you really recall the details? Which ones?
3. What was the patient's appearance?
4. Relate the history you took from the patient that helped you in making your diagnosis. What questions did you ask? Were they all answered? Did you record all pertinent positives and negatives, or are some findings assumed normal because they are not recorded in the medical record?
5. Did you note subjective symptoms and objective signs related to the patient's condition in the chart? What were they?
6. What physical examinations and laboratory tests were performed in the course of your examination? What were the findings of your examinations?
7. What was your differential diagnosis at this point? What possibilities seemed most likely?

8. Were x-rays or any type of radiological tests performed? Where were they done? How many? Were they examined by a radiologist? When? Did you depend upon the radiologist's interpretation? Did you agree with the radiologist's interpretation?
9. What consultations, if any, were called? Did you follow their advice? Why? Do you usually ask for consultations in such cases?
10. On what did you base your diagnosis? Did you have any reason to doubt your diagnosis?
11. What treatment was prescribed?
12. What is your opinion concerning the nurse's notes that stated the patient continued to have pain despite your treatment? Did the treatment work? Why did you select the treatment given?
13. Did you see any reason to change your diagnosis or differential diagnosis at a later time? If so, indicate when and why you made your new diagnosis. What actions did you take as a result?
14. How often do you get the complication which occurred? What determines whether this complication can be expected? How do you get the complication which occurred?
15. How do your statistics compare to those of other surgeons?
16. What precaution could have prevented the complication?
17. In your opinion, was it a departure from accepted medical practice not to have performed more a CT scan?
18. Was the patient cooperative with the treatment?
19. Did the patient cause or contribute to the poor outcome?
20. Does the PDR list contraindications of the drugs you used that would make them inappropriate in this case?
21. What medically recognizable factors could possibly explain the events in dispute?
22. Was any other person negligent in the care of this patient?
23. Did you continue to treat and examine the patient?
24. Identify and describe all blood vessels that lead to the area of interest.
25. Further describe the anatomy of the region of interest. Were the nerves and blood vessels identified? How, and by whom?
26. Is it not a surgical error to incise the nerve that was damaged? Isn't it a fact that severing that nerve will lead to permanent paralysis?

Establishing Damages and Liability

1. Will you state the name of each person who assisted in or witnessed the care of the patient?
2. Did you observe or were you ever informed that any person assisting in the care of the plaintiff was inefficient or negligent in the performance of his or her duties at that time? Please describe the irregularity.
3. What anesthesia was administered to the patient? Was it local or general? Who administered the anesthesia? Did this person remain with the patient throughout the operation? Who supervised the person administering the anesthesia? What was the nature of the immediate supervision?

4. When did you last examine the patient?
5. What is the current mental and physical condition of the patient?
6. What is the prognosis of the patient?
7. At the time you treated the patient, were you the member of a partnership or professional corporation? What was its nature? What past partnerships have you belonged to? What physicians were members of those partnerships?

Difficult Questions

1. In preparation for this deposition, what documents did you review, including records, book, notes, bills deposition of other, films and journals?
2. With whom did you speak to in preparation for this deposition? What was the content of your conversation? Did you make an effort to have your statements agree with those of your colleagues?
3. Has this case been the subject of correspondence, article, formal lecture, or discussion with other physicians? Please describe them.
4. What are the titles and authors of the last three journal articles you have read?
5. Is your memory clear about these events? Are you certain about that?
6. What publications do you own or subscribe to that discuss this subject? These are authoritative, are they not? Why do you subscribe to them?
7. Did the patient suffer any complications from your medical treatment? If so, what are your explanations for the complications? Are the complications, normally anticipated with this type of procedure?
8. Was the possibility of this complication explained to the plaintiff prior to the procedure? Did the patient understand the explanation? How do you know he was medicated?
9. Do your hospital bylaws require you to record information in the medical record that you omitted? When were your chart entries written and dictated? Why was there a delay?
10. What recent meetings have you attended that covered the kind of case your patient had? Why did you feel the need to attend these meetings?
11. Name each prior deposition examination you have attended. Were you a defendant, witness, or expert? What were the medical issues? What was the result of your depositions?
12. Have you ever been disciplined, had your license revoked, or had your hospital privileges limited or revoked?
13. Have you ever been reprimanded, censured, punished, or suspended from practice by any society or institution?
14. Have you ever been accused of malpractice, misfeasance, or malfeasance?
15. In what hospitals do you currently have privileges? Have you ever had an application for privileges rejected?
16. Do you teach? What subjects? How many hours a week do you teach? What is your compensation?

17. What insurance coverage do you have for this event? What is your insurance carrier: dollar amounts; limitations on coverage applicable to this case?
18. Have you ever been denied insurance coverage of any kind? Why?
19. What lawsuits have been filed against you in the past?
20. Do you have a criminal record?
21. Do you consider any texts authoritative?
22. What texts or websites did you use in training?

Talking with the Press: Why Bother?

Linn Meyer, BA

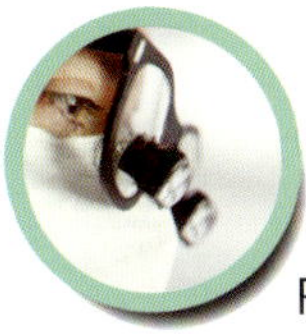

Let's face it. When it comes to the media, reporters all like a good story, and they have a reputation for often manipulating facts to keep the story interesting. Their job is to create content that sells, whether it's a newspaper, magazine or television station. Reporters and editors measure "good stories" by asking.

Does the story:

- show conflict
- appeal to human interest
- involve prominent individuals
- affect a large number of people
- have the power to determine what is and what is not newsworthy, or
- present an accurate, balanced report?

Is the story:

- new and current
- unusual
- local – affecting people in a particular area
- controversial?

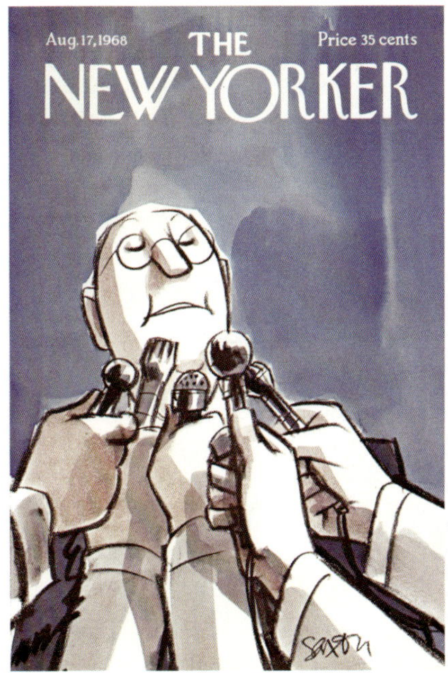

Illustration by Charles Saxon/Copyright 1968 Conde Nast Publications, Inc.

GROWING INTEREST IN HEALTH & MEDICINE

In the last 25 years we've seen a steady increase in the amount of media coverage involving health-related topics. In addition, with widespread use of the Internet, anyone can access information on just about every known malady.

As interest in health topics has increased across patient populations, even smaller stations have started to assign reporters to medical or health beats. In many instances these reporters may not have a background in health care, but decide what stories from the national networks, medical journals (early release) and wire services are published or get air time. They will be the ones you talk to most often. Do not assume these reporters know anything about your field.

Unfortunately, there may come a time when you will be facing media scrutiny about the outcome of a particular case. This is especially true if your patient is considered a VIP or is well known for his or her notable activities. After going a few rounds with the press, you may find yourself asking, "Why should I even try?"

Silence is not golden. Keeping mum about the facts of the case, and even your own involvement, isn't the answer. While you don't necessarily have to seek out the press to tell your story, providing an up-front response to inquiries from a reporter gives you an opportunity to influence the outcome of the news reports. It is your responsibility to set the record straight, speaking candidly about issues upon which you may be approached. You have a chance to:

- Clear up misconceptions
- Present the real facts
- Explain why the quality of health care is important to the quality of life.

First Line of Defense – Establish Trust

The best approach to working with the media is to develop good relationships with members of the press. Regardless of whether you are working on a newsworthy case or foresee one coming down the road, it is always beneficial to create positive working relationships with reporters. In doing so, you have already established a trust with them, and you will be more confident when speaking to someone you know.

Reporters also need to know that you're interested in working with them. Again, establish a relationship with them by making yourself available to respond to their inquiries. If a reporter calls and you are not available, be sure to return the call and follow up with him or her. Start out by offering the reporter assistance with soft stories involving medicine, research, etc. It may be as simple as pointing the reporter to the best resources, or helping him or her to make a connection within your hospital. Any effort will be a positive step in building a good rapport.

The first contact

The first contact gives the reporter an opportunity to know who you are and what you can do for them on certain topics. You may be able to interpret a NEJM story, or give her the slant for a particular procedure within your community. For instance, you may simply be saying that patients no longer have to travel to Boston or Denver for this new procedure, that it's available locally. Or, you may find yourself qualifying data about your state as an outgrowth of a national story. It is important to keep the lines of communication open. The goal is to generate an association in which there is give and take on both sides.

What you should know about reporters?

Industry-specific publications will have journalists who are fairly knowledgeable about the topics on which they are writing, and you may in some cases actually encounter reporters from these publications at some point in your career. However, it is more likely that you may be in contact with a general assignment reporter who handles a myriad of stories and topics. She may have been covering the local school board meeting the night before and contacting you today regarding the latest trend in hernia surgery. You can be sure that this type of reporter won't have the background on the issues and that you will find yourself filling her in on the basics.

There are two kinds of reporters:

- **Print**

  Print journalists take cryptic notes; therefore, the notes usually can't be subpoenaed without the reporter to interpret them. Their bureau chiefs give them a deadline to finish the story. Once you meet or talk with the reporter, remember that nothing you say is off the record, unless you both stop and agree that the next item is for background purposes only, before you divulge any secrets.

- **Electronic**

  If you are wearing a microphone, assume that anything you say while the microphone is on is on the record. Your comments will be edited. (Long silences will usually be edited out since they don't play well on air time with the exception on a purposeful reaction time latency adjustment)

  Just because the cameras aren't pointed at you, doesn't mean the microphones aren't on. Many microphones are wireless, and what you say at a distance maybe recorded clearly.

Reporters are neither "friend nor foe"

You may have dinner or lunch, perhaps cocktails, often with a specific reporter. Always remember that their job is the reason behind your relationship. If a reporter is assigned a story about you, your practice or your institution that isn't going to be good, he will do his job. If you have a relationship, he will do everything possible to be sure the story is 'fair."

Reporters:

- Distrust people who are too self-promotional or not straightforward
- Check their information
- Work on tight deadlines
- Know either a lot about one topic or a little about a lot of topics

They can be:

- Aggressive
- Belligerent
- Confused or panicked
- Friendly
- Obsequious
- Laid back (Aw, shucks!) (Columbo effect.) Some very good writers use this effect to make you think they aren't sophisticated, when in fact they are quite sharp.

What you should know about media relations.

- Cooperative give and take is the key
- They appreciate your help
- Please be patient
- Your are a reputable source
- They may go elsewhere
- Rigid deadlines
- Friendship doesn't count

PREPARING FOR AN INTERVIEW

Get the Facts First

Do some due diligence and get to know who you're dealing with. Familiarize yourself with the local news sources, ask colleagues who may have dealt with the local media already, read the daily papers, and get to know the writing styles of the journalists. Which papers are known to spin poor angles, and which are the ones you can trust? The Internet is a great resource for this type of research. All of the major news wires and most local media resources have websites where you can search for reporters and read their work.

Speak with the reporter ahead of time and learn as much as possible about what is expected. What topic(s) will be covered – and what's the angle?

For instance, if the reporter is working on a story on laparoscopic surgery, find out if the purpose of the story is to highlight the benefits of this type of procedure for the patient, or if it is to find out the likelihood of injury because of the laparoscopic approach.

Ask the reporter to submit a list of questions to you before your meeting so that you can prepare your comments. Also, inquire as to who else may be interviewed and how long the interview is expected to take. You may want to ask the reporter if you will have a chance to review the article before it goes to print; however, in most cases deadlines prevent an opportunity for review.

What to Wear?

Projecting a professional image is always the best bet for establishing credibility. This is true for your meeting with the reporter, as well as for any pictures that may be taken. Remember that a white lab coat with a white shirt and conservative tie or a business suit will play best with the national image of a surgeon. Wearing a stethoscope around your neck says "in training."

Print reporters can wear whatever they are comfortable in, so don't be swayed by casual attire. Remember that if the story is going into your local Sunday edition magazine, the reporter may describe what you are wearing and your environment in detail and take a few pictures.

Handling the Interview

When speaking with reporters, keep in mind that you only have one chance to share your viewpoint, story, knowledge, etc. Be concise, use positive examples, and if you don't know the answer to a question, don't be afraid to say so. The old adage "Honesty is the best policy" should always apply when speaking to the press.

Keep in mind that your role always is to be a patient advocate. Speak only for yourself, and do not share others' views unless they have given consent for you to do so. Know the points you want to make. If you don't have expertise on the subject – say nothing. Also, it is best to avoid medical jargon.

"Off the Record"

Do not assume if you say "off the record" before or after you comment on something, that the information will not be used. If your comments are interesting from a news perspective, the reporter may give a tip to a colleague who may pursue the story!

Be Careful with Numbers

When citing numbers, whether they are in reference to dosages, incisions, port sizes, financial figures, etc., be extremely careful to check the information. The difference between a decimal placement or measurement can have a devastating impact on the outcome of the news story and your credibility.

Be cool

Reporters employ a variety of tactics in teasing out information for their stories. Be aware of the following techniques and how to negotiate them during any interviews.

- Leading questions:

  For example, the reporter might say, "Dr. Smith used the wrong operation for this patient's condition, right?" Don't react to the assumption when it is a misstatement of fact and intended to generate controversy.

- The rapid-fire approach:

  This technique is similar to an interrogation. Normal reaction time latency is eliminated. Next question happens before three seconds have expired. Then the important question is asked and you pause for more than three seconds. This makes you look as if you are either guilty or hiding something.

  "Dr. Chicago, how many nurses work at Redwoods Hospital full time?"

  "Part-time?"

  "Number of beds?"

  "Number of bypass cases a year?"

  "Number of bypass surgeons on staff?"

  "Number of deaths in bypass cases a year?"

  Pick out one question you feel comfortable handling and provide an answer. If there is time, you can go back and address another question. Chances are good that the reporter will then move on and not go back to the other questions on the list that was thrown at you.

- Putting words in your mouth:

  Typically, a statement is made and you are asked whether you agree with the statement.

  For example, the reporter might say, "Community hospital is a dangerous place for patients. Yes or no?" Don't get drawn into the trap of providing a one-word answer.

Correct any misstatement of the facts right away before providing a more in-depth response to the question.

- The negative or incorrect opening:

  For example, the reporter erroneously says, "Yesterday it was announced that all doctors at XYZ Hospital are going on strike. Will you participate in that job action?" Simply correct the inaccurate information provided in his or her opening comment and then go on to clarify the situation.

- The pregnant pause:

  When the reporter asks you a question and then pauses for five seconds, perhaps giving you more eye contact and nodding his or her head, it makes you feel as if you are expected to say more. Instead, wait for the next question.

- The bully technique:

  Perhaps the reporter will get physically closer to you than you expected. A pen or microphone may be pointed toward you while he or she is talking. Perhaps the question will be shouted. Perhaps the reporter follows you asking questions while you are walking. The key is for you to make a decision as to whether to answer the question based on the topic, not the reporter's nonverbal aggressiveness.

What to do if you get burned

- Call or write the reporter, but remember anything in writing is a permanent record.
- Send a copy of the letter to his bureau chief
- Request a follow-up story
- Write a 'Letter to the Editor'

Who writes the headlines?

Most reporters have copy editors who read the story and assign a headline that fits with their paper's image. The purpose of the headline is to grab attention. Therefore, it may not always meet with your approval. Don't complain about the headline to the reporter you spoke with — he or she doesn't have control. However, be aware that certain headlines can have an impact on your practice.

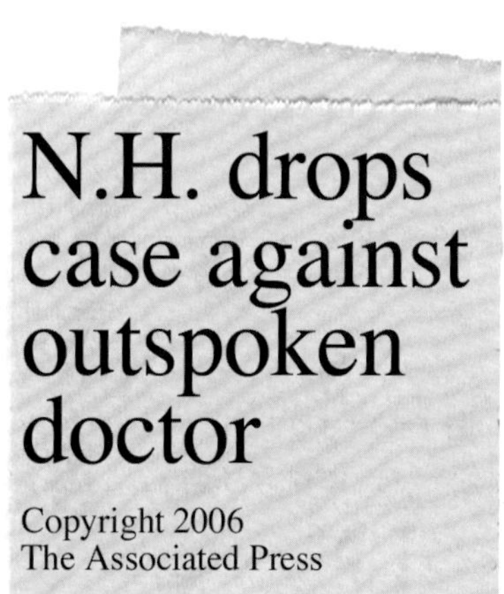
N.H. drops case against outspoken doctor

Copyright 2006
The Associated Press

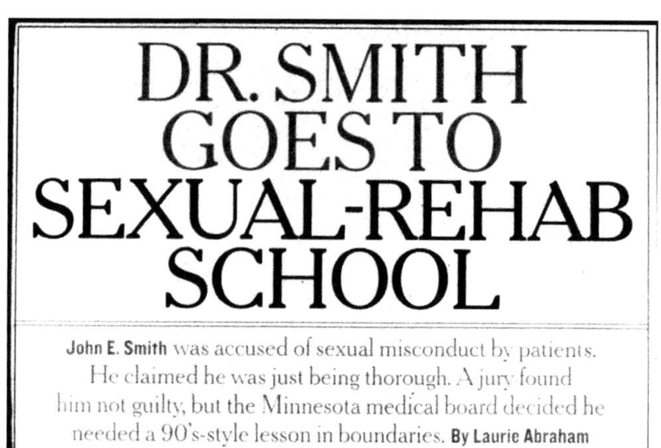
DR. SMITH GOES TO SEXUAL-REHAB SCHOOL

John E. Smith was accused of sexual misconduct by patients. He claimed he was just being thorough. A jury found him not guilty, but the Minnesota medical board decided he needed a 90's-style lesson in boundaries. By Laurie Abraham

ACTION POINTS

- Local Community

  In-house media relations departments in local hospitals or medical centers are created to promote a positive image of your institution within your community. The staff usually do not have the experience to handle national press.

- National Stories

  Current members of the American College of Surgeons may request support through the American College of Surgeons Media Office to assist them with national press. The Media Office staff is familiar with national print and broadcast press.

  Fellows of the American College of Surgeons may contact:

  Media Relations Office

  American College of Surgeons

  Chicago, Illinois

  312-202-5409

  Linn Meyer

  lmeyer@facs.org

Remember that most reporters want to be accurate.

Residency, Fellowship and Employment Interviews: Important Impressions

Joseph Jensen, MD, FACS

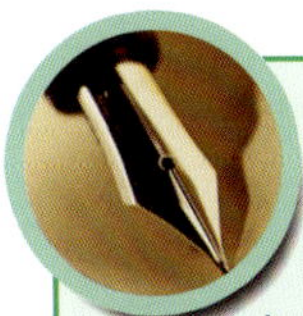

> At the end of the residency interviewing season and just prior to ranking, pictures of the interviewees were shown for additional comments to the all of the residents and attendings after M&M by the program director. One candidate looked as if the photographer said "Smile!" However, she did not. In a style typical of a two-year-old temper tantrum, the medical student did everything in her power not to smile, actually curling her lips inward. Compared to all the other applicants, the question was whether someone like this was a team player. She didn't match.

Clearly, initial impressions are made throughout the interviewing process. You may have been greeted by a resident and introduced to the residency coordinator. A secretary walks you to the next interviewer, you meet the chairman, then you attend a social get-together. Understand that you are being evaluated during each of these encounters.

Each year, about 14,000 United States senior medical students and about 6,000 physicians or other medical graduates are "matched" into PGY-1 positions in the National Resident Matching Program (NRMP). By far, this is the most common method for selection of resident physicians in the United States. The interview is a critical factor in a student's ranking and opportunity for selection. In this section we will consider an overview of the match process, and discuss specific interview techniques. Although this information is oriented to participants in the NRMP Residency Match, the concepts will also be helpful to those who participate in specialty matches or who seek residency positions outside the match. Finally, understand that these principles remain very relevant when you seek a practice opportunity on completion of your formal training.

RESIDENCY SELECTION AND THE NRMP MATCH

The NRMP Match was started in 1952 to replace a chaotic "non-system" of intern and resident selection that poorly served applicants and institutions. Virtually all PGY-1 positions in the United States are offered, and most are filled through the Match. Here is a brief overview of the match process for a typical United States senior medical student:

Step 1 During the third year of medical school, the student selects the specialty he or she wishes to pursue.

Step 2 Early during the senior year of medical school, the medical student submits an application to a number of residency training programs in his specialty. The vast majority of these applications are sent using the Electronic Residency Application

Service (ERAS) of the Association of American Medical Colleges (AAMC). Each application package consists of an application, relevant academic information and letters of recommendation.

Step 3 Residency programs review ERAS applications submitted to them and invite qualified applicants to interviews.

Step 4 Applicants interview at residency programs where they have been invited to interview. Interview season is generally November through January of each year.

Step 5 In mid-February, applicants submit to the NRMP a "rank order list" listing each program where they would like to match, and in what order of preference. Programs submit to the NRMP a "rank order list," listing the applicants they would like to match, and in what order of preference.

Step 6 The NRMP uses a sophisticated computer algorithm to match applicants to the program ranked highest on the applicants list who will offer the applicant a position.

Step 7 In mid-March, applicants are notified where they have matched for their PGY-1 year. Programs are notified of the applicants who they have matched. Unmatched applicants participate in the scramble, where a very brief, chaotic process is used to place them into programs with available positions that did not fill in the Match.

Step 8 On July 1, applicants begin the PGY-1 year of training in the program in which they have matched.

Getting Invited to Interview

Before a medical student can excel in the interview, the student must secure an invitation to interview. Interview invitations will be based almost entirely on information submitted as part of the ERAS application package. Some important points regarding selection for an interview include:

- ERAS application packets should be submitted in exactly the format requested by the program to which you are applying and in advance of the deadline. Attention to detail is a key attribute to most medical specialties, and not ensuring that your ERAS package is correct could exclude you from consideration for an interview.
- Your application should be easily readable. It is a good idea to find someone with an English or professional writing background to critique your writing before submitting it to ERAS.
- If you have a research background, be sure that all your relevant publications are listed and quoted correctly. Few applicants have a research background, and those who do should expect their research work to be examined closely.
- Your personal statement should be relatively brief, but concise and readable.

A personal statement should only be one page long.

Your personal statement should outline your goals and reasons for entering your chosen surgical specialty. This is your opportunity to write something about yourself that won't be reflected elsewhere on your application. This is the time to sell yourself to surgeons that don't know you. Any blemish in your academic record will need to be addressed.

- Your letters of recommendation will be carefully read. They should usually be from well known academic physicians in the specialty in which you are seeking a position. Letters from prominent private practice physicians are very valuable in the local or regional community, but may not be helpful to programs in other regions. The key is that letters should say that the writer knows and has worked with you personally and can comment on your suitability for postgraduate training from direct personal contact or observation. Such a letter from a Chairman or Residency Program Director is very valuable. A letter from a Chairman or Program Director that is clearly based only on a review of the file and recommendations from other faculty members is much less valuable. Letters from Members of Congress or similar civic officials are not helpful; unless they note that they have worked with you personally in a substantial professional capacity and are personally commenting on your professional suitability. For example, once I received a letter of recommendation from the president of a prestigious university with an associated medical school. I expected an unhelpful generic "I have reviewed the file" letter, but instead the letter described that the applicant, while maintaining a very good academic record in medical school, worked directly for the university president managing a multi-million dollar student government project. This letter was very well received as evidence that this applicant could handle a very responsible and rather complex student government project while also excelling in medical school.
- Federal law allows you to review all information in your academic record, including letters of recommendation, unless you waive that right. Unless there are very unusual circumstances that you have carefully discussed with a trusted academic advisor, you should always waive your right to review your letters of recommendation. Right or wrong, not waiving your right to review your letters of recommendation often invites unfavorable attention to your application.
- Dean's letters are released on November 1 of each academic year. Often interview decisions are made before the release of the Dean's letter. The narrative of the Dean's letter is not usually helpful, as they rarely contain anything more than general comments from junior student evaluations. The dean's letter does, however, usually have some objective measure of the student's academic standing.
- USMLE Step 1 (and if available, USMLE Step 2) scores will be closely scrutinized, as this is the only item in the ERAS packet that is standardized among all applicants. Many programs use a specific USMLE Step 1 score as a "cutoff" line for interview invitations. Applicants with poor USMLE Step 1 scores should take USMLE Step 2 as early as possible (so programs will have the score to consider when making a decision to interview) and obviously should make the best possible score on USMLE Step 2.

A Picture Is Worth a Thousand Words

- Early in the application process you should have a professional photograph made with a fresh, conservative haircut or hairstyle and a nice and well-fitted coat and tie (or equivalent professional attire for women). A nice smile is always appropriate for a professional photograph. Casual or clinical attire, yearbook photos, I.D. card type photos or other types of "less than professional" photos should not be a part of your application packet.
- Your photograph should be in color and conform to the exact specifications published by ERAS. Photographs that do not meet ERAS specifications may have unpredictable results when submitted to the ERAS system, such as being extremely small with scanner hardware in the background, having gray "dead-space" around portions of the photograph or having a portion of the photograph automatically "cropped" out because it is too large. It is helpful if your Dean's office will allow you to review your photograph after it is scanned into the ERAS system.
- You will submit your photograph as part of your ERAS application package. The ERAS system will allow you to permit programs to see your photograph, or to mask your photograph to prevent any personal characteristics from influencing an interview decision. Although the intent of the AAMC is understandable, the author's opinion is that there is little risk in allowing a high-quality professional photograph to be seen as virtually all initial interview decisions are made on academic criteria. However, there is probably no downside to masking your photograph until the time of your interview. The photograph is primarily for identification purposes during the interview process, and you will likely be asked to unmask it at the time of your interview if you haven't already done so. Often the photograph is also used to help the program to remember you when the program's rank order list is finalized. You may recall the fraternity candidate selection scene from the classic movie "Animal House." Although rank order list finalization is sometimes more dignified, the same concepts apply to the professional photograph.

Scheduling Your Interviews

You may have a choice of dates when you may interview at a program. There is probably no significant difference if you interview at a given program early in the season or late in the season. The most important thing is how the scheduling of the interview fits into your overall interview and travel schedule.

Some programs have specified interview dates, but will interview students on "off dates" as well. You should make a serious effort to interview on a scheduled date, but if offered an off date for your interview, it is appropriate to accept if it is impossible to interview on a scheduled date.

Obtaining Letters of Recommendation

Before reading this section, go back and reread the section above about letters of recommendation. Letters of recommendation are always carefully reviewed both before and after the interview process. Here are some important points in obtaining letters of recommendation:

- Do not be afraid to ask for letters of recommendation, and do not think you are bothering a medical school faculty member by doing so. The preparation of letters of recommendation is a normal part of academic life. Virtually all faculty members truly enjoy recommending good students, and they will expect you to ask them to do so.
- It is a good idea to make a formal appointment with a faculty member to request a letter of recommendation. Treat this visit as a "mini-interview." Be early, be professionally dressed, have a CV or ERAS application ready to leave with the faculty member and silence your cell phone or pager for the meeting. You may have a similar meeting with a representative of the Dean's office to prepare your Dean's letter. Treat this visit with the same respect.
- You will have a document from ERAS to leave with the faculty member outlining the specifics of an ERAS letter of recommendation. In summary, they will title the letter as "Dear Program Director." The letter should be sent to your Dean's office, which will then enter it into ERAS.
- If you waive your right to review your letters of recommendation (which you usually should), then you will not see your letters. ERAS does, however, allow you to select which letters you want to be sent to which program. Some students have more than the required number of letters of recommendation (usually three) and strategically choose whose letter they want sent to which program. For example, you might want a junior faculty member who is a recent graduate of a program to recommend you specifically to that program.
- Some students may apply for positions in the match in more than one specialty. This is possible by knowing which faculty member will be recommending you to which type of program, and selecting the letters to be included with your application. If you do this, be absolutely sure that you are sending the correct letters to the correct program. If you send a letter that says you will be a great radiologist to a surgery program, you will probably not be regarded seriously. By the same token, if you are going to apply to two different specialties in the same match, you should ask your Dean's office to ensure that your Dean's Letter is generic enough to accommodate this.
- Rarely should there be a question as to whether a faculty member or other individual should write a recommendation for you. If there is any question in your mind, simply make a formal appointment and during the interview ask: "Would you be willing to write a favorable letter of recommendation for me?" This will usually leave an opening for the faculty member to politely decline if so inclined. If there remains a concern, either do not submit the letter to any programs via ERAS, or seek counsel from your academic advisor (who may have access to review the letter and can then advise you accordingly).

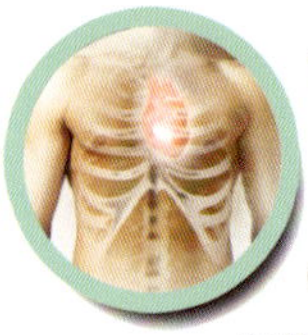

THE INTERVIEW PROCESS

There are many variations on the interview process for residency selection. Certain concepts, however, will be relevant for all residency selection interviews. The usual purposes of the interview are to assess your interpersonal and communications skills, to further explore information contained in your ERAS application and to assess your fit in the given residency program.

- There will be an opportunity to meet faculty members from the program.
- There will be an opportunity to meet current residents in the program.
- There will likely be the opportunity to meet the senior leaders (Chairman and Program Director) of the program.
- You will likely have the opportunity to meet the administrative staff of the program.
- There will generally be a tour of the clinical and educational facilities.
- There will frequently be an opportunity to participate in a social event related to the program.

The interview should be considered the only opportunity you will have to sell yourself in person. Resident candidates are, to some extent, under a microscope for the entire interview visit. Here are some important tips regarding the actual interview process:

- Travel arrangements must be carefully planned. An interview delayed or cancelled because of an airline connection problem or other similar problem can usually be re-scheduled, but keep the program informed. An unexplained no-show for a residency program interview is rude, unprofessional and immediately excludes you from consideration. If there is no other way to contact someone from a program to report a travel delay, call the main teaching hospital for the program and ask to speak with the intern on call for the department. They will usually get you in touch with the right person.
- If traveling by air, consider transporting your interview clothes as carry-on. Although understandable, you will be uncomfortable if forced to interview in your finest traveling blue jeans due to a loss of your luggage by the airline.
- The same clothing and grooming rules that apply to your professional photograph also apply here. A neat, professional and somewhat conservative haircut or hairstyle is expected. The formal interviews call for a conservative suit and tie (or equivalent for women). For social events, business casual is very appropriate. Please note that business casual is dress slacks, shirt and jacket but no tie for males, no shorts, t-shirts, etc. The exception might be a poolside event, which should be clearly marked on the invitation. If there is a question about attire, discretely ask the residency or interview coordinator.
- Spend some time determining exactly where you will need to be at what time. Modern hospital campuses are large and you may need some preparation to determine where on campus you need to be.

- Some programs will recommend a convenient and inexpensive hotel. If there are problems with your accommodations, address them in a polite and cooperative manner. One recent interviewee to our program stayed at a hotel in the medical center complex. She had a problem with her room, and the hotel management offered to fix the problem right away or move her to another room. The candidate declined both offers, but then refused to pay her bill the next day. Since the hotel provided the candidate's transportation to our department for her interview, guess who they called to report her behavior? Does this leave a positive impression on the department?
- Plan on being 10 minutes early to every appointment. If you are kept over during an interview (which will make you tardy for the rest), politely let you interviewers know. They will usually be sure you are on time for your next interview, or explain on your behalf if they have kept you late.
- Remember, resident candidates are being evaluated by everyone they meet (and some they don't meet). Be polite to everyone. The person handling the administrative details of the interview may be the Chairman's secretary.
- The interview will often involve a group of other candidates. Use this time to compare notes about other programs you may have already visited. You will see many of the same candidates at other interviews, and often a camaraderie forms among interviewees of a given academic year.

Meals and Refreshments

The interview schedule may offer the opportunity for meals, coffee or other refreshments with faculty or residents. If so, feel free to partake but do so in moderation. There is no reason to add self-consciousness after having a large coffee spill on your new shirt to the other stresses of the process. Most programs that have a meal as part of the interview process will have choices for those with dietary restrictions. In some instances, alcoholic beverages may be offered at a reception or dinner. Again, it is perfectly acceptable to partake in moderation, but you should never feel obligated to do so. If alcoholic beverages are offered, non-alcoholic beverages will also be available.

The Formal Interviews

There will always be at least one and often several formal interviews during your visit. Usually you will be brought to the interview area by the interviewer or an assistant. The usual rules of common courtesy apply. Smile, offer a handshake and introduce yourself. Make every effort to remember your interviewer's name (if you don't know it already) and use it occasionally during the interview. It is always polite to stand until you are invited to be seated.

There are certain questions that are commonly asked of resident candidates. Many of these are listed later in the chapter in the section written for programs (obviously you should also read that section as well). Expect to be asked to explain why you have chosen the specialty and why the program can expect you to excel in your residency. Often you will be asked simple, open-ended questions such as "Tell me about yourself and your professional goals." You may be asked about items in your personal statement, and you likely will be asked about any research you have listed on your ERAS application. If you have any academic blemishes on your record, you will likely be asked about them.

The interview really is an exercise to determine if you can think on your feet and communicate effectively. While you will likely have carefully thought out possible answers to many questions, others may come out of the blue. While it is wise to prepare in advance to answer common questions, you should avoid scripted answers. At a minimum, you should have well thought out, prepared (but not scripted) answers to these common questions:

- Why did you choose to become a physician?
- Why do you want to be a surgeon?
- Why should we rank you above the other applicants here today?
- What has been your greatest achievement?
- What has been your worst failure?
- Tell me about a role model in your life.
- Why did you get a (undesirable grade) in (medical school course)?
- Have you continued working in your research field?
- How would you describe an ideal training program for you?
- What questions may we answer for you?

Here is good advice for answering any question: Smile, speak clearly, answer the question directly but completely and be yourself! A pleasant, polite and engaged candidate is almost always remembered favorably.

In addition to formal interviews with program faculty, you may have a formal or informal interview with a current resident of the program. You may also meet other residents in the social setting. Do make a point of visiting with some residents out of earshot of the program faculty. Most residents will be happy to give you a frank assessment of their thoughts about their residency program, but they may be more comfortable doing so during a private conversation away from their faculty. Most programs will select the residents you will meet, but beware of a program that allows you to see only one or two residents, or none at all.

Illegal or Offensive Interview Questions

Unfortunately, it is very possible that you may be asked an inappropriate or illegal question at some point in your residency program experience. How should these questions be handled? Most of them are asked innocently as part of a conversation by surgeons who don't know they are illegal. This is why the nonverbal and verbal signals must be closely observed. Fortunately for the surgical community the incidence of this regrettable problem seems to be on the decline. You should read the advice for interviewers to avoid inappropriate or illegal questions later in this chapter.

If you are asked an inappropriate or illegal question, you have at least eight choices:

1) Answer the question directly and politely.

2) Tell the interviewer that asking such things is not allowed but you don't mind answering the question. The latter approach risks embarrassment or even anger of the interviewer. The candidate must decide if it's worth risking by weighing how much he or she wants the residency position.

3) Confront the question and ask, for instance, "what marital status has to do with whether you will be ranked."

4) To be more challenging, ask the interviewer to explain *why* marital status is a criterion to being ranked by the department.

5) Say, with a smile, that they wouldn't mind answering the question, but only after you've been ranked. Or you may say, "My children have nothing to do with my ability to complete my call or the program in five years."

6) Ignore the question like a politician and emphasize your qualifications.

7) Skip to something else discussed already in the interview such as what the department is looking for in a resident, and ask the interviewer to elaborate on that attribute.

8) However, if the question is completely offensive, you have the option of simply leaving the room.

It is entirely your choice how to respond, and you will likely need to make this decision "on the spot." If you encounter this conduct, please inform the director of the program after the rank order deadline. The program director cannot monitor every interview, and may not know there is a problem unless you let the program know what happened.

Couples Match Situations

There are special considerations that apply to those who are seeking to match as a couple with another student (or physician). Most of these situations are handled in the NRMP Couples Match. A few arise when one candidate has already matched in an early match, and the partner is seeking a match in the same city. An important principle, however, is to be sure the program where you are interviewing knows that you are in the couples match and knows who your couples match partner is. The program may not ask you about this, so it is important information for you to communicate.

Women – shake the back of the hand. Press in the web space at the bottom of the thumb, rather than squeeze fingers.

After the Interviews

After the interviews, a simple thank you note is always appropriate and tasteful. You may verify the name of your interviewers with the interview coordinator before you leave. On some occasions, a follow-up telephone call may be appropriate (especially if invited). Usually this will be to the coordinator or to a resident whom you met. If you feel that a telephone call to the program director might be helpful, a good way to do this is to ask a faculty mentor at your current school to make the call on your behalf. On the other hand, if the program director has specifically invited return phone calls, the door is open. Be pleasant and brief. DO NOT BE A PEST.

Second Interviews

A second interview is when a student visits a program for a second time, usually for a more in-depth look or an opportunity to meet additional people from the program. Most program directors have mixed feelings about second interviews. In my experience, second interviews don't usually have any effect on one's final position on the rank order list. Second interviews may be very helpful, however, if the candidate needs to know more about the program or the locale to decide where to rank the program. You may or may not have the opportunity to meet again with the program director or other program leaders. You usually will meet with more residents, and may have an opportunity to participate in rounds, conferences or other educational activities. A request for a second interview would ordinarily be directed to the program coordinator.

Discussions with the Program after your Interview

Sometimes there are discussions between you and the program director or coordinator regarding your placement on the rank order list, and the placement of the program on your rank order list. First you should understand that any discussion is absolutely non-binding. That is why the match is a confidential system. You should also know that some comments made by candidates, and some made by programs, may be made in a way that seems to imply more than the comment means. Understand that comments like "We expect to rank you highly..." and "We hope to work with you soon..." are not commitments. It is important that you understand the NRMP requirements in this regard: You may volunteer to tell a program where you will rank them, but you are not required to and may not be asked to do so. A program may volunteer to tell you where they will rank you, but they are not required to and you may not ask them. It is probably best to exchange pleasantries such as, "You have a wonderful program and I appreciate very much the opportunity to interview" and to take whatever the program tells you with a grain of salt. Programs are unlikely, however, to volunteer to tell you your actual position on the rank list unless they are telling you the truth and they want you to know your position on the rank list. By the same token, you may certainly tell a program where you will rank them but if you do so, you should tell the truth. At the end of the match, programs are notified of the final match destination of all candidates that they ranked. If you tell a program that you have ranked them number one, and they rank you in a position that guarantees you a match in that program and then you don't match there, the program will know you didn't actually rank them number one and they will know where you actually matched. The surgical community is a small world. This is an excellent reason to be truthful but politely non-committal in any discussion regarding your rank order list.

Preparing your Rank Order List

The beauty of the match system is that you may prepare the rank order list in privacy, and you may rank programs wherever you wish to rank them for whatever reason you find important. The specific reasons that are important for ranking programs are beyond the scope of this book, but do know that there is no system that works for gaming the match. The match will assign you to the program highest of your choice that has a position available for you. Simply rank the program you want to go to the most as #1, the program you want to go to second as #2, and so forth. Do not rank any program where you do not wish to go. If the program is on your rank order list, there is a chance that you may match there. If you do match there, you are obligated to go there for at least one year.

Match Week and the Scramble

Match week is always in mid-March. Students who match find out where they will be going for their intern year at the same time across the country. Students who do not match find out at the start of Match week, and they will then participate in the medical education equivalent of speed-dating, the "Scramble." This is a brief period (usually about 48 hours) where Dean's offices work to arrange last minute placement of unmatched students in programs with unfilled positions.

We hope that the guidance we have provided you will help you avoid the Scramble. However, if you become a Scramble participant, here are some helpful tips.

- If you are scrambling in Surgery, there are many details you need to know about Surgery categorical positions versus Surgery preliminary positions. You should seek advice from an experienced surgical faculty member as soon as you know you will be in the scramble.
- The interviewing will be done by telephone. All of the same interviewing and communications skills apply. A basic, but critical point: If you will be doing a telephone interview, try to do the interview from a standard (land-line) telephone. If you must do the interview on a cell phone, be sure you are in an area of good service and have a charged battery. This is a particularly inopportune time for dropped calls.
- You may need to fax your application. A copy of your ERAS application is fine. Be sure it is a good quality copy that will fax well. Many programs now ask you to simply send your application to them electronically by ERAS during the Scramble. If you are given instructions regarding your application, follow them exactly. Attention to detail is important in Surgery and failure to follow straightforward instructions in the application process reduces the chances of matching.

Avoid covering the "family jewels" with your arms or hands as it serves as an indicator of how uncomfortable you feel.

A Summary for Residency Candidates

Resident applicants are seeking an appointment to a position of great responsibility that includes providing for the care of fellow human beings. The application packet and interview should reflect your respect of the responsibilities inherent in the position you are seeking. An excellent application and interview will not overcome a poor academic record, but optimizing the application and interview with excellent communications skills will provide the best opportunity to be selected at your choice of training programs.

POST-RESIDENCY FELLOWSHIP APPLICATIONS

The application process for post-residency fellowship is similar to that for residency. Most fellowships now participate in a match program, either through the NRMP or a specialty match. The applicant pool is smaller. Competitiveness varies widely. At the writing of this monograph, pediatric surgery is the most competitive surgical fellowship with only 50% of all candidates securing a position.

The principles above are all applicable to the fellowship application process. In addition, personal contacts to selected programs from your mentors are often of great importance.

Interviewing for Practice Positions

As you approach the completion of your post graduate medical education, you will likely face a strange new environment into which many medical students have never entered – seeking a real job. Most of the advice given above is valid, but there are several things that are quite different.

- There is no match.
- There are numerous professional recruiters who will seek your attention.
- There are many more options to be considered.
- Your negotiating power is much greater than when you were seeking a residency.

Initial (Pre-Interview) Considerations

A complete application generally includes only an introductory letter from you, a Curriculum Vitae (C.V.) and letters of reference. More information will be obtained later if there is mutual interest. Here are some important points:

- Your letter and your C.V. will be the only way that your potential employer can initially evaluate you. They should be of the highest quality, carefully screened for spelling and grammatical errors. They should also be printed on good-quality paper, possibly a lightly textured off-white parchment or similar.
- It may be helpful to enclose a quality professional photograph as described above. Some photographers can incorporate your photograph onto your C.V.
- Your letter should be one page only, and if possible your C.V. should be no longer than two or three pages. A longer C.V. is acceptable for those with an extensive bibliography.

- As with your residency application, select the writers of your recommendation letters carefully. The best letter is from someone of accomplishment who worked directly with you in the professional setting and is willing to strongly support you. The rules for letters of recommendation for professional placement are less defined than for residency placement, but it is still very helpful to, if possible, know what will be in your recommendation letter before it is sent.
- In this setting it is very likely that the author of the letter will be called for additional information, which is often the most valuable information obtained in the entire process.
- Be prepared for a telephone interview, which may be either scheduled or impromptu. Candidate recruitment for surgical positions is time-consuming and expensive, and a brief telephone interview, often loosely disguised as just a friendly chat, will determine if a candidate is given further consideration.

The Interview Process

If there is mutual interest after the first contact, then a series of interviews will follow. Commonly there will be a first interview, which will consist of a series of meetings with potential partners and others with whom you might practice. Often you will be asked to make a formal presentation, such as a Grand Rounds, on a topic of interest.

A serious candidate will likely be interviewed a second time. Often the spouse is invited for the second interview. The purpose of a second interview is more often to negotiate an offer and to allow an opportunity for the spouse to explore the community, meet realtors and the like.

The principles for success in these interviews are exactly the same as for your interviews for medical school and residency:

- Your interviewers are evaluating you as a potential practice partner and neighbor, and you will be evaluating the practice situation as a potential permanent professional home, as well as a home for your family.
- You should ask any question you need to ask to make an informed decision, and you should truthfully answer questions asked of you by your interviewers.

Evaluation of a practice opportunity is a complex task, and a complete review is beyond the scope of this text. There is, however, some information that will be critical for you to obtain to make a good decision.

- Do you see yourself being able to work with your future partners?
- Do your future partners seem happy with their practice situation?
- Is the practice one where you will be able to use your skills?
- Will your family be happy in the community?
- Where does the practice fit in your personal career plan?

Details such as monetary opportunity and fringe and professional benefits are important but can be negotiated after you are satisfied that the major requirements above are satisfied.

Physician Employment Contract Review

Usually the practice agreement will be in the form of a contract. The American Medical Association publishes an annotated model physician employment contract that is very useful, and many state medical societies have arrangements for review of physician employment contracts for a very reasonable fee. Here are some critical points to address before sending the contract on to your attorney:

- Understand the exact practice model being proposed.
- Understand the opportunity, if any, for partnership (or tenure in academic settings).
- Carefully review details of professional expenses (i.e. malpractice insurance, CME, office overhead) and fringe benefits (401K or equivalent, malpractice insurance, health/dental/disability insurance).
- Understand the obligations of the group to retired or "about-to-retire" partners.
- Determine if there is a non-compete clause in the contract.
- Without fail, have the contract reviewed by an attorney licensed in the state of the proposed practice. Many issues in employment contract law vary considerably from state to state.

Few contracts have "deal-killer" provisions, but you should know the details of these critical points before you sign.

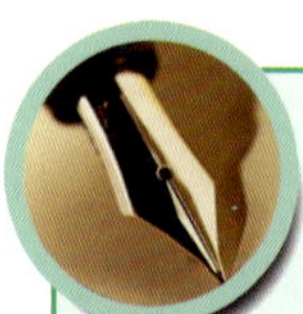

A surgical specialist is asked by the university to leave private practice and return to academic surgery. He is very excited about the opportunity and makes plans to close down his practice during the following three months. His office manager reminds him that he signed a contract with the local hospital one year ago that guaranteed him 100K per year as compensation for providing care to uninsured patients and providing emergency room coverage. He decides at this point to have an attorney look at the contract and is shocked to find that he has signed a contract that binds him for five years with an automatic five-year extension that he can get out of only by paying the hospital one year's salary. While the legal advice to him is that the contract is illegal because it is a model of indentured servitude, he is concerned about the cost of fighting the contract. This has suddenly completely disrupted his plans to return to academic surgery.

REFERENCES

1. Jolly P. Charting Outcomes in the Match – Characteristics of Applicants Who Matched to Their Preferred Specialty in the 2005 NRMP Main Residency Match. The National Resident Matching Program and the Association of American Medical Colleges July, 2006. Available at http://www.nrmp.org/matchoutcomes.pdf.
2. Employment Contracts: What Residents Need to Know American Medical Association Resident Physicians Section. JAMA. 1998; 279(14):1138.
3. Double DL. The Physician in Transition: Managing the Job Interview. American Medical Association; 1997.
4. Edwards JC, Currie ML, Wade TP, Kaminski DL. Surgery resident selection and evaluation: A critical incident study. Eval Health Prof .1993; 16(1):73-86.
5. NRMP Match Statistics available at http://www.nrmp.org/res_match/data_tables.html.

Index

O

P

T

U

V